Art Therapy and Clinical Neuroscience

Edited by Noah Hass-Cohen and Richard Carr

Jessica Kingsley Publishers
London and Philadelphia

First published in 2008
by Jessica Kingsley Publishers
116 Pentonville Road
London N1 9JB, UK
and
400 Market Street, Suite 400
Philadelphia, PA 19106, USA

www.jkp.com

Library of Congress Cataloging in Publication Data
Art therapy and clinical neuroscience / edited by Noah Hass-Cohen and Richard Carr ; foreword by Frances F. Kaplan.
p. ; cm.
Includes bibliographical references and index.
ISBN 978-1-84310-868-9 (pbk. : alk. paper) 1. Art therapy. 2. Neurosciences. I. Hass-Cohen, Noah. II. Carr, Richard, Psy.D.
[DNLM: 1. Art Therapy. 2. Brain--physiology. 3. Mind-Body Relations (Metaphysics)--physiology. 4. Neurosciences--methods. 5. Psychophysiology--methods. WM 450.5.A8 A783873 2008]
RC489.A7A767 2008
616.89'1656--dc22
2008002230

British Library Cataloguing in Publication Data
A CIP catalogue record for this book is available from the British Library

ISBN 978 1 84310 868 9

Printed and bound in the United States by
Thomson-Shore, 7300 Joy Road, Dexter, MI 48130

Dedicated to our families,

Amit, Nimrod, Lina
and Hamutahl Cohen

and

Martha, Tim and Alicia Carr

Contents

FOREWORD   13
Frances F. Kaplan, Marylhurst University

Introduction   **15**
Noah Hass-Cohen, Phillips Graduate Institute
and Richard Carr, Phillips Graduate Institute

Part 1: The Framework

1   **Partnering of Art Therapy and Clinical Neuroscience**   21
    Noah Hass-Cohen

2   **Sensory Processes and Responses**   43
    Richard Carr

3   **The Cortex: Regulation of Sensory and Emotional Experience**   62
    Darryl Christian, California Family Counseling Center and Family Service Agency

4   **Neurotransmitters, Neuromodulators and Hormones: Putting It All Together**   76
    Richard Carr

5   **Visual System in Action**   92
    Noah Hass-Cohen and Nicole Loya, Child Saving Institute

6   **The Stress Response and Adaptation Theory**   111
    Kathy Kravits, City of Hope National Medical Center, and Phillips Graduate Institute

Part II: The Ideas

7   **The Neurobiology of Relatedness: Attachment**   131
    Kathy Kravits

8   **The Influence of Attention Deficit Problems**   147
    Darryl Christian

9   **Memory and Art**   159
    Robin Vance, Phillips Graduate Institute, and Kara Wahlin,
    Youth and Family Enrichment Services Daybreak Shelter

10   Couples Art Therapy: Gender Differences
      in Neuroscience   174
      Jessica Tress Masterson, Phillips Graduate Institute

Part III: In Praxis

11   **Circles of Attachment: Art Therapy Albums**   191
      Joanna Clyde Findlay, Centre de Psychothérapie et Art Thérapie de Provence,
      Margarette Erasme Lathan, Los Angeles Child Guidance Clinic, and Noah Hass-Cohen

12   **Immunity at Risk and Art Therapy**   207
      Joanna Clyde Findlay

13   **Art Therapy, Neuroscience and Complex PTSD**   223
      Erin King-West, Phillips Graduate Institute, and Noah Hass-Cohen

14   **Alzheimer's Disease: Art, Creativity and the Brain**   254
      Anne Galbraith, Phillips Graduate Institute, Ruth Subrin, Psychological Trauma
      Centre, and Drew Ross, Creative Counseling for Elders and Families

15   **Art Therapy and Acquired Immune Deficiency Syndrome (AIDS):**
      A Relational Neuroscience Case Conceptualization   270
      Terre Bridgham, Family Service Agency of Burbank, and Noah Hass-Cohen

16   ***CREATE*: Art Therapy Relational Neuroscience Principles (ATR-N)** 283
      Noah Hass-Cohen

      GLOSSARY   311
      NOTES ON CONTRIBUTORS   324
      SUBJECT INDEX   327
      AUTHOR INDEX   332

List of figures

Figure 1.1   *How Can Participation in Art Therapy Arouse Positive Feelings, Help*
              Therapists and Clients Understand Complex Material, and Contribute to the
              Understanding of Self in the World? By Elizabeth Park.   22
Figure 1.2   Central nervous system and the peripheral nervous system.   23
Figure 1.3   Cortex, central brain and brainstem.   25
Figure 1.4   The neuron image shows the basic neuron structure.   27
Figure 1.5   Learning about learning: a group collage allows students to understand
              and express dendritic connections symbolically. By Jacqueline Camacho,
              Tania Sabljic, Barbara J. Mosteller, Ladan Safvati and Cynthia Niell Knezek. 28
Figure 1.6   Central brain and limbic system.   32
Figure 1.7   Structures and functions.   34
Figure 1.8   Does this picture stimulate your desire to pick a pastel and follow along? 37

Figure 1.9   *Self-Portraits: From Expression To Mindfulness* by Noah Hass-Cohen.   39
Figure 2.1   The cerebral cortex, the outermost brain layer, has changed significantly
               during human evolution.   44
Figure 2.2   Sensory paths to the brain. The smell path differs from the touch
               and temperature paths.   46
Figure 2.3   Brain cross-section showing location of structures.   47
Figure 2.4   Thalamic nuclei connections to brain structures along with the superior
               colliculus are essential in blindsight and visually orienting.   49
Figure 2.5   Cross-section of the brain showing lateralization of structures.   51
Figure 2.6   Low road-high road.   52
Figure 3.1   Lateral view of cortical lobes and specialized areas.   63
Figure 3.2   Medial view indicating locations of subcortical structures.   64
Figure 3.3   Projection pathways convey sensory information from lower regions
               to the posterior portion of the brain, and action messages from the
               frontal cortex to lower regions.   65
Figure 3.4   *A Folk Tale Tells of a Farmer who Falls Asleep and has his Basket of Goods
               Taken Over by a Band of Monkeys* by Robin Vance.   69
Figure 3.5   Prefrontal cortex areas.   70
Figure 4.1   Neurons, synapses, and neurotransmitters.   77
Figure 4.2   Chemical neurotransmitter relationships.   80
Figure 4.3   Dopamine circuits.   83
Figure 5.1   The visual system with enlarged view of the thalamus.   93
Figure 5.2   LGN six layers of quick and slow processing.   94
Figure 5.3   Visual information processing.   96
Figure 5.4   *My Mom* by Nicole Loya.   101
Figure 5.5   *The Greebles* were created for researchers Michael J. Tarr and Isabel Gauthier.   102
Figure 5.6   Separate and convergent neurocorrelates of fearful, angry and disgusted
               facial expressions.   106
Figure 6.1   Limbic related structures.   113
Figure 6.2   Direct and indirect pathways.   114
Figure 6.3   Divisions of the nervous system.   116
Figure 6.4   Primary structures activated during a response of the SAM axis.   117
Figure 6.5   Hypothalamus-pituitary-adrenal axis.   118
Figure 6.6   Impact of the stress response on the body.   119
Figure 6.7   Social engagement.   120
Figure 6.8   Polyvagal system and stress response.   121
Figure 6.9   Stress and attachment.   122
Figure 6.10   Reticular activating system (RAS).   124
Figure 7.1   "*I see you.*" by Kathy Kravits   136
Figure 7.2   "*I see you, too.*" by Kathy Kravits   137
Figure 7.3   Mutual engagement of attachment dynamics.   138
Figure 8.1   Brain structures involved in the attentional systems.   149
Figure 9.1   Hemispheric lateralization of memory.   160
Figure 9.2   *Dance* by Robin Vance.   161
Figure 9.3   Mechanisms of long-term potentiation.   162
Figure 9.4   *Juggler* by Robin Vance.   164
Figure 9.5   *Butterfly* by Robin Vance.   165
Figure 9.6   *Jumping Through* by Robin Vance.   167
Figure 9.7   Detail of *Figure Group* by Robin Vance.   170

Figure 9.8	*Ocean Selves 1 and 2* by Robin Vance.	171
Figure 10.1	Midbrain and limbic diagram.	175
Figure 10.2	*Me ←—→ Thee*: male's drawing.	179
Figure 10.3	*Alone*: female's drawing.	180
Figure 10.4	Two-dimensional bridge image.	182
Figure 10.5	Three-dimensional bridge image.	182
Figure 10.6	Seating arrangements.	184
Figure 11.1	Final image from attachment album by Jessica Tress Masterson.	194
Figure 11.2	House attachment album by Andrea Lewis.	196
Figure 11.3	Flowers attachment album by Marissa Raderman.	196
Figure 11.4	Secure attachment style by Andrea Lewis.	197
Figure 11.5	Secure attachment style by Jessica Tress Masterson.	197
Figure 11.6	Insecure resistant-ambivalent attachment by Andrea Lewis.	199
Figure 11.7	Insecure resistant-ambivalent attachment by Jennifer Lathrope.	199
Figure 11.8	Avoidant attachment by Jennifer Lathrope.	200
Figure 11.9	Avoidant attachment by Andrea Lewis.	200
Figure 11.10	Disorganized attachment by Jennifer Lathrope.	203
Figure 11.11	Disorganized attachment by Andrea Lewis.	203
Figure 11.12	Disorganized attachment by Lee Ignacio.	203
Figure 11.13	Disorganized attachment by Georgina Marshall.	203
Figure 12.1	Effects of the stress response.	208
Figure 12.2	*The Death of a Cancer Cell* by Joanna Clyde Findlay.	209
Figure 12.3	Immune system summary chart.	211
Figure 12.4	*Safe Place*, with red-tumor-dot.	216
Figure 12.5	*Self Portrait*, terrified self-portrait.	216
Figure 12.6	*Enhanced Safe Place*.	216
Figure 12.7	*Sunlight*, early oil pastel image of healing light, with anxious dark lines in the center.	218
Figure 12.8	*Healing Light*, three-dimensional sun with yellow clay and green construction paper.	218
Figure 12.9	*Three Stages of Healing*, the visual story of the penetration and consumption of Jim's tumor in colored clay.	218
Figure 12.10	*All is One*, a circle of small colored clay balls assembled from multiple tiny colored balls.	218
Figure 12.11	*Illumination*, Jim's reflection, colored clay, four years after end of treatment.	220
Figure 13.1	Flashbacks of bloody hands and knives (years 1–3).	223
Figure 13.2	Food (year 9).	224
Figure 13.3	Illustration of the day Jo's brother lured her to be raped by a cousin (year 1).	226
Figure 13.4	Various self-representation images (years 3–7).	228
Figure 13.5	Examples of Jo's anxiety (years 2–9).	229
Figure 13.6	Depression (years 4–5).	231
Figure 13.7	Watching the abuse from the ceiling (year 4).	232
Figure 13.8	Nightmare, cleansing her face with gasoline (year 2).	233
Figure 13.9	Visual flashes: Bloody knives and in the coffin (years 1–3).	234
Figure 13.10	Pleasant dream (drawing unfinished, year 7).	236
Figure 13.11	Some of Jo's split off parts (year 1).	237
Figure 13.12	Protecting her parts from the outside world (year 3).	238
Figure 13.13	No safety (year 2).	239

Figure 13.14   The series of images reflects (a) the process of exposure to the trauma,
                (b) turning the anger upon herself, (c) owning the anger and directing
                it back towards mother, (d) the two sides of father (years 3-14).   242
Figure 13.15   A friend pushing pills on her (year 2).   243
Figure 13.16   Processing safety in relationships (year 2).   244
Figure 13.17   Comparison of Jo's boundaries before and after she stated her desire
                to a friend (year 10).   245
Figure 13.18   Processing fear experiences in groups (year 2).   245
Figure 13.19   Hiding from Erin (year 2).   247
Figure 13.20   Jo's internal experience at the beginning of treatment, at termination and her
                fantasized future (year 14).   249
Figure 14.1   Psychoeducational drawing of working memory space.   256
Figure 14.2   Working memory boxes.   257
Figure 14.3   *Chasm.* Members draw away from the problem side of the chasm
                to the solution side. Group drawing by Alzheimer's patients.   258
Figure 14.4   Using pre-cut shapes to support visuospatial functioning.   260
Figure 14.5   Creating a community.   262
Figure 14.6   BRC-CR hand directive.   263
Figure 14.7   Psychoeducational drawing of plaque formation.   266
Figure 14.8a   Healthy neuron.   266
Figure 14.8b   Breakdown of tau protein collapsing the neuron.   266
Figure 15.1   Dillon's art therapy clinical neuroscience art therapy protocol.   271
Figure 16.1   The cerebral cortex, central brain and brainstem.   284
Figure 16.2   Motor control system.   287
Figure 16.3   How art therapy supports the consolidation of self-memories.   291
Figure 16.4   *Lee Recalled the Nature of a Transitional Object* by Lee Ignacio.   292
Figure 16.5   Location of the superior temporal sulcus.   294
Figure 16.6   Conditioned amygdala responses by Juli Ann Martinez.   297
Figure 16.7   Two Mandala-like flowers by Andrea Lewis.   300
Figure 16.8   Stress response.   301

List of tables

Table 2.1   Right and left amygdala contribute different aspects to early
              stimulus appraisal.   53
Table 5.1   Updated art media psychological continuum of safety and mastery.   100
Table 5.2   Non-familiar, familiar and self-face processing advantages.   101
Table 5.3   How to present faces.   104
Table 6.1   Allostatic levels.   112
Table 7.1   Attachment developmental milestones.   134
Table 7.2   Infant/child attachment styles.   141
Table 7.3   Adult attachment styles.   143
Table 10.1   Questions for therapeutic inquiry.   186
Table 11.1   Grice maxims.   204
Table 12.1   Imagery principles can assist the art therapist in forming diagnostic impressions
              and in furthering mental health outcomes.   215
Table 13.1   Trauma-based clusters.   227
Table 13.2   Neurobiology of C-PTSD-CSA.   230
Table 15.1   Analysis of drawing characteristics.   273
Table 15.2   Neurocorrelate correspondences in broad strokes.   274

Foreword

Back in the 1970s when I was receiving my training in art therapy and through much of the 1980s when I was working in psychiatric settings, the mind-body problem was truly a problem. There were the mind camps ("depression is caused by anger turned inward") and the body camps ("depression is caused by a chemical imbalance"). As a result, those in the mental health professions who attempted to put mind and body together often took an either-or position; they might decide that, in one case, the source of the problem was the mind while, in another case, the source was the body. There was an uneasy sense that somehow we therapists were missing the point, but there was no clear understanding of how to put things right.

As brain science began to advance, along with a deepening understanding of genetics, it became harder to maintain that mind and body were separate entities. I can remember telling a group of art therapy students that we now know mind and body constitute a whole; however, we have been thinking in dichotomous terms for so long that we don't yet know how to talk about this whole in a meaningful way.

It is with great pleasure and excitement that I can say that we are increasingly less hampered in this regard – we are rapidly acquiring the knowledge and accompanying language that promotes dialogue about how "mental ills" can be helped and healed by taking an integrated mind-body perspective. The twenty-first century has seen the publication of several works on neuroscience as it relates to psychotherapy. And following on the heels of these, we now have this groundbreaking volume that brings clinical neuroscience and art therapy together. Something that a number of us in the field of art therapy have been advocating for a while – a true melding of art and science – is exemplified here. It is enough to make someone like myself, nearing the end of a career in art therapy, wish that beginning again were possible.

Art Therapy and Clinical Neuroscience provides basic information concerning the structures and functions of the various areas of the brain, relates this information to the process and product of art and art therapy, and offers some practical suggestions for the clinician. In so doing, it also lays down tentative outlines for a scientific theory of art therapy. This is an impressive accomplishment, and editors Noah Hass-Cohen and Richard Carr are to be both thanked and commended for having taken on and successfully completed what must have initially seemed an exceedingly daunting task.

13

Although we may still ask if the mind-body problem has been thoroughly solved (we have barely begun to show how doing art affects the brain and hence the mind), we should no longer question the existence of mind-body unity. Hass-Cohen and Carr and their contributors have blazed a trail for us to follow. Helping professionals who use art would be wise to put on their hiking boots and begin the journey. It starts on the next page…and ends where we collectively take it.

Frances F. Kaplan, Marylhurst University

Introduction

Noah Hass-Cohen and Richard Carr

> The scientific theory of art therapy must take into account the findings of evolutionary biology and anthropology concerning mankind, the findings of neuroscience and psychology concerning the workings of the human brain and the findings of the physical sciences concerning the laws of nature. (Kaplan 2000, p.94)

The burgeoning of neuroscience findings has revolutionized clinical psychology, making it necessary to update art therapy perspectives. The book's contributors have collaborated in order to articulate the application of interpersonal neurobiology to art psychotherapy. In this endeavor, we are privileged to join pioneering art therapists who have taken on this contemporary challenge. Frances Kaplan, Vija Lusebrink, Cathy Malchiodi, Gussie Klorer, Linda Chapman, Caroline McNamee, the late Shirley Riley, and other art therapists have expressed in their writings the need to extend art therapy practices using functional information about the brain and nervous system. Our team of writers elucidates ideas linking human behavior, mental events and underlying neural systems that can stimulate more attuned art therapy techniques. Many of the art therapy ideas presented in the chapters highlight the connections between the immune, the endocrine and the nervous systems, most notably the visual and the motor systems.

The book is divided into three sections: the *framework*, the *ideas* and *in praxis*. The framework introduces neuroscience language and concepts needed for art therapists to participate in this paradigm shift. In *Chapter 1*, Noah Hass-Cohen describes basic neuroscience with examples illustrating how art therapists can interface clinical neurobiology with art therapy mind-body approaches. She surveys human development and neuroscience concepts and perspectives that reveal how art therapy practices can contribute to positive excitation, affect regulation and the well-being of a relational self, such as brain plasticity. In *Chapter 2*, Richard Carr discusses the interplay of the sensory system, specifically the thalamus, with responses in several emotion regulating structures in the brain. He suggests that art therapy applications may utilize higher brain structures to inhibit and extinguish conditioned fear and anxiety responses created in lower brain regions. In *Chapter 3*, Darryl Christian delineates executive, connective, supervisory, inhibitory and integrative functions provided by the four cortical centers in the most evolved region of the brain. The chapter focuses on how cortical functions help develop relational abilities during the processing of sensory experiences. *Chapter 4* discusses how chemical messengers adjust brain/body emotions and behaviors over a lifetime. Richard Carr hypothesizes that, during art therapy, chemical messengers from the nervous, endocrine and immune systems promote specific functions that advantage psychosocial functioning. *Chapter 5* is dedicated to understanding how the visual system transforms sensory stimuli and internal imagery. Noah Hass-Cohen and Nicole Loya articulate a neuroscience-based media continuum that addresses multiple dimensions, such as movement, novelty and thinking as they underscore the significance of utilizing images of the face and self. In *Chapter 6*, Kathy Kravits addresses adaptation and stress responses from a neurobiological perspective. Using examples from her work with cancer patients, her informative chapter reflects upon whether stress responses are always detrimental to our lives. And, with that, the framework section concludes.

The book's mid-section, the *ideas*, is dedicated to specialized topics that further the discussion of the information presented in the *framework*. In *Chapter 7*, Kathy Kravits writes about the way in which early brain development interfaces with child and adult attachment styles. To tell the story intimately, she includes pictures showing her grown, married children interacting with their babies. In *Chapter 8*, Darryl Christian suggests that our capacity for attention influences how we process information, sense identity and form flexible, adaptable, interpersonal relationships. He explains the neurobiology of attention deficit problems and suggests modifications to art therapy approaches that assist children whose attentional difficulties propel them away from others. *Chapter 9* brings together memory processes and the creation of fine art. Robin Vance and Kara Wahlin introduce the central role that memory plays in defining personhood. Vance illustrates how implicit and explicit memory processes are expressed in her work as a practicing artist. In *Chapter 10*, Jessica Tress Masterson explores gender differences from an evolutionary and brain-based perspective and suggests appropriate modifications for traditional couples art therapy directives.

In praxis, the last section of the book, showcases art therapy practices that clarify how art therapy relational neurobiology principles can be used. The evolving concepts, processes, and approaches provide opportunities for increased clinical efficacy and improved therapeutic outcomes. In *Chapter 11*, Joanna Clyde Findlay, Margarette Erasme Lathan and Noah Hass-Cohen combine attachment theory with clinical examples and reflections that use tactile albums to illustrate the advantages of attachment training for art therapy trainees. Included is a unique application of the MARI© mandala approach to the illustrated attachment stages. In *Chapter 12*, Joanna Clyde Findlay uses psychoneuroimmunology research to describe an immune-compromised, clinical art therapy case. She reviews the literature on health psychology and imagery and suggests neurobiological-based imagery principles for medical art therapy work. *Chapter 13* unfolds a case of complex post-traumatic stress disorder (C-PTSD). Erin King-West describes a long-term trauma case that involves a history of sexual abuse, dissociation, and relational difficulties, illustrated with art sequences and accompanied by her reflections. Noah Hass-Cohen highlights relevant clinical neuroscience findings and reflects upon interventions that mediate the long-term effects of trauma. In *Chapter 14*, Anne Galbraith, Ruth Subrin, and Drew Ross share rich directives developed by them at Older People in a Caring Environment (OPICA). The art illustrates how enlisting procedural memory and right hemisphere functions can compensate for the explicit memory losses associated with Alzheimer's disease. In *Chapter 15*, Noah Hass-Cohen and Terre Bridgham provide a blueprint for integrating clinical neuroscience with an art therapy protocol. Terre Bridgham showcases artwork from an AIDS-HIV participant, while she and Noah Hass-Cohen discuss the case from attachment theory and stress response perspectives. *Chapter 16* proposes an art therapy relational neuroscience (ATR-N) framework. Noah Hass-Cohen describes how interpersonal neuroscience helps tie art therapy expressions to critical moments in a person's life journey. She proposes six art therapy relational neuroscience principles: Connectivity in Action, Relational Resonance, Expressive Communication, Adaptive Responses, Transformation, and Empathy, that form a cohesive framework called *CREATE*. This completes the journey.

We believe that including the saliency of clinical neuroscience research to the theory and practice of visual- and sensory-based therapies has led to a new way of thinking about art therapy. This new approach has increased our appreciation of art therapy. We also invite you to share our appreciation of the contributions that art-making provides to the understanding of complex brain information. In order to facilitate this new approach we have included a basic glossary at the end of the book. Our hope in introducing this model is to inspire a dialogue about the integration of complex neurobiological information into art therapy practices.

Acknowledgements

The editors want to express their heartfelt gratitude to the wonderful contributors to this book – faculty, alums, and students at Phillips Graduate Institute in Encino, California, who collaborated in the learning process in order to facilitate the writing and conveyance of their ideas. They pursued answers to difficult questions that captured our attention for endless hours as all of us attempted to digest the incredible amount of research that contributed to this book. Of course, our debt to the neuroscience researchers who published their research on human functioning is immeasurable. Their ever unfolding data and expositions invite us and others to gain insight, hypothesize and seek a better comprehension of art therapy and human functioning.

Many thanks go to Dr. Lisa Porché-Burke, for supporting the project, and to Jessica Kingsley for inviting Noah Hass-Cohen to publish her ideas. We are deeply indebted to Robin Vance for so generously contributing her art to the book's cover and for her chapter. Thanks to Gabriela Acosta, Britta Amundsen, Jacqueline Camacho, Tise Chao, Lee Ignacio, Jennifer Kirk, Jennifer Lathrope, Andrea Lewis, Georgina Marshall, Juli

Ann Martinez, Jessica Tress Masterson, Barbara J. Mosteller, Cynthia Neill Knezek, Elizabeth Park, Tania Sabljic, and Ladan Safvati for their contributions, illustrations and art. The authors want to thank Sonja Wilson, Lina Cohen, Sylvia Cary and Leyla Gulen for editorial assistance and Linda Folsé at Phillips Graduate Institute library and Mirian Hicks, the librarian, and her assistant, Sujatha Bhuvanaraj, at Cleveland Chiropractic College in Los Angeles for research support. This project would have not been possible without the support of our commissions editor, Steve Jones. Our gratitude goes also to two very special people: Caroline Elman, former library director at Phillips Graduate Institute, who made her extensive expertise available to us, and Jessa Forsythe-Crane, who provided us with daily administrative support, and diligent, excellent editing of our many drafts. We also want to recognize the many clients and students who have taught us so much over the years. Finally, our heartfelt thanks goes to our families for seeing us through the many, long hours of writing and editing.

July 2008

Reference

Kaplan, F. (2000). *Art, Science and Art Therapy: Repainting the Picture.* London and Philadelphia, PA: Jessica Kingsley Publishers.

Part 1

The Framework

1

Partnering of Art Therapy and Clinical Neuroscience

Noah Hass-Cohen

Art therapy is poised to take advantage of the abundance of information from clinical neuroscience research. We can draw from clinical neuroscience to describe and enhance the therapeutic advantages of arts in action and further illuminate the unique contributions of art therapy to well-being and health.

Clinical neuroscience is the application of the science of neurobiology to human psychology. Human and animal empirical research is revealing the dynamic interplay of the nervous system, particularly the brain, with a person's environment. Neuroimaging studies allow clinical neuroscientists to hypothesize about structural, functional and environmental correlations that connect observable human activity with measurable brain activity. The connections between the nervous system, the endocrine system and the immune system all shed light on the intrapersonal expressions of the relational self.

In art therapy, the artwork is a concrete representation of such mind-body connectivity, which contributes to internal feelings of mastery and control (Camic 1999; Malchiodi 1998; Naparstek 1994). In the art therapist's presence, the artwork is an expression of how the self organizes internally as well as in relationship with others. It is a visual reiteration of the interplay between the person and their environment. An understanding and appreciation of mind-body connectivity and interpersonal neurobiology (Siegel 2006) can also facilitate a dialogue about potential contributions of clinical neuroscience to art therapy (Lusebrink 2004). Art therapy practices, research, and theory-building can be updated to suggest a new framework of art therapy relational neurobiology principles (ATR-N) (Hass-Cohen 2008; Figure 1.1).

Mind-body connectivity

The interplay of experiences, emotions, behavior and physical health characterize the study of mind-body connections (Achterberg *et al.* 1994; Cousins 1979). Mind-body approaches link nervous, endocrine and immune systems with physiological and psychological changes. Psychoneuroimmunology (PNI) is the discipline that studies these

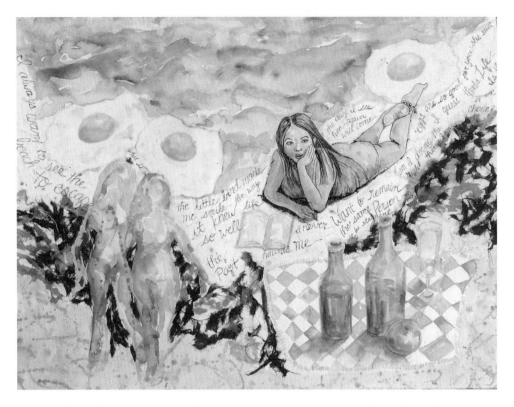

Figure 1.1 How Can Participation in Art Therapy Arouse Positive Feelings, Help Therapists and Clients Understand Complex Material, and Contribute to the Understanding of Self in the World? *By Elizabeth Park.*

complex, chemical, bodily connections. Understanding the neurobiological connections between the mind and body furthers therapeutic utility rendering the dualistic separation of mind and body a futile Cartesian endeavor (Damasio 1994).

Mind-body connectivity manifests in the nervous system's organization. The central nervous system consists of the brain and the spinal cord, which innervates the body organs and their extremities through the peripheral nervous system. The peripheral nervous system produces involuntary and voluntary responses to environment. It has two branches: the autonomic nervous system, which controls involuntary responses to stimuli, maintains normal functions, and restores homeostasis; and the somatic nervous system, which conveys sensory information to the central nervous system and controls voluntary muscular or motor actions (Carlson 2004). Information is received (afferent) and sent (efferent), allowing physiological and psychological changes to unfold. The autonomic nervous system further divides into the sympathetic (SNS) and parasympathetic (PNS) nervous systems. The SNS's functioning helps a person quickly adapt to relational and environmental situations. The SNS enhances everyday functioning. Governed by the brain, the sympathetic function propels us into action, such as running away from an environmental danger or struggling with the impulse to avoid a psychosocial conflict. The flight or fight response is associated with SNS activation. In contrast the parasympathetic returns a person to more relaxed, ordinary functioning. If we are able to resolve a stressful problem successfully, the parasympathetic nervous system re-establishes a balance that allows the sympathetic to diminish its flight or fight response. In response to daily circumstances, the SNS and PNS functions complement each other and mildly shift a person between mild variations of excitation and relaxation states (Figure 1.2).

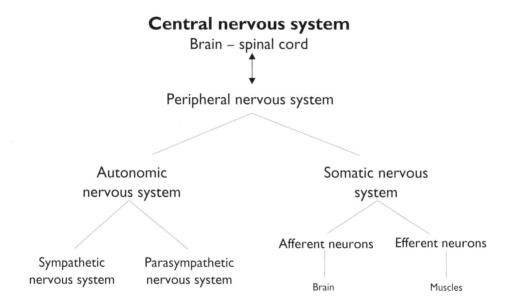

Figure 1.2 Central nervous system and the peripheral nervous system. The central nervous system includes the brain and spinal cord. The peripheral nervous system divides into the autonomic and somatic nervous systems. The autonomic nervous system contains the sympathetic (SNS) and parasympathetic (PNS) nervous systems. The sympathetic system is excitatory and the "para" (meaning over) sympathetic attempts to restore normal function by counterbalancing the sympathetic. The somatic/sensory nervous system responds to incoming afferent sensory messages and carries efferent messages to the major voluntary muscle groups.

Initially, the strain of a novel demand, such as art-making, can be experienced as a SNS excitement and emotionally anticipated. However, if the task is not mastered and the client's sense of control is challenged, the SNS stress response might increase. For example, Mary, a 60-year-old client struggling with leukemia and loneliness, reported that she was initially excited about the fine art class recommended by her church counselor. She hoped to gain some support as well as express some of what she was going through. Mary reported that she was discouraged by her lack of art skills, and she left the course after a couple of classes. She did not feel safe in the judgmental fine arts environment. Recognizing her need to create art in a non-threatening and supportive environment, she successfully sought out an art therapist.

At times, psychosocial stressors may not be able to be resolved by leaving the situation or finding new ways of coping, which contributes to a sense of fear and loss of safety (Sapolsky 1998) often expressed by clients. In order to regain a measure of safety and control, art therapists encourage clients to practice taking action in session. Actions such as drawing or sculpting in the face of difficult issues can express the voluntary function of the somatic nervous system and provide clients with the opportunity to participate in pleasurable kinesthetic experiences. Doing so can bring the somatic nervous system's afferent and efferent nerves into play. Afferent nerves carry incoming sensory information from touching the art materials (soft or sharp, warm or cold), which may elicit emotional reactions such as pleasure, discomfort or distaste. At the same time, efferent nerves cause the necessary muscle contraction needed for drawing, painting and sculpting. Art therapy activities, grounded in affective-sensory experiences, assist in keeping clients in touch with their therapeutic surroundings and can also provide relief through the expression of emotions and the kinesthetic and voluntary actions required to make and complete the art. For example, upon touching the velvety wet clay, a female client became quiet and quickly wiped her hands. She reported recoiling from the cold quality of the clay. Another client reported that the smell of the brown clay reminded her of fond childhood memories creating mud-pies. Such art therapy experiences may help provide a sense of control and mastery, which is mediated by sympathetic-parasympathetic balance (Hass-Cohen 2003, 2007).

An example of mind-body connectivity is the social function of the vagal nerve (the tenth cranial nerve), which has connections to the brain as well as to the chest and abdominal areas. "Gut feelings" can be partially attributed to the vagal nerve's connections with, and influences on, the digestive system (Carlson 2004). The vagus is also implicated in social engagement functions (Porges 2001) such as described below.

Vagus function was associated with death from the "Voodoo Curse." Walter Cannon described this freeze response in 1929, and was first to show the connectivity of physical and emotional/psychological stressors (Sapolsky 1998). Cannon hypothesized that the tribesmen's belief in the witch doctor's curse caused a prolonged stress response that could sometimes result in death. Believing that the shaman has supernatural healing powers that can give life or take life away creates a complicated cascade of mind-body reactions. Situations appraised as unsafe do not support proactive social interactions and can result in stress, isolation, mobilization and in immobilization (Porges 2001; Kravits 2008).

It is important to share with art therapy clients how a person's response to stress may be affected by how he/she perceives, emotes and thinks about the situation (Barlow 2001). Thoughts are governed by the functioning of the cerebral cortex, the top part of the brain. Also known as the newest brain, the neocortex covers the limbic system structures located in the central brain and most of the brainstem. Responsible for sophisticated social cognitions, the cortex is considered the seat of thought, emotional appraisal, and voluntary movement. The cortex has two hemispheres, right and left; each side is divided into five lobes (Figure 1.3).

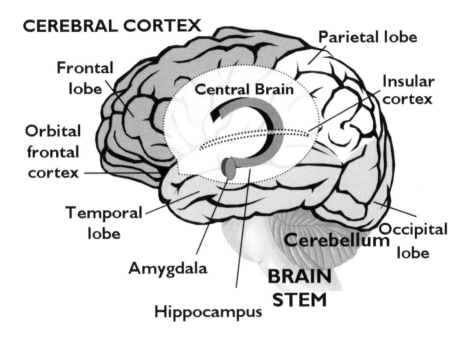

Figure 1.3 Cortex, central brain and brainstem. The brainstem and the cerebellum are important for motor reactions and basic body processes. The limbic system within the center brain regions is responsible for social emotional processing. The amygdala triggers the fear response and the hippocampus holds emotional experiences in memory. The cortex is responsible for sophisticated social cognitive functions. It includes the occipital lobe, the parietal lobe, the temporal lobe, the frontal lobe, the orbital frontal cortex, and the insular cortex (located within the sulcus that separates the temporal lobe and inferior parietal cortex. The insula conveys bodily states to the cortex. The orbital frontal cortex is an area above the eyes and behind the forehead (also see Figure 1.7).

The cortex is responsible for linking information from the body, the brainstem and the limbic system. The frontal lobes integrate visual data from the occipital lobes and temporal lobes, along with a sense of space and navigation from the parietal lobes. The temporal lobes are involved with auditory and visual processing. They associate visual social information, such as faces, with meaning and assess it for familiarity. Connections between the temporal lobes and the limbic system allow emotion, recognition and memory to influence the meaning of visual information. The right temporal lobe is associated with nonverbal response-oriented activities.

Chronic stress experiences shift the person away from the integrated feelings and thoughts associated with the function of the frontal lobes towards a limbic-based survival reaction (Henry and Wang 1999). This survival shift stimulates hormonal and neurotransmitter responses that can over time diminish immune system functioning. The limbic system is sensitive to the kind of interpersonal threats demonstrated by the Voodoo death reports. When an immediate threat is not resolved, long-term stress may occur. PNI studies indicate that, to survive, central brain regions signal the endocrine and the immune system to slow down and alter everyday functions. As a result, the effects of chronic stress can be devastating not only to well-being and health but also to memory and cognitive functions (Bremner 2006; Sapolsky 1998).

Art therapy is recognized as an intervention that facilitates the expression of mind-body connectivity through the remediation of acute and chronic stress (Achterberg *et al.* 1994; Hass-Cohen 2003; Kaplan 2000; Lusebrink 2004). Mind-body-based interventions are also characteristic of health psychology, medical arts, sports psychology and shamanic practices. Treatment interventions in the later modalities include biofeedback, EMDR (eye movement desensitization and reprocessing), relaxation techniques, sensory-motor sequencing, mindfulness meditation, imagery/guided imagery, hypnosis, rituals, myths and prayer. Most mind-body approaches are intrapersonally oriented. They focus on the remediation of stress and restoring a sympathetic-parasympathetic balance by teaching clients experiential practices. Art therapy differs in that it includes expressive and relational foci. At the same time that art therapists assist clients in reducing the effects of stressors, they also encourage self-expression and promote a sense of intra/interpersonal connectivity through the therapeutic relationship. The advantages are that clients gain more support for generalizing in the outside world what they have experienced in session.

Establishing connectivity: development and learning

The earliest therapeutic relationship between the primary caregiver and infant directly shapes the infant's emotional brain. From birth, the subcortical regions of the central brain, responsible for emotional processing, are actively making neural connections. Consequently, the infant/caregiver affective relationship has a large impact on neural networks' connectivity thus shaping brain development and maturation (Diamond and Hopson 1998; Perry 2001; Schore 2001).

The basic building blocks of relational connectivity are neurons, which are electrically excitable cells. The basic structure of a neuron includes the cell body and nucleus, axon, axon terminals and dendrites. Some neurons are covered by myelin sheathing which facilitates faster communication (Figure 1.4).

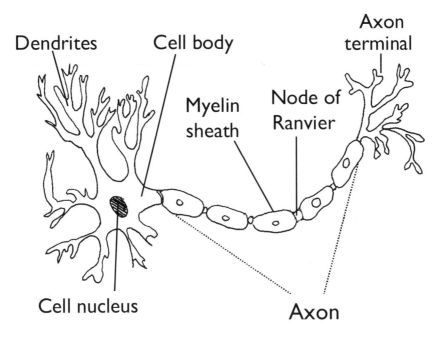

Figure 1.4 The neuron image shows the basic neuron structure: dendrites, cell body, cell nucleus, axon, Node of Ranvier, axon terminal and myelin sheath (Nodes of Ranvier are not myelinated).

Shaped like tree branches, dendrites communicate messages from other neurons to the cell body of their neuron. Once a threshold of activation occurs, the neuron activates and fires. Firing causes the cell body to send a single impulse along the axon, a long nerve bundle, to axon terminals. This signal has the potential to activate subsequent neurons. The impulse causes the release of chemical messengers into the space between neurons. Chemical messengers called neurotransmitters negotiate synapses or spaces between the axon terminal of the sending neuron and the dendrites of the receiving neuron. Neurotransmitters stimulate dendrites to convey the information they receive to the cell body. The process starts all over again in the next neuron in the sequence. Neurons that fire together rely upon chemical signals that cross the synapses that connect an axon terminal of one nerve to a dendrite of the next. Frequently repeated sequences of neuronal firing establish learning and memory formation (Bishop 1995), which thickens dendritic connections. Repeated sensory art experiences contribute to the formation and strengthening of memories (Vance and Wahlin 2008). Creating art about how our brains learn and change assists in retaining complex information in memory (Riley 2004; Figure 1.5).

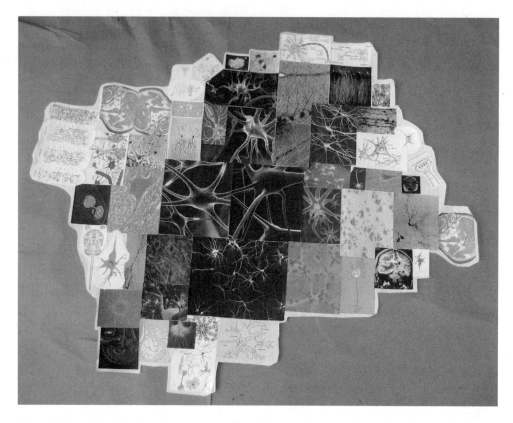

Figure 1.5 Learning about learning: a group collage allows students to understand and express dendritic connections symbolically. Jacqueline Camacho, Tania Sabljic, Barbara J. Mosteller, Ladan Safvati and Cynthia Neill Knezek.

Synaptic pruning is another way that the brain communicates, learns and shapes. Synaptic pruning involves the removing of unused neuronal connections and damaged neurons. Disruptions in synaptic pruning can be damaging to effective circuitry communication (Abitz *et al.* 2007). For example, synaptic pruning deficiencies in the autistic brain seem to result in too many ineffective neural connections (Courchesne 2004).

The effectiveness of neuronal communication is also assisted by myelination. Myelin is an insulating white sheath around axons that facilitates unimpeded electrical communication. Unlike dendritic connectivity and the pruning of synapses, myelination is mostly genetically wired (Eliot 1999). Myelination occurs sequentially from the back to the front of the brain. Synaptic shaping and the myelination of neurons contribute to brain weight and volume, and processing efficiency (Eliot 1999).

From a developmental perspective, synaptic shaping and myelination contribute directly to brain maturation and growth (Eliot 1999). Experience-dependent brain maturation and change is especially characteristic of the first two years of life (Bear,

Connors, and Paradiso 2006). In the first two years, neuronal connections are preserved or pruned to enable efficient hearing, seeing, moving, emoting and thinking. The two-year-old cerebral cortex contains a thousand trillion synapses which progressively organize neural connections from latency through age 25 to lower, more efficient adult levels (Eliot 1999).

As stated earlier, non-verbal communications between mother and infant organize neurobiological systems (Schore 1994). The baby's social brain matures in accordance with a developmental timeline of critical periods. The development of the infant's self-regulation organizes the growth of the human nervous system, linking subcortical areas with the developing cortex. Art therapists working with mothers and caregivers may want to share how somatosensory regulatory experiences of holding, touching and gazing help organize their child's nervous system. The interactive brain is social (Cozolino 2002; Perry 2001) as mothers and babies continue to soothe each other and grow in shared contexts of emotion and behavior.

Relational art activities can increase mother-child trust and attachment (Gillespie 1994). The pleasure associated with therapeutic art-making may also help mitigate postpartum and/or clinical depression shown by Tronick (2007) to reduce mothers' capacity for attuned non-verbal response. Sharing the knowledge that consistent and responsive care and early childhood interventions correlate with positive development trajectory (National Research Council of Medicine 2000) can be helpful for primary caregivers. Caution must also be taken in order not to overwhelm and bombard developing brains with too much somatosensory stimuli (Ahlander 2002). Most importantly, the focus of intervention should be preventing and treating severe child abuse and neglect, both of which can result in deprivation of brain stimulation resulting in neuronal death (Ahlander 2002; Perry 1996). The neurobiological consequences of childhood physical, emotional and cognitive abuse and neglects often contribute to enduring states of personal fear that can lead towards perpetuating violence on to others later in life (Perry 1997) and/or to being adult victims of violence.

The brain continues to develop during the adolescent years and young adulthood as the frontal lobes, areas responsible for attention, concentration and sophisticated decision-making, myelinate and reorganize. Fifteen years of imaging studies have shown increases in myelination and further pruning of dendritic connections and neurons during adolescence (Giedd 2004; Giedd et al. 1999). These extensive synaptic changes contribute to the social-emotional turmoil characteristic of the preadolescent and adolescent age. However, these changes eventually contribute to increased planning and self-regulation associated with mature functioning in the frontal areas of the cortex. As the adult frontal cortex further develops and higher cortical functions are acquired, the brain continues to organize and change throughout the lifespan by means of social-emotional experiences.

Connectivity throughout the lifespan: brain plasticity

Brain plasticity is the ability of the brain to strengthen, renew and, to a certain degree, rewire to compensate for developmental, learning and traumatic brain deficits (McEwen and Lasley 2002). Evidence is mounting that brain plasticity once thought to be limited to early development is now being more extensively explored as an experience-dependent adult phenomenon (Kandel 1998; May and Gaser 2006). The phenomena of brain plasticity is perhaps one of the most significant outcomes of neuroimaging as it has potential clinical applications: "a very important recent finding of magnetic resonance-based morphometry is the discovery of the brain's ability to alter its shape within weeks, reflecting structural adaptation to physical and mental activity" (May and Gaser 2006, p.407; review). Greater brain usage increases neuronal activity, which increases dendrites and synaptic activity, thickening brain gray matter and resulting in heavier brains (Mechelli *et al.* 2004; Stein *et al.* 2006). Heavier brains are less vulnerable to neurogenerative diseases, such as Alzheimer's, and can better compensate for brain injury (Allen, Bruss, and Damasio 2005; Satz 1993). In older adults, aerobic exercise increased brain volume and function while reducing the normal cortical atrophy associated with aging (Colcombe *et al.* 2003). Cognitive behavioral therapies also modified neural circuitry function (Lazar *et al.* 2005; Prasko *et al.* 2004; Straube *et al.* 2006), suggesting that altering how people think about other people triggers changes that affect brain function. Perhaps the repeated practices involved in making art and consistently communicating with others through art forms may have similar, positive effects.

Medical students in their mid-twenties studying for an exam showed significant neuroimaging-based increases in gray matter (non-myelinated neurons) in the posterior (back) hippocampus (Figures 1.3 and 1.6) and in the bilateral posterior and lateral (side) parietal cortices. Scans three months later revealed that these structural changes persisted in each area, and that in fact posterior hippocampal areas continued to increase (Draganski *et al.* 2006). Responsible for acquiring new information, the hippocampus holds short-term memory for about two years before embedding it into long-term memory. In 1998, it was discovered that adult neurons could regenerate in the hippocampus, a seahorse-shaped structure in the brain's limbic system responsible for learning and memory (Eriksson *et al.* 1998). Hippocampal neurogenesis occurs during physical exercise in an enriched environment and while learning new memory-dependent tasks (Elder, De Gasperi, and Gama Sosa 2006). Hippocampal neurons respond poorly to long-term, chronic stress (Bremner 2006) yet pharmacological and non-pharmacological treatments for depression can successfully enhance hippocampal neurogenesis, as well as assist in the treatment of mood disorders (Malberg and Schechter 2005).

At the core of mood disorders, such as depression and anxiety, are problems with the regulation of affect. From infancy throughout the lifespan, the social brain is governed by the ability to express and self-regulate emotional experiences. Affect regulation is a functional expression of connectivity between subcortical, limbic and cortical brain activity. The circuitry of the brain integrates limbic, bottom-up expression and cortical top-down regulation of affect (Baumeister and Vohs 2004). Art therapy practices provide a unique opportunity for expression of emotions and practicing the regulation of affect. Colors and textures easily arouse affectively laden limbic memories while purposeful art-making provides a here and now opportunity to express, understand and integrate emotional reactions.

Affect expression

Understanding how the brain evolved and organized clarifies when and how strong emotional reactions propel people into action. The ascending order of brainstem to central brain to right hemisphere and then across to the left hemisphere (Figure 1.3) is associated with increased integration of emotions with cognitive functions resulting in complex social function. In comparison, central brain areas closely connected with limbic function are associated with survival-based emotions. During times of crisis, function reverts to older regions of the brain as they are more strongly connected; strong neural connections between the limbic and cerebellum motor areas are accompanied by much weaker neural connections to cortical regions (Panksepp 1998). The result is that under stress fear and anger guide more complex emotions and cortical cognitions.

The basic core emotions associated with pleasure and discomfort are happiness, surprise, fear, anger, disgust and sadness (Tamietto *et al.* 2007). Basic emotions categorized as unpleasant or pleasant inform the person that his or her environment is "helpful or harmful, rewarding or threatening, calling for acceptance or rejection" (Barrett *et al.* 2007, p.377; review). The arousal of displeasure and pleasure builds upon autonomic reflexes mediated by the brainstem and the basal ganglia, which is involved with the brainstem motor activation. The innate human tendency to revert to emotions is expressed in the organization of the brain. The one-on-top-of-the-other organizational structure of the brain model is functionally expressed in bottom-up and top-down neural pathways. Bottom-up, sensory cues and incoming visual information are relayed by the thalamus and are assessed for danger by the amygdala. The amygdala is responsible for the fear response (LeDoux 2000). This bottom-up process may activate the short-term flight or fight stress response or the long-term endocrine stress response. The flight or fight response involves the sympathetic nervous system response discussed earlier. The long-term endocrine stress response includes activation of the hypothalamus and of the pituitary gland, the master gland of the endocrine system. The hypothalamus, which sends signals to the endocrine system, is also a bodily regulator of sleep, appetite and other endocrine functions (Figure 1.6).

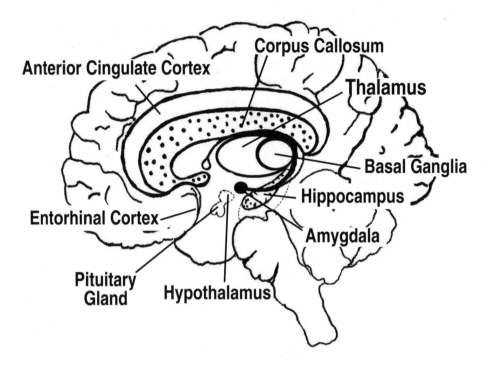

Figure 1.6 Central brain and limbic system. Hippocampus: a seahorse-shaped structure responsible for learning. Amygdala: almond-shaped structure responsible for fear and emotional responses. Thalamus: egg-shaped structure responsible for the relay of sensory and motor information. Hypothalamus: bodily regulator of sleep, appetite and other endocrine functions. Basal ganglia: part of the motor system. Anterior cingulate cortex: amygdala regulator and mediator of conflicts and anxiety.

The cortex regulates excitatory bottom-up emotional and sensory messages. Top-down cortical dampening reactions are associated with conscious decisions that are controlled by the frontal cortex. Emotional experiences are held in short-term memory by the hippocampus, a seahorse-shaped structure implicated in learning. The regulation of emotional experiences is also facilitated by the function of the anterior cingulate cortex (Figure 1.6), which helps mediate conflicts and anxiety and connects the limbic and the central brain to the lower part of the cortex. Bottom-up core affects form the basis from which more complex social affects arise. The orbital frontal cortex regulates complex emotions (Figure 1.3). Examples of complex social affects are pride, guilt, shame, pity and jealousy, as well as cognitive affects like curiosity and surprise, and moral effects such as righteousness.

Experiences of core affects, such as anger, give rise to mental representations of anger. Drawn from memories of similar experiences, a mental appraisal of the current experience also accounts for current relational and situational contexts (Barrett *et al.* 2007; review). These kinds of connections are integral to the managing and regulation of affect. Referring to our earlier example, the client who recoiled from the velvety wet clay reported a shaming memory of her mother reprimanding her for getting dirt under her fingernails. The art therapist paused and encouraged her to experience what she had revealed. Together they noted the differences between who she is and who she was in her memory. With this, the client calmed. She created a pot named "Many Togethers," which she explained as representing her relationship with her self, her sister, her mother and the therapist. She carefully signed her name to the pot, claiming authorship.

Crisis puts the higher verbal regulatory functions in the cerebral cortex out of reach, possibly rendering a person without words (Hull 2002) and making it necessary to work directly with non-verbal, emotional systems (Schore 2007). As emotionally salient information emerges in color and shapes, art therapy provides the advantages of accessing non-verbal emotions through the art (Malchiodi 1998). Understanding the social and emotional role of the limbic brain underscores the applicability of non-verbal therapies: "Art expression could be useful in the treatment of trauma, particularly for individuals who were unable to communicate their experiences with words alone" (Collie *et al.* 2006, p.159). However, it is incumbent upon art therapists to realize that the non-verbal power of the art can work both ways (Chapman and Klorer 2004). Activating visual images of traumatizing memories and talking about trauma can be emotionally overpowering and may reawaken amygdala fear responses. Neuroimaging reviews suggest the centrality of the amygdala to the processing of basic emotions (Barrett *et al.* 2007). Primarily responsible for the fear response, the amygdala is connected to both sensory and motor systems (LeDoux 2002). One of the advantages of art therapy is that it can provide relief by pairing fear-arousing emotions with positive, new sensory experiences. The pot maker example illustrates how the client's shaming memories were updated to include a successful experience. Successfully coping with fear helps regulate and integrate affective experiences.

Affect regulation and integration

Affective neuroscience (Panksepp 1998) emphasizes the importance of connecting limbic emotions with right prefrontal cortex communication (Schore 1999). According to a review of neuroimaging studies, the common significant area of activation for both core and social affects is the orbital frontal cortex (OFC) (Barrett *et al.* 2007). The lower portion of the prefrontal cortex, called the OFC, is located above the eyes and just behind the forehead. The OFC is considered the pinnacle of emotional processing (Schore 2007). As shown in Figure 1.7, its location just above the central brain is central to its role of connecting limbic emotions with the frontal cortex.

Circuitry in the right OFC inhibits sympathetically induced, defensive behavior stimulated by the amygdala (Phelps *et al.* 2004) and responds to rewarding visual stimuli. Abstract and patterned visual stimuli activate the right OFC area located in the right prefrontal lobe (Petrides, Alvisatos, and Frey 2002). Lower OFC regions

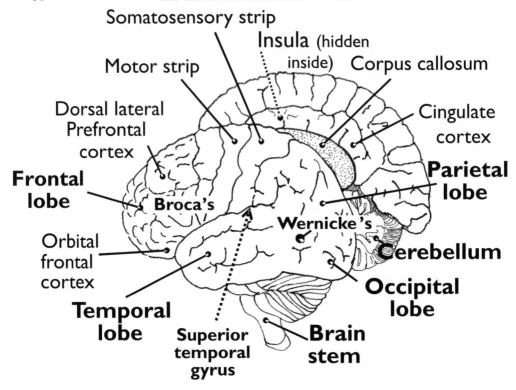

Figure 1.7 Structures and functions. The left prefrontal lobe includes Broca's expressive language center. Corpus callosum: bridges left and right hemispheres. The left temporal cortex includes Wernicke's area responsible for language comprehension. Superior temporal gyrus: polymodal ridge of sensory information integration, bounded by the sulci folds above and below it. Somatosensory strip: holds a map of the body. Motor strip: associates motor activity with visual spatial. Insular cortex: located within the sulcus, which separates the temporal lobe and inferior parietal cortex. The insula conveys bodily states to the cortex.

(ventromedial) have been shown to inhibit autonomic, endocrine and behavioral responses associated with fear and stress caused by unexpected and/or frightening stimuli (Phelps *et al.* 2004). In comparison, frontal areas of the OFC regions activate when people look at expected visual stimuli (Petrides *et al.* 2002). For example, looking at Sonia Delaunay's expected patterns in the Rythme Couleur series (undated) most likely activates the frontal areas of the OFC. In contrast, Wassily Kandinsky's art, where bold strokes interrupt even and smooth patterns, more likely activates the back, lower areas of the OFC (Kandinsky Image 1; Improvisation 26, Oars, 1912).

When participants were asked to make a decision, whether the abstract pattern was familiar or not, a frontal area above the OFC involved in hierarchically higher cognitive processing was also activated (mid-dorsal prefrontal). Broad inferences from this research can explain the advantages of collaging. Based on the research described above it seems likely that, even without words, inspecting, sorting and choosing preferred imagery assists in initiating emotional and cognitive function integration.

The OFC processing of limbic emotions is helped by anterior cingulate cortex (ACC) functioning. The ACC is a brain structure that mediates affect regulation and mind/body conflicts like anxiety that can be aroused by unfamiliar patterns. The OFC also receives information about the body from the insular cortex. The insular cortex is located within the lateral sulcus, a fold that separates the frontal lobe from the temporal lobe and parietal cortices (Figures 1.3 and 1.6). The insular cortex contributes to a sense of self through embodied cognitions. It transmits visceral bodily events associated with emotions transforming them into conscious feelings (Damasio 1999). Further contributing to the connections between the body and the brain are the somatosensory cortex and the motor strips. The somatosensory strip, also called the primary somatosensory cortex, holds a map of the body, and the motor strip associates motor activity with visual spatial information. For children, engaging in sensory-based activities provides a crucial foundation for later, more complex learning and behavior (Roseann, Schaaf, and Miller 2005; review).

"Art as therapy" activities have the potential to activate neural pathways related to tactile and kinesthetic sensations associated with the primary somatosensory cortex. Sensory experiences include touch, movement, visual and sound. Junctures where different areas in the brain meet, such as the superior temporal gyrus (Figure 1.7), are areas of polymodal integration. Expressing, experiencing and learning how to regulate affects can perhaps happen more easily through sensory integration activities and kinesthetic movement associated with art therapy activities. As described earlier in the pot maker example, sensory art-making processes can encourage vertical integration of brain function and result in complex feelings such as authorship. The non-verbal exploration and expression of emotions may entrain the expression of more complex cortical feelings such as a determination to problem-solve or the anticipation of pride or shame if the task is or is not completed according to expectations.

Achieving stable mental states also requires integrating left and right hemispheres function (Schore 2007), which can potentially be facilitated by therapeutic art-making (McNamee 2003). The connections between the left and right hemispheres are facilitated by the corpus callosum, a broad band of neural fiber. While the right and left hemisphere share more functions than popularly thought, there are dominant lateralized trends associated with each hemisphere. The right hemisphere is described as more emotional, avoidant oriented, intuitive and non-verbal, whereas the left hemisphere is more sequential, problem-solving oriented, positive, approach oriented and is lateralized for language (Carter 1998; Goulven and Tzourio-Mazoyer 2003; Harmon-Jones 2007). McNamee suggested that a neurologically based bilateral art protocol can possibly facilitate a systemic integration of hemispheric right-left functions. The protocol assists clients in exploring conflicting choices, cognitions or emotions. The therapist provides a page divided by a midline. The client determines which hand connects to which conflict or aspect of it and decides which conflict (aspect) should be drawn first with that hand and on which side of the page. The therapist also places art materials on the corresponding right or left side of the page. After completing one drawing, the client is invited to revisit the page. This second transposed drawing is a response to the first drawing and is drawn with the opposite hand and/or with both hands (for a full and precise description of the protocol and case study see McNamee 2003, p.285).

Art therapy practices can assist in regulating limbic affects by engaging left cortical functions. For example, art therapists may be able to do so by asking clients to title the artwork and talk about their feelings with the therapist. The left hemisphere specializes in the reception of language and the production of speech. Relative to other mammals the human cortex has expanded to accommodate our unique language abilities (Kalat 2004). Language and social communication directly contribute to necessary affect regulation. There are two main language centers in the human brain, Wernicke's and Broca's. Wernicke's area, responsible for language comprehension, is located in the left temporal lobe. The temporal lobe is also responsible for receptive language and auditory processing. While receptive language is primarily located in the left temporal lobe, speech and expressive language are located in the Broca's area close to the motor strip in the left prefrontal lobe. Thus talking about the art seems to engage cortical shifts: "Putting feelings into words is an effective strategy for regulating negative emotional responses" (Lieberman 2007, p.270; review). Asking clients always to title and talk about the art may result in them routinely doing so. Automatically talking about and labeling feelings has been shown to reduce amygdala activity and increase prefrontal activation (Lieberman 2007).

Expressions of relational empathy and mindfulness

Affect regulation is mediated by relationships with others. Interpersonal relationships can arouse as well as alleviate stressful emotions and humans are more likely to turn to others at times of distress (Zeanah 2002). The therapist's and the client's brains and their nervous system reciprocate and synchronize (Siegel 1999). The therapeutic goals of interpersonal neurobiology are to recruit the other's mind in order to increase flexible, adaptive, coherent, energized and stable states of mind (FACES) (Siegel 2006). As people respond to each other, networks from similar brain areas respond and fire, evoking empathic resonance (Gallese 2006; Gallese, Keysers, and Rizzolatti 2004). Facilitated by mirror neurons, humans can learn through empathic imitation and observation of another's actions, observing and recognizing that someone else's action is something that we can do also (Gallese 2003). First discovered in the brains of Macaque monkeys, mirror neurons fired when the monkeys performed purposeful hand and feet actions, as well as in response to their recognizing or even anticipating purposeful and successful acts performed by others (Buccino, Binkofski, and Riggio 2004; Rizzolatti *et al.* 1996). For the art therapist, this may represent an exciting representation of empathic connectivity. In anticipation of the therapist's hands purposefully offering soft oil pastels, the client reaches out to take them (Figure 1.8).

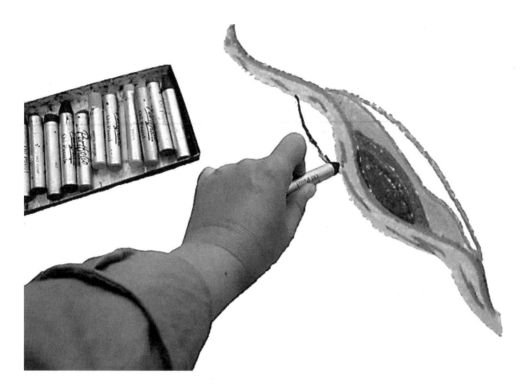

Figure 1.8 Does this picture stimulate your desire to pick a pastel and follow along? The artist is left-handed, which will modulate the impact for right-handed viewers.

While originally it was thought that using tools for purposeful actions did not demonstrate mirror neuron firing, more current research supports that, at least in Macaques, mirror neurons fire in response to using tools for purposeful actions (Iacoboni and Dapretto 2006; review). The impact of recognizing that *I can do what you can do*, and *make what you make*, reflects an emotional resonance that can be experienced by art therapy clients and art therapists. Artists learning from the masters also report a similar reaction as they are inspired by works of art. When looking at the client's artwork, the therapist's empathy is aroused by recognizing how she could have made what the client made.

In humans, research has shown an observation/executive function mirror system close to Broca's area suggesting an evolutionary link to language development (Buccino *et al.* 2001, 2004; Figure 1.7). Perhaps that is why the manipulation and purposeful grasping of art therapy media can often be experienced as a non-verbal language (Hass-Cohen 2007).

The planning and execution of purposeful choices, decisions and actions requires controlling affective response and self-regulation (Banfield *et al.* 2004). The prefrontal lobes are associated with executive functions such as perceiving, verbalizing, motivating, attending and coordinating (Faw 2003) and they mediate a higher order of control used in willed actions such as making art. Carefully made media choices help regulate essential expressivity and integrate affect with willful action. Traditionally, structured art therapy media are advocated for control (Malchiodi 1998). However, the use of very structured media, such as pencil, may stifle affective expressivity and may not provide sufficient impetus for the integration of affects and cognitions. Considering more subtle media differences may help solve this problem. For example, Lark (2007) advocates using tempera paint rather than acrylic in her art therapy painting approach. She described how the flat tempera paint requires more mindful efforts whereas "acrylic does the work" for her highly emotive and severely traumatized clients. Sometimes she switches between the two paint media encouraging the necessary expression of emotions. Similar parallels can be made to painting with pastels; a range of soft to hard pastels, color restrictions and the paper gradations help structure and integrate emotional experiences.

In the first of the three self-portraits in Figure 1.9 (left portrait), the gliding of soft pastels on very fine sandpaper allows for immediate expression of emotional conflict on the portraiture of the author's face. Dark and white areas clash expressively while naked pixel sizes of the black sand paper disturb the visual flow. The use of soft and hard pastels in the middle portrait slowed the artist down, allowing for more reflection and a recognizable face to emerge. The final portrait is affected by the restricted color palette and traditional pastel paper. Here, there is more space on the page for the figure portrait and the visual reiteration of the facial shadowy feelings in the background begins a new dialogue within the artist. The effortful experience in the last portrait should not be confused with realism. Rather, it allows for a more mindful expression of the self (Figure 1.9 a–c).

Summary

The art therapy approach outlined in this chapter highlights a mind-body practice that can help organize, integrate and enhance the complexity of people's intrapersonal and interpersonal interactions. Key to the development of interpersonal neurobiology sensitive art therapy directives is finding out how our clients may have adapted to life stressors and appreciating that unresolved adaptations may have created emotional residue. The action of art-making is a unique way in which art therapy helps clients resolve, in the here and now, responses to residual fears and memories of disturbing events. Therapy interventions that have the potential to rewire the brain also have the power to recondition such traumatic residues. For art therapists, it makes sense that the excitatory and pleasurable effects of art-making and the ability to distance oneself from a tangible image can mitigate the fear of being re-traumatized.

In doing art therapy, "the challenge is to learn enough about the mechanisms of plasticity to be able to guide them, suppressing changes that may lead to undesirable behaviors while accelerating or enhancing those that result in a behavioral benefit"

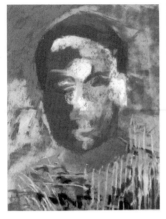 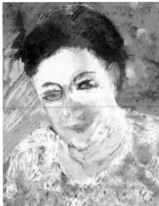 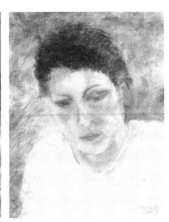

Figure 1.9 Self-Portraits: From Expression to Mindfulness. *Pastels, Hass-Cohen, 2005.*

(Pascual-Leone 2006, p.315). Art activities, which can be novel and challenging, provide stimulating and kinesthetic activities that have been associated with an enriched environment (Jensen 1996, 2001; Nithianantharajah and Hannan 2006). In the future, interpersonal, sensory-based art therapy interventions may prove to be a way of creating change in the brain. Sharing information about how the brain changes with therapists and with clients can also generate powerful art therapy psychoeducational interventions.

People's functions range from physiological arousal, appraisal, subjective experience to expression which ultimately lead to intentional actions and relational interactions. Completing the art therapy task requires the integration of higher cortical thinking, such as planning, attention, and mindful problem-solving with social-emotional investment. The support and skills of an attuned art therapist helps recruit, express and hold the relational self in mind while allowing for the expression of needed emotions and motivations. The realization of emotions in the artwork becomes a natural accompaniment to completing higher cortical tasks. Emotions, such as frustration and joy, which emerge in the artwork, are experienced whilst learning to trust another person, in our case, the art therapist.

References

Abitz, M., Nielsen, R. D., Jones, E. G., Laursen, H., Graem, N., and Pakkenberg, B. (2007). Excess of neurons in the human newborn mediodorsal thalamus compared with that of the adult. *Cerebral Cortex, 17*(11), 2573–2578; doi:10.1093/cercor/bhl163. Cerebral Cortex Advance Access originally published online on January 11, 2007.

Achterberg, J., Dossy, L., Gordon, J. S., Hegedus, C., Herrmann, M. W., and Nelson, R. (1994). *Mind-body Interventions.* Panel report to the National Institutes of Health on Alternative Medical Systems and practices in the United States. Washington, DC: U.S. Government Printing Office.

Ahlander, N. R. (2002). 'The Science of Infant Brain Development: Insights on the Nature/Nurture Debate', *World Family Policy Forum*: 78–82.

Allen, J. S., Bruss, J., and Damasio, H. (2005). The aging brain: the cognitive reserve hypothesis and hominid evolution. *American Journal of Human Biology, 17*(6), 673–689. Review.

Banfield, J., Wyland, C. L., Macrae, C. N., Munte, T. F., and Heatherton, T. F. (2004). The cognitive neuroscience of self-regulation. In R. F. Baumeister and K. D. Vohs (eds), *The Handbook of Self-Regulation* (pp.62–83). New York: Guilford Press.

Barlow, B. (2001). *Clinical Handbook of Psychological Disorders* (3rd edition). New York: Guilford Press.

Barrett, L. F., Mesquita, B., Oschner, K. N., and Gross, J. J. (2007). The experience of emotion. *Annual Reviews, Psychology 58*, 373–403.

Baumeister, R. F., and Vohs, K. D. (2004). *Handbook of Self-regulation*. New York, London: Guilford Press.

Bear, M. F., Connors, B. W., and Paradiso, M. A. (2006). *Neuroscience: Exploring the brain* (3rd edition). Philadelphia, PA: Lippincott Williams & Wilkins.

Bishop, C. M. (1995). *Neural Networks for Pattern Recognition*. New York: Oxford University Press.

Bremner, J. D. (2006). Stress and brain atrophy. *CNS Neurological Disorders Drug Targets, 5*(5), 503–512. Review.

Buccino, G., Binkofski, F., Fink, G. R., Fadiga, L., Fogassi, L., Gallese, V., *et al.* (2001). Action observation activates premotor and parietal areas in a somatotopic manner: an fMRI study. *European Journal of Neuroscience, 13*, 400–404.

Buccino, G., Binkofski, F., and Riggio, L. (2004). The mirror neuron system and action recognition. *Brain and Language, 89*, 370–376.

Camic, P. M. (1999). Chapter 2: Expanding treatment possibilities for chronic pain through the expressive arts. In C. Malchiodi (ed.), *Medical Arts Therapy with Adults*. London and Philadelphia, PA: Jessica Kingsley Publishers.

Carter, R. (1998). *Mapping the Mind*. Los Angeles, CA: University of California Press.

Carlson, N. R. (2004). *Physiology of Behavior* (8th edition). Boston, MA, New York, San Franscisco, CA: Pearson.

Chapman, L. and Klorer, P. G. (2004). Cumulative trauma and art therapy: Neurodevelopmental advances in theory and practice (with Linda Chapman). Proceedings of the 35th Annual Conference of the American Art Therapy Association, Mundelein, IL: AATA Inc.

Colcombe, S. J., Erickson, K. I., Raz, N., Webb, A. G., Cohen, N. J., McAuley, E., and Kramer, A. F. (2003). Aerobic fitness reduces brain tissue loss in aging humans. *Journal of Gerontology: Series A: Biological and Medical Sciences, 58*, M176–M180.

Collie, K., Backos, A., Malchiodi, C., and Spiegel, D. (2006). Art therapy for combat-related PTSD: Recommendations for research and practice. *Art Therapy: Journal of the American Art Therapy Association, 23*(4), 157–164.

Courchesne, E. (2004). Brain development in autism: early overgrowth followed by premature arrest of growth. *Mental Retardation and Developmental Disabilities Research Reviews, 10*, 106–111.

Cousins, N. (1979). *Anatomy of an Illness as Perceived by the Patient*. New York: W. W. Norton and Company.

Cozolino, L. (2002). *The Neuroscience of Psychotherapy*. New York, London: Norton.

Damasio, A. R. (1994). *Descartes' Error: Emotion, Reason, and the Human Brain*. New York: Harper Perennial.

Damasio, A. (1999). *The Feeling of What Happens: Body, Emotion and the Making of Consciousness*. Heinemann: London.

Diamond, M. and Hopson, J. (1998). *Magic Trees of the Mind: How to Nurture Your Child's Intelligence, Creativity, and Healthy Emotions from Birth through Adolescence*. New York: Penguin Putnam.

Draganski, B., Gaser, C., Kempermann, G., Kuhn, H. G., Winkler, J., Büchel, C., *et al.* (2006). Temporal and spatial dynamics of brain structure changes during extensive learning. *Journal of Neuroscience, 26*(23), 6314–6317.

Elder, G. A., De Gasperi, R., and Gama Sosa, M. A. (2006). Research update: Neurogenesis in adult brain and neuropsychiatric disorders. *Mount Sinai Journal of Medicine 73*(7), 931–940. Review.

Eliot, L. (1999). *What's Going On in There? How the Brain and Mind Develop in the First Five Years of Life*. New York: Bantam Books.

Eriksson, P. S., Perfilieva, E., Bjork-Eriksson, T., Alborn, A. M., Nordborg, C., Peterson, D. A., *et al.* (1998). Neurogenesis in the adult human hippocampus. *Nature Medicine, 4*(11), 1313–1317.

Faw, B. (2003). Pre-frontal executive committee for perception, working memory, attention, long-term memory, motor control, and thinking: A tutorial review. *Consciousness and Cognition, 12*, 83–139.

Gallese, V. (2003). The roots of empathy: the shared manifold hypothesis and the neural basis of intersubjectivity. *Psychopathology, 36*, 171–180.

Gallese, V. (2006). Intentional attunement: A neurophysiological perspective on social cognition and its disruption in autism. *Brain Research. Cognitive Brain Research, 1079*, 15–24.

Gallese, V., Keysers, C., and Rizzolatti, G. (2004). A unifying view of the basis of social cognition. *Trends in Cognitive Sciences, 8*(9), 396–403.

Giedd, J. N. (2004). Structural magnetic resonance imaging of the adolescent brain. *Annals New York Academy of Sciences, 1021*, 77–85.

Giedd, J. N., Blumenthal, J., Jeffries, N. O., Castellanos, F. X., Liu, H., Zijdenbos, A., *et al.* (1999). Brain development during childhood and adolescence: a longitudinal MRI study. *Nature Neuroscience, 2*(10), 861–863.

Gillespie, J. (1994). *The Projective Use of Mother-and-Child Drawings: A Manual for Clinicians.* New York: Brunner/Mazel Publishers.

Goulven, J. and Tzourio-Mazoyer, N. (2003) Review: Hemispheric specialization for language. *Brain Research Reviews, 44*, 1–12.

Harmon-Jones, E. (2007). Asymmetrical frontal cortical activity. In E. Harmon-Jones and P. Winkielman (eds) *Social Neuroscience, Integrating Biological and Psychological Explanations of Social Behavior.* New York, London: The Guilford Press.

Hass-Cohen, N. (2003). Art therapy mind body approaches. *Progress: Family Systems Research and Therapy, 12*, 24–38.

Hass-Cohen, N. (2007). Cultural arts in action: musings on empathy. GAINS *Community Newsletter: Connections and Reflections,* Summer 2007, 41–48.

Hass-Cohen, N. (2008). *CREATE:* Art therapy relational neuroscience principles (ATR-N). In N. Hass-Cohen and R. Carr (eds) *Art Therapy and Clinical Neuroscience.* London and Philadelphia, PA: Jessica Kingsley Publishers.

Henry, J. P. and Wang, S. (1999). Effects of early stress on adult affiliative behavior. *Psycho-neuroendocrinology, 23*(8), 863–875.

Hull, A. (2002). Neuroimaging findings in post-traumatic stress disorder, systematic review. *British Journal of Psychiatry, 181*, 102–110.

Iacoboni, M. and Dapretto, M. (2006). The mirror neuron system and the consequences of its dysfunction. *Nature Reviews Neuroscience, 7*(12), 942–951.

Jensen, E. (1996). *Brain-Based Learning.* Del Mar, CA: Turning Point Publishing.

Jensen, E. (2001). *Arts with the Brain in Mind.* Alexandria, VA: Association for Supervision & Curriculum Development.

Kalat, J. W. (2004). *Biological Psychology* (8th edition). Belmont, CA: Wadsworth/Thomson Learning.

Kandel, E. (1998). A new intellectual framework for psychiatry. *American Journal of Psychiatry, 155*, 457–469.

Kaplan, H. H. (2000). *Art, Science and Art Therapy: Repainting the Picture.* London, Philadelphia, PA: Jessica Kingsley Publishers.

Kravits, K. (2008). The stress response and adaptation theory. In N. Hass-Cohen and R. Carr (eds) *Art Therapy and Clinical Neuroscience.* London and Philadelphia, PA: Jessica Kingsley Publishers.

Lark, C. (2007). Personal communication.

Lazar, S. W., Kerrb, C. E., Wasserman, R. H., Gray, J. R., Greved, D. N., Treadwaya, M. T., *et al.* (2005). Meditation experience is associated with increased cortical thickness. *Neuroreport, 16*(17), 1893–1897.

LeDoux, J. E. (2000). Emotion circuits in the brain. *Annual Reviews Neuroscience, 23*, 155–184.

LeDoux, J. E. (2002). *The Synaptic Self.* New York: Viking Penguin.

Lieberman, M. (2007). Social cognitive neuroscience: a review of core processes. *Annual Reviews of Psychology, 58*, 259–289.

Lusebrink, V. B. (2004). Art therapy and the brain: An attempt to understand the underlying processes of art expression in therapy. *Art Therapy: Journal of the American Art Therapy Association, 21*(3), 125–135.

Malberg, J. E. and Schechter, L. E. (2005). Increasing hippocampal neurogenesis: a novel mechanism for antidepressant drugs. *Current Pharmaceutical Design, 11*(2), 145–155. Review.

Malchiodi, C. A. (1998). *The Art Therapy Sourcebook.* Los Angeles, CA: Lowell House.

May, A. and Gaser, C. (2006). Magnetic resonance-based morphometry: a window into structural plasticity of the brain. *Current Opinion Neurology, 19*(4), 407–441.

McEwen, B. and Lasley, E. N. (2002). *The End of Stress as We Know It.* Washington, DC: National Academies Press.

McNamee, C. M. (2003). Bilateral art: facilitating systemic integration and balance. *The Arts in Psychotherapy, 30*, 283–292.

Mechelli, A., Crinion, J. T., Noppeney, U., O'Doherty, J., Ashburner, J., Frackowiak, R. S., *et al.* (2004). Neurolinguistics: structural plasticity in the bilingual brain. *Nature, 14*, 757.

Naparstek, B. (1994). *Staying Well with Guided Imagery.* Boston, MA: Warner Books.

National Research Council of Medicine (2000). *From Neurons to Neighborhoods: The Science of Early Childhood Development.* Washington, D.C: National Academies Press.

Nithianantharajah, J. and Hannan, A. J. (2006). Enriched environments, experience-dependent plasticity and disorders of the nervous system. *Nature Reviews/Neuroscience, 7*, 607–709.

Panksepp, J. (1998). *Affective Neuroscience: The Foundations of Human and Animal Emotions.* New York: Oxford University Press.

Pascual-Leone, A. (2006). Disrupting the brain to guide plasticity and improve behavior. *Progress in Brain Research, 157*, 315–329.

Perry, B. D. (1996). *Maltreated Children: Experience, Brain Development and the Next Generation.* New York and London: W. W. Norton.

Perry, B. D. (1997). Incubated in terror: neurodevelopmental factors in the "Cycle of Violence". In J. Osofsky (ed.) *Children, Youth and Violence: The Search for Solutions* (pp.124–148). New York: Guilford Press.

Perry, B. D. (2001). The neurodevelopmental impact of violence in childhood. In D. Schetky and E. Benedek (eds) *Textbook of Child and Adolescent Forensic Psychiatry* (pp. 221–238). Washington, D.C.: American Psychiatric Press.

Petrides, M., Alvisatos, B. and Frey, J. (2002). Differential activation of the human orbital, mid-ventrolateral, and mid-dorsalteral prefrontal cortex during the processing of visual stimuli. *Proceedings of the National Academy of Sciences, 99*(8), 5649–5654.

Phelps, E. A., Delgado, M. R., Nearing, K. I., and LeDoux, J. E. (2004). Extinction learning in humans: Role of the amygdale and vmPFC. *Neuron, 43*, 897–905.

Porges, S. W. (2001). The polyvagal theory: phylogenetic substrates of a social nervous system. *International Journal of Psychophysiology, 42*, 123–146.

Prasko, J., Horacek, J., Zalesky, R., Kopecek, M., Novak, T., Paskova, B., *et al.* (2004). The change of regional brain metabolism (18FDG PET) in panic disorder during the treatment with cognitive behavioral therapy or antidepressants. *Neuroendocrinology Letters, 25*(5), 340–348.

Riley, S. (2004). The creative mind. *Art Therapy Journal of the American Art Therapy Association, 21*(4), 184–190.

Rizzolatti, G., Fadiga, L., Gallese, V., and Fogassi, L. (1996). Premotor cortex and the recognition of motor actions. *Cognitive Brain Research, 3*, 131–141.

Roseann, C., Schaaf, R. C., and Miller, L. J. (2005). Occupational therapy using a sensory integrative approach for children with developmental disabilities. *Mental Retardation and Developmental Disabilities: Research Reviews, 11*, 143–148.

Sapolsky, R. (1998). *Why Zebras Don't Get Ulcers.* New York: W. H. Freeman and Company.

Satz, P. (1993). Brain reserve capacity on symptom onset after brain injury: A formulation and review of evidence for threshold theory. *Neuropsychology, 7*, 273–295.

Schore, A. N. (1994). *Affect Regulation and the Origin of the Self: The Neurobiology of Emotional Development.* Hillsdale, NJ: Lawrence Erlbaum.

Schore, A. N. (2001). Contributions from the decade of the brain to infant mental health: An overview. *Infant Mental Health Journal, 22*(1–2), 1–6.

Schore, A. (2007). The Science of the Art of Psychotherapy [Conference], Skirball Cultural Center, Los Angeles, CA. 02 Feb. 2007–03 Feb. 2007.

Schore, A. (1999). *Affect Regulation and the Origin of the Self.* London: Lawrence Erlbaum Associates.

Siegel, D. J. (1999). *The Developing Mind: Towards a Neurobiology of Interpersonal Experience.* New York, London: The Guilford Press.

Siegel, D. J. (2006). An interpersonal neurobiology approach to psychotherapy: Awareness, mirror neurons, and neural plasticity in the development of well-being. *Psychiatric Annals, 36*(4), 248–256.

Stein, M., Dierks, T., Brandeis, D., Wirth, M., Strik, W., and Koenig, T. (2006). Plasticity in the adult language system: A longitudinal electrophysiological study on second language learning. *Neuroimage, 33*(2), 774–783.

Straube, T., Glauer, M., Dilger, S., Mentzel, H. J., and Miltner, W. H. (2006). Effects of cognitive-behavioral therapy on brain activation in specific phobia. *Neuroimage, 29*(1), 125–135.

Tamietto, M., Adenzato, M., Geminiani, G., and de Gelder, B. (2007). Fast recognition of social emotions takes the whole brain: Interhemispheric cooperation in the absence of cerebral asymmetry. *Neuropsychologia, 45*, 836–843.

Tronick, E. (2007). *The Neurobiology and Social-emotional Development of Infants and Children.* New York: Norton & Company.

Vance, R. and Wahlin, K. (2008). *Memory and Art.* In N. Hass-Cohen and R. Carr (eds), *Art Therapy and Clinical Neuroscience.* London and Philadelphia, PA: Jessica Kingsley Publishers.

Zeanah, C. H. (2002) *Handbook of Infant Mental Health.* London, New York: Guilford Press.

2

Sensory Processes and Responses

Richard Carr

Introduction: from past to present

Humans process and sense the internal and external world in ways shaped over an incredibly long evolutionary journey. During the last two to three million years, we attained a brain to body mass ratio (measured on a logarithmic scale to eliminate overall animal size effects) of six to seven times the average in the animal kingdom (Dawkins 2004; Schoenemann 2006). Brain to body ratios seem to correlate with a species' need to inhibit impulses consciously (Finley, Darlington, and Nicastro 2001; McKinney 2000), and to regulate affect with intuitive awareness (Schore 1994). For humans, the neocortex or new brain embodies many of these changes. The larger neo or cerebral cortex shown with major divisions in Figure 2.1 reflects the brain's ability to cortically govern impulses otherwise controlled by subcortical instinct or drive states.

Within the neocortex's frontal lobe (Figure 2.1), the prefrontal cortex (PFC) (Figure 2.2) lies just behind or posterior to the forehead. Determining PFC ratio to brain volume on a logarithmic scale establishes humans as having the largest such ratio in the animal kingdom (Schoenemann 2006). For mammals, including humans, this ratio correlates with the size of typical social groups in which the species congregates (Sapolsky 2004). From this we might surmise that during evolution regulating psychosocial awareness became more critical than regulating survival moments. Consequently, priorities within sensory processes shifted somewhat from those driven by survival needs that are defined by nature to those defined by psychosocial determinants. Over time, instead of chasing, attacking, or running from those who angered or threatened us, we learned to manipulate vocal cords in order to talk or yell—sometimes even managing to reduce threats through psychosocially sensitive expressions of empathy. Organizing around psychosocial cues continues to reprioritize complex human perceptions of and interactions with the world.

Our prefrontal cortex has become specialized in executive functions: problem-solving, anticipating events that affect us, conjuring how to reconfigure perceptions, and deciding how to direct actions. The PFC helps us alter and diversify our living environment. Human hand manipulations, reflecting over 3,500,000 years of

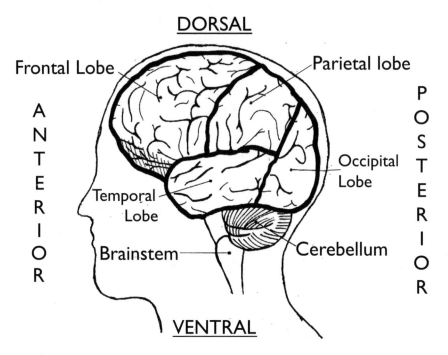

Figure 2.1 The cerebral cortex, the outermost brain layer, has changed significantly during human evolution. The dark outlined area shows the cerebral (neo) cortex. Orienting directions: dorsal, ventral, anterior and posterior are also shown. Illustration by Tise Chao.

specialization, exhibit greater dexterity and sensitivity to touch than every other species. It is quite possible that our abilities to gesture, take aim and throw elevated us from prey to predator, strengthening goal orientations while weakening our survival orientation (Sapolsky 2004). Confidently saying, "I can handle this!" might stir deep feelings of being superior that unconsciously acknowledge the shift away from being prey.

Sophisticated hand gestures also integrate many brain functions that contribute to making art. Red and black pigments found in 400,000-year-old early human sites suggest body art or tool decoration. A female stone figure from 3 to 400,000 years ago, the earliest known art piece, while possibly a by-product of nature, appears to have been humanly enhanced and reddened with ocher. It represents a significant shift towards externalizing or objectifying our mental experience during our psychological evolution (Potts 2007). The archeological record reveals that humans increasingly manifested their inner life by making visibly concrete, symbolic creations that exposed human emotion and thought (Bradshaw 2001). Further innovations that made gathering food easier, life safer and more comfortable, convenience more obtainable continue to show artistic adornment.

Did art-making embody a primal process for expressing and accessing awareness of self and other? Archeology suggests that cave painting and rock art from around 18,000 years ago may have captured spiritual or early empathic attempts to become one with animals critical for human survival (Potts 2007). These artistic expressions arose from the artists altering their state of mind so that attunement with the habits of prey or with illnesses shared with prey became easier to understand. Flowers strewn over a gravesite, decorations on bone and shell necklaces, cave paintings, Egyptian murals, and eventually modern art and architecture command that we acknowledge repeated and spirited attempts to understand, represent, change, share and define a world altered by psychosocial sensory and emotional creations.

Sensing the world

Sensory prompts subliminally continue to shape and influence verbal and non-verbal communication processes. Note how your senses and attention shift when you imagine hearing and seeing the following: While gesturing, he exulted, "The sun, a flaming orb, descends until only a rosy ball slinks beneath the silvery, ink blue surface, bringing the graying land towards a peaceful slumber." This gestured, spoken, concrete, abstract, metaphorical and emotional descriptive invites complex, organized activation in our newly evolved neocortex.

Neural pathways and mechanisms facilitate humans sensing their environment. Specialized sensory receptors reacting to specific types of stimuli, like light, sound, heat, cold, odor, taste, texture, proprioception, and interoception occupy the body's most likely places for encountering these stimuli: the eyes, ears, lips, tongue, hands, feet... Stimulated sensory receptors react by activating neurons that cause sensation-creating energy bursts to energize subsequent neurons in a follow-the-leader fashion. Incoming signals are directed into discrete information-carrying neural networks destined to reach more evolved brain areas. Passing the message from neuron to neuron continues until specific brain areas receive and start a response to the sensations (Figure 2.2).

If strong enough, a stimulus replicates many times on its way towards awareness or reaction. When neocortical areas engage, complex, conscious responses awaken that can lead to subtle experiences such as feeling enveloped by music or poetry.

However, sensory signals traversing and neuronally engaging specialized brain structures do not always attain awareness. The brain recorded our evolutionary journey by stacking later evolving brains on top of early ones. Sometimes this evolutionary hierarchy prevents stimuli responses from reaching awareness, as earlier evolutionary adaptations found in our reptilian or earlier mammalian brains usurp the processing. Blindsight, for instance, stimulates even blind people to respond to certain movements not visually conscious (Ramachandran 2004). Beneath the thalamus (Figures 2.2, 2.3 and 2.4), a structure called the superior colliculus (Figure 2.4) retains a reptilian ability to respond to motion without engaging the visual centers. Thus, a moving, unidentified object can orient self-protective reactions that protect us from unseen stimuli, such as turning or blinking without our knowing why (Ramachandran 2004). Structures that

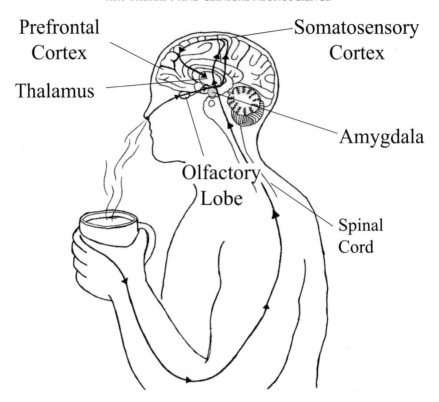

Figure 2.2 Sensory paths to the brain. The smell path differs from the touch and temperature paths. Illustration by Tise Chao.

facilitate survival responses, like the superior colliculus, reduce energy expenditure and the time-consuming conscious effort needed to form a reaction.

How a stimulus becomes conscious is determined by which brain structure—the new and specifically human neocortex; the less changed, mammalian limbic cortex; or the ancient, reptilian brain–regulates behavior. When lower brain centers exclusively engage, responses range from reflexive to affective, typical in reptiles, non-primate mammals (Panksepp 1998), and frightened people. For example, the subcortically driven, startle response remains outside of consciousness until after the body reacts.

Lateralization of the brain's two hemispheres (Figure 2.5) further divides the functional orientation used to process a stimulus. Dominance in the right or the left hemisphere alters conscious awareness. Right hemisphere processing generates more intuitive or "gut" feelings through direct, preconscious awareness of and impact upon bodily change (Schore 1994). Processing in the left hemisphere increases explicit awareness as conscious memory activates and influences perception, communication, and behavior. Both right and left hemispheric neocortical orientations enact perceptions proven advantageous throughout evolution. Perhaps if humans had evolved by obtaining food nocturnally, "darkness" might strike us differently and "shadows" might offer solace.

Ontogeny, environment, genes, and responses built from learned patterns of attention selectively modify brain structures, functions and interactions within neural pathways. Exceptionally vulnerable and malleable critical and sensitive developmental periods, such as learning to walk and talk, occur when specific structures and neural networks initially link and become refined. These influences combine ultimately to define later abilities with which a person imagines and anticipates the world.

Early unconscious or preconscious processing engages neuroanatomical structures like the thalamus, the amygdala, the somatosensory cortex, the anterior cingulate cortex, the insula, and the prefrontal cortex displayed in Figure 2.3.

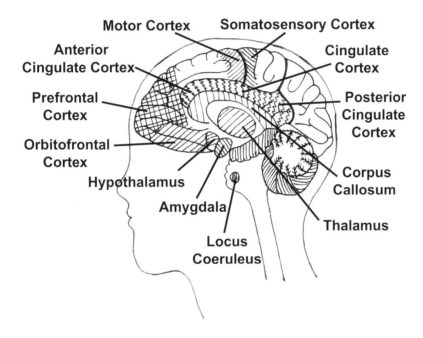

Figure 2.3 Brain cross-section showing location of structures. Illustration by Tise Chao.

The thalamus, functioning as the brain's sensory gateway from the body and brainstem (Figure 2.1) to higher brain centers, spreads its information over large areas of the cortex (Castro-Alamancos and Calcagnotto 2001). It "represents a hub from which any site in the cortex can communicate with any other such site or sites" (Llinás *et al.* 1998, p.1841; Figure 2.4). Feedback loops between the thalamus and reciprocal structures dynamically alter interactions, so that as we become aware of something, it is as if different brain areas simultaneously gain access (Edelman and Tononi 2000). For instance, experiencing pain sensitizes awareness and anticipation of similar subsequent possibilities. When anticipation of pain increases, the thalamus, insula, anterior cingulate cortex, prefrontal cortex, and other brain regions increase intercommunication. If decreased pain is anticipated, activity in these structures decreases reducing nearly 25 percent of the subjective pain experience (Koyama *et al.* 2005). Thus, "consciousness arises from a continuous 'dialogue' between the thalamus and the cortex" (Llinás and Ribary 2001, p.167). Anticipating meaningful occurrences causes brain areas to refine incoming sensory information and shift awareness. Feedback and "dialogue" critically mainipulate conscious sensory awareness and therefore experience.

Sensory journeys take milliseconds to blend stimuli responses rapidly in higher and/or lower brain structures. Consequently, interesting blends of evolutionary and brain/body responses occur. Imagine the expressive outcome as portions of the neocortex direct some body parts to respond in a uniquely human fashion, while others, directed by reptilian brain areas, respond more reflexively, similar to a lizard. In the end a single outcome or behavior needs to achieve coherency. Imagine an orchestra composed of different musical sections. Each combines their effects, creating a harmonious, meaningfully conscious, personal experience of reality. If misattunements occur, like those that accompany drug-induced hallucinations, head trauma or psychopathology, the experienced reality becomes distorted. Responses and response patterns misalign and trouble follows.

The thalamus: sensation and action gateway between body and brain

Nearly all the senses, except the olfactory, initially route their neurons to the thalamus. This structure, consisting of two walnut-sized, egg-shaped masses centrally situated in the brain, forms the key relay station of sensations from the body to the rest of the brain (Figure 2.2). Sensory input is assembled there and sent to multiple processing destinations in the brain. Stimulation destined to become conscious connects with specialized neural networks linking the thalamus to specific sensory processing areas in the cerebral cortex (Castro *et al.* 2002; Figure 2.4). Stimulation needing to affect consciousness indirectly is sent to nearby, more rapidly processing limbic structures in the central brain region beneath the neocortex (Figure 2.6). The thalamus, potentially subject to overwhelm and imbalance, very actively facilitates communication with and between cortical sites.

Cortical feedback to the thalamus, more than twice the sensory input from the body, brakes the flow of incoming thalamic information as needed. Imagine quick, terse messages—redundant, enough, or more—dynamically feeding back to the thalamus and helping to regulate distribution of sensory information further (Castro-Alamancos and Calcagnotto 2001). Corticothalamic communication creates a complex, constant dialogue about stimuli inhibition and simultaneous occurrences (Figure 2.4).

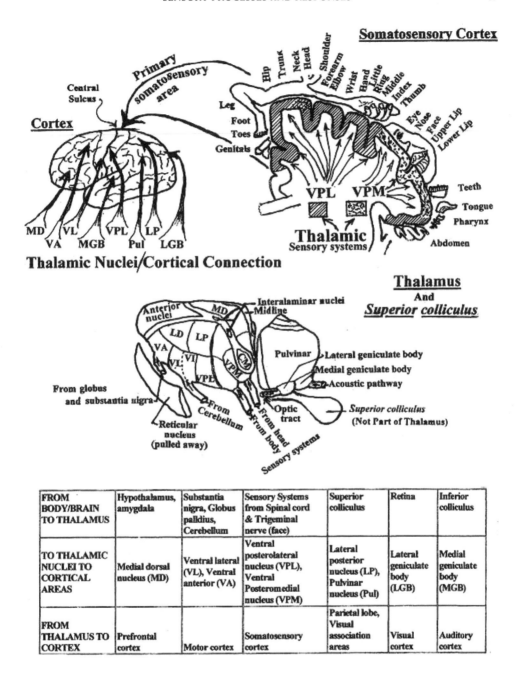

Figure 2.4 Thalamic nuclei connections to brain structures along with the superior colliculus are essential in blindsight and visually orienting: Thalamic nuclei: AN: Anterior; LD: Lateral dorsal; LP: Lateral posterior; Pul: Pulvinar; MD: Medial dorsal; Mid: Midline; VA: Ventral anterior; VL: Ventral lateral; VPL: Ventral posterolateral; VPM: Ventral posteromedial; LGB: Lateral geniculate body; MGB: Medial geniculate body; IL: Intralaminar; CM: centromedian. The LGB and MGB respectively convey visual and sound stimuli. The VPL conveys body sensations from the spinal cord to the somatosensory cortex, while the facial trigeminal nerve conveys facial information to the somatosensory cortex.

The somatosensory area (SSA, Figure 2.4) in the brain's parietal lobe (Figure 2.1) is a prime area for sorting sensory stimuli. The central sulcus (a groove separating the front and back portions of the neocortex) delineates the anterior motor cortex (discussed in Chapter 3) from the posterior sensory cortex (Figure 2.3), home of the SSA. The SSA contains representational areas for the body's entire surface: hand, foot, tongue, lips, and so forth. Each representational area is proportional to the receptor density in its respective body part. Therefore, the highly sensual lip and tactile hand areas are large in the SSA when compared with the less sensual stomach or tactile calf and forearm areas.

Stimulating body areas initiates thalamic activation in the corresponding SSA areas (Figure 2.4). Specifically, the activated SSA hand area matches proportionately the quantity of stimulation experienced at the hand. From the SSA, this information transfers to more refining cortical areas until awareness of the hand touching something becomes conscious. Cortical feedback helps diminish awareness of irrelevant sensations, like a hand resting on an armrest. Diminishing irrelevant awareness facilitates conscious processing of other relevant stimuli, perhaps a steering wheel held by the other hand. Binding shifting quantities of input from the thalamus with the qualitative output needed for higher processing requires attuned feedback loops that adjust thalamic and cortical interactions on a moment-to-moment basis (Llinás and Ribary 2001).

Cortical control over the thalamus essentially coordinates widespread impacts from body sensations coherently (Destexhe 2000). Signals to the thalamus about basic body functions like arousal, breathing, heart rate, and so forth can be disrupted by very high or low intensity brainstem stimulation (Castro-Alamancos and Calcagnotto 2001). Either "bottom-up," affect-driven, or "top-down," cognition-driven dysregulation can result in neuropsychiatric conditions (Llinás and Ribary 2001).

Overwhelming trauma leading to PTSD (post-traumatic stress disorder) and disso-ciation displays significant thalamic inactivation (Lanius et al. 2001, 2005), as does sensory deprivation in severe childhood neglect. In neglect, insufficient stimulation of thalamic circuits during critical developmental periods minimizes the creation of effective feedback loops (Schore 2001b). During trauma, overpowering sensory stimuli test the strength of feedback loops to decrease cortical input and to recover quickly when traumatic stimuli stop. Weakened or diminished corticothalamic feedback creates a vulnerability culminating in various brain dysfunctions and increased prioritizing of subcortical, survival-based brain functions.

Sensory art therapy practices stimulate thalamic connections to and from cortical and subcortical brain regions. Frequently engaged, these regions may be tested, tuned, and strengthened. Sensory enriched, multi-modal, self- and other-regulated environ-ments are known to help "bottom-up" and "top-down" approaches coordinate and reregulate thalamic gateway functions that shift affective awareness, attention and con-sciousness (Cozolino 2002; Schore 1994).

The amygdala: gateway of emotions

The amygdala in the lower limbic, central brain region is one of the first respondents to thalamic output (Figures 2.3 and 2.6). It reacts long before conscious awareness begins, between approximately 20 and 100 milliseconds (ms) after a stimulus (Repa *et al.* 2001). This speedy response dramatically alters important brain and body functions through connections to the sympathetic nervous system (SNS), the fastest nervous system in the body. Rapid amygdala initiation of the SNS's flight or fight response enables reactivity and it is hoped, recovery during stress, crises or survival situations.

By comparison, conscious actions like pushing a button after seeing a flashed light generally take individuals about 220 ms. More discriminating tasks, like pushing a button in response to a flashed red stimulus but not a white one, require nearly half a second (420 ms; Kosinski 2006). The difference in reaction times reflects cortical decision-making needed to inhibit rapid impulses that begin non-conscious reactions.

A pair of almond-shaped bodies creates the brain's amygdala. One amygdaloid resides in the right hemisphere and the other in the left. Almost all brain structures share the lateral division seen in Figure 2.5.

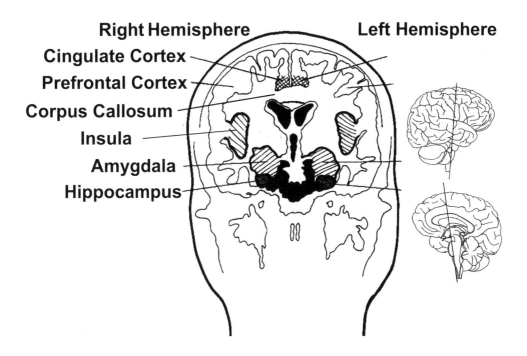

Figure 2.5 Cross-section of the brain showing lateralization of structures. Dark areas are ventricular spaces. The central dark space, the third ventricle, has no twin like the other brain ventricles. The axis for this brain section is shown to the right. Illustration by Tise Chao.

Each amygdalae in the pair engages all stages of affect-related information processing: encoding, storage, and retrieval. Experiential cues become charged with positive or negative valances so that memory in emotional contexts can be more easily and effectively searched and activated (Adolphs, Tranel, and Denburg 2000; Atkinson and Adolphs 2005). Non-conscious, aversive or fear-causing stimuli frequently activate the amygdala (Schore 2001b; Zald 2002, review). However, it also activates during appetitive learning, recognition of members of the same species (Izquierdo and Murray 2004), happiness (Haman *et al.* 2002), and while recognizing social cues and emotionally valenced facial expressions (Suslow *et al.* 2006). The right amygdala reacts more to angry faces than the left, while both react to discern fearful faces consciously (Suslow *et al.* 2006). Amygdala evaluations and mediation during emotionally experienced events and their encoding and consolidation into memory affects any subsequent body/mind processing (Markowitsch 1999).

Thalamic input to the right amygdala is assessed for shape and movement that might signal stimulus threat potential. Further evaluation occurs as the right amygdala references imprinted experiences and a very rudimentary and potentially genetic memory system. The results are conveyed to the hypothalamus (HY), an endocrine gland in the brain (Sapolsky 2005). If fear-inducing, the amygdala immediately signals via the "low road" through the HY to the SNS, for creation of a stress response. The SNS connects to all of the organs in the body, causing preconscious rapid, global, emotional, and bodily arousal

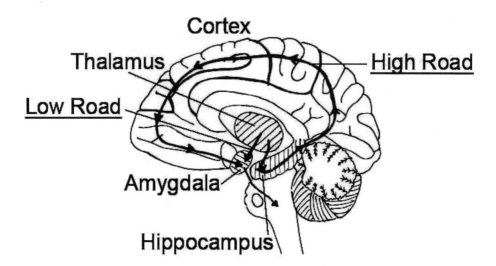

Figure 2.6 Low road-high road: Sensory stimuli quickly travel the low road from the thalamus to the amygdala. The response ensures rapid response to survival threats as the amygdala stimulates the hypothalamus, which in turn engages the sympathetic nervous system. They also travel the high road from the thalamus through the hippocampus to cortical sites where evaluations based upon memory and cognitive processes consciously determine which actions need inhibition or initiation. Illustration by Tise Chao.

(Gläscher and Adolphs 2003). The low road and its companion, the "high road," illustrated in Figure 2.6 are discussed later in the text.

Quick right amygdala evaluations of potential threats prevent death or damage. Imagine being startled. You jerk back and freeze as the thalamus processes more information. Heart rate, blood pressure, respiration rate, and energy to large muscles increase because the right amygdala has sensed movement signaling a potential threat. Action before thought is its credo. "Flight or fight" reactions continue to unfold until awareness of what's "spooked" you dawns. If no actual danger materializes, then your heart and other organs were exercised.

In the left amygdala, arousal reflects reactivity to stimuli details that need decoding (Table 2.1). The left amygdala helps consolidate declarative memory for emotionally arousing events (Adolphs *et al.* 2000), especially if stimulated by a high interest, ambiguous, visual image or during visually elicited positive emotions (Haman *et al.* 2002). The left amygdala's evaluations show refinement related to language-based threats (Phelps *et al.* 2001; Williams *et al.* 2004) as it restructures memory to incorporate lexical and visual knowledge (Adolphs *et al.* 2000). This more articulate sensing of arousing stimuli before consciousness reflects left amygdala evaluations (Gläscher and Adolphs 2003; Markowitsch 1999). Once consciously appraised, the startle produced by the right amygdala may prove irrelevant. The left amygdala may help redirect flight or fight impulses as your spouse emerging from the shadows speaks. The ensuing relief could shift impulses to flee towards laughter. The amygdala's right and left sides dynamically and rapidly alter body and mind differently while consorting with other brain structures. See Table 2.1 for more details on those differences.

Table 2.1 Right and left amygdala contribute different aspects to early stimulus appraisal.

	Right amygdala	*Left amygdala*
Facial expressions	Angry, fearful, in men happy	Fearful, in women happy
Stimulus threat potential	Shape, motion, imprinted memory, genetic memory	Stimulus details decoded, language-based threats incorporated into lexical and visual knowledge
Arousal	Startle or SNS: flight, fight, freeze response, in men activates for emotion stimulating visual stimuli, in women activates for increases in hemisphere activation	High interest, ambiguous visual images or visually elicited positive emotions, in women increases in hemisphere activation, depression and irritable bowel syndrome
Memory	Imprints threats, builds implicit emotional memory, integrates stimuli, emotion and body functioning during first three months, influences potential attachment	Memory consolidation for emotionally arousing events, helps connect tone of voice and language function

While "low road" alterations in body state and interoceptive information occur, a slower "high road" brings neural impulses from sensory receptors to thalamus to hippocampus to cortical sensory structures, like the SSA, auditory, visual, and parietal cortices; and to action-oriented cortical areas, like the motor areas, the prefrontal (PFC) and the orbitofrontal cortex (OFC). Conscious evaluation of high road communication ends in the PFC, which contains the OFC, for emotional assessments, and the dorsolateral prefrontal cortex (DLPFC), for working memory and more contextual memory processing. Input from the sensory cortices to the OFC and DLPFC allows comparisons of the situation to previous events and the body's readiness to respond. Emotion- and fact-based memory-informed processes inhibit the limbic system as needed and direct the thalamus, the muscles, and the organs in the body towards more refined action (Schore 1994).

Psychosocially stimulating stressors ignite current amygdala responses more often than nature-based, survival threats. While ideally adapted to our "wild" evolutionary past, the amygdala can be conditioned to respond to modern un-past-like fears, such as being evaluated by others. Conditioned memories merge and store within the amygdala's crude unconscious repository of potential precursors to danger, creating cues that increase fear and anxiety reactions. Movie images of people rushing or sounds of background music in a minor key paired with unexpected, aversive stimuli, like blood-curdling screams, startle us. Though produced for our entertainment, this illusion causes an amygdala response, despite foreknowledge. Adrenaline-based entertainment delights our later occurring consciousness, which relishes the chance to practice "roping in" the amygdala's overly quick response. Pleasure sometimes consciously follows half to a second later as higher neocortical structures assemble sensory details and discover the illusory threat. Fear becomes relief—laughter discharges muscle tension and hypervigilance diminishes as the slower, more cautious, refined inhibitory, cortical feedback arrives. If conditioned cues repeat often, the amygdala habituates or ceases responding to the stimuli. Thrill-seekers and moviegoers endlessly seek new twists to prevent amygdala habituation or de-conditioning.

Psychosocial uncertainties or thoughts anticipating them frequently kindle fear, anxiety, and stress, in which case, flight or fight responses don't protect us, and can injure long-term brain and body functioning (McEwen 2003). Conditioned, amygdala-based, unconscious memory forms more rapidly and efficiently during dangerous and emotional situations than during non-threatening and neutral events. Startle and patterned unconscious anxiety and fear-based reactions reveal conditioning to stressful and psychosocially threatening memories from a person's earlier life.

Paired or conditioned stimuli like those mentioned above may not reflect external stimuli. Blends of memory, patterned responses, schemas, fear-based assumptions, feelings, and reactive thoughts can combine to create seemingly irrational or nonsensical implicitly conditioned responses. Superstitions often vary with cultures and regions. Cardiac deaths increase 7 percent on the fourth of each month for Japanese and Chinese

Americans. The number four, which sounds like the word for death in Mandarin, Cantonese and Japanese, excites unconscious fear (Phillips *et al.* 2007). Americans may eliminate the unlucky thirteenth floor of a building, while Britons, who also fear Friday the thirteenth, endure statistically reported increases in traffic accidents on that day.

The amygdala's reaction to perceived or imagined threats causes intense body changes. The conscious calm needed to sort out different perspectives and meanings slips away. Consequently, a "look," a "tone of voice," a metaphor, an idiom, a gesture, a "vision" or an image may strike a reactive person more strongly than another. Privately formed and unconsciously held interpretations of events motivate and create internally held psychosocial stressors that predispose stress responses. If startle or flight or fight responses happen too often, they escalate aging, deplete energy resources, dysregulate the thalamus, cause chronic stress and autoimmune illnesses, and establish response patterns that occur too fast or too slow (McEwen 2003).

During development and functional integration into the nervous system, the amygdala, like all forming structures, displays significant vulnerability to many influences. The right amygdala, active both during late pregnancy and after birth, seems to lead in integrating stimuli and body functions during the first three months of postnatal life (Schore 2001a, 2001b). Animal research on rats, cats, and chimps during the prenatal period found that a mother's extreme or prolonged stress responses cause increased density of amygdala neurons and interconnectivity. This outcome seems to apply to humans also (Salm *et al.* 2004). As a result, future conditioning to aversive stimuli occurs more easily predisposing amygdala-enhancing, emotion-based interaction patterns like those shaping later attachments between mother and child (Lemche *et al.* 2006). Mother/child fear-based and joy-based high arousals strongly influence personality formation during infancy and early childhood (Schore 1994). A valence attached by the amygdala modulates perceptual processes in perpetuity, especially visual processes (Hendler, Rothstein and Hadar 2002). Propensities towards fear, anxiety, or soothing oneself vary from person to person; often reflecting conditioned responses placed by the amygdala into procedural memory during formative developmental periods. Right/left hemispheric dominance switches as developmental periods and circumstances where reasoning (cause and effect learning) skills predominate versus other periods where emotion-based (psychosocial) behaviors organize. Yet, all subsequent developmental stages reflect and build upon limbic amygdala-based reactivity patterns.

Gender differences express during amygdala functioning. For instance, a male's right amygdala shows more activity during emotional memory processing, particularly related to visual images, whereas in females the left is more active (Cahill 2006, review). Men's right amygdala and women's left react to happy faces and activity increases in the corresponding hemisphere. Women show increased left amygdala activation during depression and irritable bowel syndrome (Cahill 2006).

The amygdala prioritizes emotional cues for the visual cortex and acts as an automatic orchestrating force during affective learning (Schupp *et al.* 2007). In art therapy, interrupting this automaticity and allowing higher cortical structures to inhibit and help recondition the amygdala is critical. Non-conscious reactions may influence choices and emotional expressions as the art is attended to and/or created. Anxiety and fear-based reactions may be stimulated while making, discussing, titling or simply looking at art that reveals previously stored amygdala-based memories. What art therapy aspect could help interrupt and recondition amygdalar processes? Schupp *et al.* (2007) note that "emotional stimuli guide selective attention during visual processing" (p.16), and that taxing emotion-attention processing with a competing visual task interferes, especially when the competing task increases demand or task load by explicitly requiring locating task relevant details (Schupp *et al.* 2007). From this, we might hypothesize that creating art in a therapeutic environment slows amygdala guidance of emotional attention. Motor coordination requirements and conscious media selection could support "high road" inhibitory advantages. A sense of safety, calm, and added time to address moments previously shaped by "low road" effects may occur, preventing the amygdala from disabling higher cortical functioning. Making artwork therapeutically may generate a sense of entering a mental space in which fear and anxiety (disruptive emotions) decrease, while action, intuition, thoughtfulness and positive emotions increase. Perhaps previously provocative memories and stimuli processing are de-conditioned or habituated.

The anterior cingulate cortex

If the amygdala alone shaped our response to the world, life would be a string of fast arousals and survival reactions with fear and anxiety more common than joy. Luckily, the amygdala's response is curtailed. Cortical structures higher in the brain, like the cingulate and the orbitofrontal cortices, assist the amygdala's subcortical neighbor, the hippocampus, in modifying amygdala impact (Figure 2.3). For most people, these modifications increase reward-based experiencing (Bechara, Damasio, and Damasio 2003).

The cingulate cortex, the largest limbic structure, rests atop the corpus callosum at the interface between the limbic area and the cortex. Many cortical and subcortical structures, like the OFC, the insula, the hippocampus and the amygdala, interconnect with the cingulate cortex (Tamminga *et al.* 2000; Figures 2.3 and 2.5). Physiologically, the cingulate cortex divides into anterior (front) and posterior (back) sections (Figure 2.1). More refined designations, like rostral (towards the mouth), caudal (back), dorsal (top) and ventral (bottom), add meaning to discussions of anterior cingulate cortex (ACC) or the posterior cingulate cortex (PCC) functions, such as affect regulation, response selection, visuospatial processing or memory access. The ACC functions during emotional self-control, focused problem-solving, error recognition, and adapting to changing conditions (Allman *et al.* 2001). The ACC detects and corrects errors during cognitive and emotional processing (Raz 2004). The PCC activates during emotion and memory retrieval functions, especially autobiographical memory retrieval (Maddock, Garrett, and Buonocore 2001, 2003).

About 100,000 years ago, human and great ape cingulate cortices evolved unique neurons called spindle cells, which connect and coordinate diverse brain regions (Allman *et al.* 2001). Spindle, or Von Economo, neuron (VEN) distribution helps solve difficult problems with fast intuitive assessments of complex situations (Allman *et al.* 2005), such as understanding large psychosocial group interactions, communicating about mental states, and sharing experiences (Frith 2002). VENs may enable a sense of agency through representations of mental and intentional states in oneself and others (Frith 2002). Integrating a multitude of sensory, memory and executive functions reflects cingulate activation. Perhaps VENs also activate during the selection of what and how to represent in the art and/or how to process meaning in the outcome.

Conscious experiencing activates many ACC functions. Experiencing negative pain affect was shown to activate the rostral ACC causing the release of endogenous opioids, the body's natural painkiller, which inhibits ACC-induced pain awareness (Derbyshire 2002). Participants given immediate feedback about their successful activation of the rostral area of the ACC gained control over chronic clinical pain (deCharms *et al.* 2005). Emotional and physical pain share areas of activation in the ACC. Being aware of an affect while focusing upon feedback may encourage changes in rostral ACC functioning. Experiences like waiting for adverse outcomes (in one case, electric shock) or feeling dread also activate the rostral ACC area (Berns *et al.* 2006). Conversely, feeling excluded (social rejection) excites the right OFC, which normally disrupts and regulates ACC activity (Eisenberger, Lieberman, and Williams 2003).

The ACC helps a person consciously sort and attend to relevant information while ignoring the irrelevant. It enables decision-making when conflicting tendencies in responding to a stimulus occur (Awh and Gehring 1999). Working memory tasks, planning, hypothesis testing, and guessing activate the ACC (Elliott and Dolan 1998). Selecting motor movements, while processing reward-based information, also excites the rostral ACC (Shima and Tanji 1998). Neuroimaging research in the future may show that the desire to produce satisfying and coherent art expressions, while conceptualizing and selecting art materials, activates the ACC in the presence of difficult or shifting emotions.

Error processing, conflict monitoring, motor control and response selection mediate bodily arousal. These responses are modulated by the dorsal ACC (Critchley *et al.* 2003). For example, during effortful cognitive and motor behavior, the dorsal ACC contributes to autonomic cardiovascular arousal. The dorsal ACC also activates during short duration failed attempts at inhibiting neural impulses, while longer inhibitory failures activate the ventral ACC, known to influence emotion regulation (Matthews *et al.* 2005). Numerous connections from the thalamus and amygdala to the ACC suggest it strongly influences affect processing (Derbyshire 2002). People whose biology predisposes them to high anxiety overactivate their ACC, even when the risk of making mistakes is very low (Paulus *et al.* 2004). Images, media, conceptions and the art product may fall short of one's expectation, creating some disappointment. In low risk art therapy contexts repeated opportunities to experience and recover from short- and longer-term failures occur. Sharing the artwork's intent and meaning can also diminish the relevance of these initial creative disappointments.

Thalamic and insula input stored in the ACC maintain representations of the body's ongoing condition that are matched against limbic input to the ACC that motivates action. If input from each source suggests the body's ability to meet the limbic demands matches the body's resources for action, then the limbic input, including that from the amygdala, is facilitated. If the contrary condition occurs, the limbic input is inhibited. Conflict and detected errors cause ACC reactions that favor habitual limbic responses to stimuli. Orbitofrontal cortex functioning supports novel responses (Schore 1994). Habituation, extinction, and memory reconsolidation processes shape coping strategies that allow ACC habitual responses and OFC novel solutions to influence amygdala reactivity and possibly art-making effectively. Gaining functional access through these processes to ACC functioning and understanding PCC influences facilitates various forms of therapy, perhaps most especially art therapy.

Summary

Humans evolved a unique ability to concretize, understand and transform their inner experiences through art long ago. Interdependence upon large social groups promoted complex interactive processes that required higher brain functions to regulate affectively driven subcortical functions successfully in both familiar and novel contexts. Rich, dynamic sensory input distributed by the thalamus flows through intricate, interlocking feedback relationships with cortical areas that shape awareness and perception. Art therapy invokes these feedback functions while revealing and engaging disruptive areas of affective expression emerging from subcortical structures, such as the amygdala. Invoking higher limbic structures, like the ACC, to inhibit amygdala impulsivity and possibly initiate more regulated and familiar processing patterns is known to help remodel internal processing errors. Art therapy practices seem to engage the ACC as well as complex regulatory centers in the PFC that utilize explicit and implicit memory to problem solve and create novel ways to diminish expressed conflicts. Multimodal contexts available during art therapy invite creative, comprehension-oriented and expressive possibilities that avoid becoming simplistically linear or impulsive. The bilateral orientation of art therapy draws upon the functional differences in both hemispheres to facilitate individualized, coherent and integrative resolutions of present, past and evolution-based disruptions in self-functioning within a safe, manageable psychosocial context.

References

Adolphs, R., Tranel, D., and Denburg, N. (2000). Impaired emotional declarative memory following unilateral amygdala damage. *Learning & Memory, 7,* 180–186.

Allman, J. M., Hakeem, A., Erwin, J. M., Nimchinsky, E., and Hof, P. (2001). The anterior cingulate. The evolution of an interface between emotion and cognition. *Annals of the New York Academy of Sciences, 935,* 107–117.

Allman, J. M., Watson, K., Tetreault, N. A., and Hakeem, A. Y. (2005). Intuition and autism: a possible role for Von Economo neurons. *Trends in Cognitive Sciences, 9,* 367–372.

Atkinson, A. P. and Adolphs, R. (2005). Visual emotion perception: Mechanisms and processes. In L. Feldman-Barrett, P. M. Niedenthal, and P. Winkielman (eds) *Emotion and Consciousness* (pp.150–182). New York: Guilford Press.

Awh, E. and Gehring, W. J. (1999). The anterior cingulated cortex lends a hand in response selection. *Nature Neuroscience, 2*(10), 853–854.

Bechara, A., Damasio, H., and Damasio, A. R. (2003). Role of the amygdala in decision-making. *Annals of the New York Academy of Sciences, 985,* 385–469.

Berns, G. S., Chappelow, J., Cekic, M., Zink, C. F., Pagnoni, G., and Martin-Skurski, M. E. (2006). Neurobiological substrates of dread. *Science, 312,* 754–758.

Bradshaw, J. L. (2001). Ars brevis, vita longa: The possible evolutionary antecedents of art and aesthetics [Electronic Version]. *APA Division 10: Bulletin.* Retrieved 6/25/06 from www.apa.org/divisions/div10/articles/bradshaw.html.

Cahill, L. (2006). Why sex matters for neuroscience. *Nature Reviews Neuroscience, 6,* 477–484.

Castro, A. J., Merchut, M. P., Neafsey, E. J., and Wurster, R. D. (2002). *Neuroscience, an Outline Approach.* St. Louis, MO: Mosby.

Castro-Alamancos, M. A. and Calcagnotto, M. E. (2001). High-pass filtering of corticothalamic activity by neuromodulators released in the thalamus during arousal: In Vitro and In Vivo. *Journal of Neurophysiology, 85*(4), 1489–1497.

Cozolino, L. (2002). *The Neuroscience of Psychotherapy, Building and Rebuilding the Human Brain.* New York: W. W. Norton & Company.

Critchley, H. D., Mathias, C. J., Josephs, O., O'Doherty, J., Zanini, S., Dewar, B.K., *et al.* (2003). Human cingulated cortex and autonomic control: Converging neuroimaging and clinical evidence. *Brain, 126,* 2139–2152.

Dawkins, R. (2004). *The Ancestor's Tale, A Pilgrimage to the Dawn of Evolution.* New York: Houghton Mifflin.

deCharms, R. C., Maeda, F., Glover, G. H., Ludlow, D., Pauly, J. M., Soneji, D., *et al.* (2005). Control over brain activation and pain learned by using real-time functional MRI. *PNAS, 102,* 18626–18631.

Derbyshire, S. W. G. (2002). Measuring our natural painkiller. *Trends in Neuroscience, 25,* 67–68.

Destexhe, A. (2000). Modeling corticothalamic feedback and the gating of the thalamus by the cerebral cortex. *Journal of Physiology, Paris, 94,* 391–410.

Edelman, G. M. and Tononi, G. (2000). *A Universe of Consciousness: How Matter Becomes Imagination.* New York: Basic Books.

Eisenberger, N. I., Lieberman, M. D., and Williams, K. D. (2003). Does social rejection hurt? An fMRI study of social exclusion. *Science, 302,* 290–292.

Elliott, R. and Dolan, R. J. (1998). Activation of different anterior cingulated foci in association with hypothesis testing and response selection. *Neuroimage, 8,* 17–29.

Finley, B. L., Darlington, R. B., and Nicastro, N. (2001). Developmental structure in brain evolution. *The Behavioral and Brain Sciences, 24,* 263–278.

Frith, C. (2002). Attention to action and awareness of other minds. *Consciousness and Cognition, 11,* 481–487.

Gläscher, J. and Adolphs, R. (2003). Processing of the arousal of subliminal and supraliminal emotional stimuli by the human amygdala. *The Journal of Neuroscience, 23*(32), 10274–10282.

Haman, S. B., Ely, T. D., Hoffman, J. M., and Kilts, C. D. (2002). Ecstasy and agony: Activation of the human amygdala in positive and negative emotion. *Psychological Science, 13,* 135–141.

Hendler, T., Rothstein, P., and Hadar, U. (2002). Emotion-perception interplay in the visual cortex: "The eyes follow the heart." *Cellular and Molecular Neurobiology, 21,* 733–752.

Izquierdo, A. and Murray, E. A. (2004). Combined unilateral lesions of the amygdala and preorbitofrontal cortex impair affective processing in Rhesus monkeys. *Journal of Neurophysiology, 91,* 2023–2039.

Kosinski, R. J. (2006). A literature review on reaction time. Retrieved 6/26/07 from Clemson University, http://biae.clemson.edu/bpc/bp/Lab/110/reaction.htm

Koyama, T., McHaffle, J. G., Laurenti, P. J., and Coghill, R. C. (2005). The subjective experience of pain: Where expectations become a reality. *PNAS, 102*(36), 12950–12955.

Lanius, R. A., Williamson, P. C., Bluhm, R. L., Densmore, M., Boksman, K., Neufeld, R. W. J., *et al.* (2005). Functional connectivity of dissociative responses in posttraumatic stress disorder: A functional magnetic resonance imaging investigation. *Biological Psychiatry, 57,* 873–884.

Lanius, R. A., Williamson, P. C., Densmore, M., Boksman, K., Gupta, M. A., Neufeld, R. W. J., *et al.* (2007). Neural correlates of traumatic memories in posttraumatic stress disorder: A functional MRI investigation. *American Journal of Psychiatry, 158,* 1920–1922.

Lemche, E., Giamietro, V. P., Suruladze, S. A., Amaro, E. J., Andrew, C. M., Williams, C. C. R., *et al.* (2006). Human attachment security is mediated by the amygdala: Evidence from combined fMRI and psychophysiological measures. *Human Brain Mapping, 27,* 623–635.

Llinás, R. and Ribary, U. (2001). Consciousness and the brain: The thalamocortical dialogue in health and disease. *Annals of the New York Academy of Sciences, 929,* 166–175.

Llinás, R., Ribary, U., Contreras, D., and Pedroarena, C. (1998). The neuronal basis of consciousness. *Philosophical Transactions of the Royal Society of London, Series B, Biological Sciences, 353*(1377), 1841–1849.

Maddock, R. J., Garrett, A. S., and Buonocore, M. H. (2001). Remembering familiar people: The posterior cingulate cortex and autobiographical memory retrieval. *Neuroscience, 104,* 667–676.

Maddock, R. J., Garrett, A. S., and Buonocore, M. H. (2003). Posterior cingulate cortex activation by emotional words: fMRI evidence from a valence decision task. *Human Brain Mapping, 18,* 30–41.

Markowitsch, H. J. (1999). Differential contribution of right and left amygdala to affective information processing. *Behavioral Neurology, 11,* 233–244.

Matthews, S. C., Simmons, A. N., Arce, E., and Paulus, M. P. (2005). Dissociation of inhibition from error processing using a parametric inhibitory task during functional magnetic resonance imaging. *NeuroReport, 16,* 755–760.

McEwen, B. S. (2003). *The End of Stress as We Know It.* Washington, DC: John Henry Press.

McKinney, M. (2000). Evolving behavioral complexity by extending development. In S. T. Parker, J. Langer, and M. McKinney (eds) *Biology, Brains, and Behavior: The Evolution of Human Development* (pp.25–40). Santa Fe, NM: School of American Press.

Panksepp, J. (1998). *Affective Neuroscience: The Foundations of Human and Animal Emotions.* New York: Oxford University Press.

Paulus, M. P., Feinstein, J. S., Simmons, A., and Stein, M. B. (2004). Anterior cingulated activation in high trait anxious subjects is related to altered error processing during decision-making. *Biological Psychiatry, 55,* 1179–1187.

Phelps, E. A., O'Connor, K. J., Gatenby, J. C., Gore, J. C., Grillon, C., and Davis, M. (2001). Activation of the left amygdala to a cognitive representation of fear. *Nature Neuroscience, 4,* 437–441.

Phillips, D. P., Liu, G. C., Kwok, K., Jarvin, J. R., Zhang, W., and Abramson, I. S. (2007). The *Hound of the Baskervilles* effect: Natural experiment on the influence of psychological stress on timing of death. *British Medical Journal, 323,* 22–29.

Potts, R. B. (2007). *Human Evolution* (Publication). Retrieved 4/20/07 from Microsoft Corporation: http://encarta.msn.com/text_761566394_0/Human_Evolution.html

Ramachandran, V. S. (2004). *A Brief Tour of Consciousness.* New York: Pi Press.

Raz, A. (2004). Anatomy of attentional networks. *The Anatomical Record (part B, New Anatomy), 281B,* 21–36.

Repa, J. C., Muller, J., Apergis, J., Desrochers, T. M., Zhou, Y., and LeDoux, J. E. (2001). Two different lateral amygdala cell populations contribute to the initiation and storage of memory. *Nature Neuroscience, 4,* 724–731.

Salm, A. K., Pavelko, M., Krouse, E. M., Webster, W., Kraszpulski, M., and Birkle, D. L. (2004). Lateral amygdaloid nucleus expansion in adult rats associated with exposure to prenatal stress. *Developmental Brain Research, 148,* 159–167.

Sapolsky, R. M. (2004). *Why Zebras Don't Get Ulcers: An Updated Guide to Stress, Stress-related Diseases, and Coping* (3rd edition). New York: W. H. Freeman and Company.

Sapolsky, R. (2005). *Biology and Human Behavior: The Neurological Origins of Individuality* (2nd edition) Chantilly, VA: The Teaching Company.

Schoenemann, P. T. (2006). Evolution of the size and functional areas of the human brain. *Annual Review of Anthropology, 35,* 379–406.

Schore, A. N. (1994). *Affect Regulation and the Origin of the Self.* Hillsdale, NJ: Lawrence Erlbaum Associates.

Schore, A. N. (2001a). Effects of a secure attachment relationship on right brain development, affect regulation, and infant mental health. *Infant Mental Health Journal, 22,* 7–66.

Schore, A. N. (2001b). The effects of early relational trauma on right brain development, affect regulation, and infant mental health. *Infant Mental Health Journal, 22,* 201–269.

Schupp, H. T., Stockburger, J., Bublatzky, F., Junghöfer, M., Weike, A. I., and Hamm, A. O. (2007). Explicit attention interferes with selective emotion processing in human extrastriate cortex. *BMC Neuroscience, 8,* 16–28.

Shima, K. and Tanji, J. (1998). Role for cingulated motor area cells in voluntary movement selection based upon reward. *Science, 828*, 1335–1338.

Suslow, T., Ohrmann, P., Bauer, J., Rauch, A. V., Schwindt, W., Arolt, V., *et al.* (2006). Amygdala activation during masked presentation of emotional faces predicts conscious detection of threat-related faces. *Brain and Cognition, 61*, 243–248.

Tamminga, C. A., Vogel, M., Gao, X. M., Lahti, A. C., and Holcomb, H. H. (2000). The limbic cortex in schizophrenia: Focus on the anterior cingulate. *Brain Research Reviews, 31*, 364–370.

Williams, L. M., Brown, K. J., Das, P., Boucsein, W., Sokolov, E. N., Brammer, M. J., *et al.* (2004). The dynamics of cortico-amygdala and autonomic activity over the experimental time course of fear perception. *Cognitive Brain Research, 21*, 114–123.

Zald, D. H. (2002). The human amygdala and the emotional evaluation of sensory stimuli. *Brain Research Reviews, 41*, 88–123.

3

The Cortex: Regulation of Sensory and Emotional Experience

Darryl Christian

Introduction

The cortex, specifically the prefrontal cortex, makes us uniquely human. The cortex links us to others by monitoring and regulating each others' internal states through eye contact, touch, body language, relational patterns, and representational narratives (Cozolino 2006; DeVries, Glasper, and Detillion 2003; Greenspan 1997). Brain structures and functions in the cortex contribute to conscious choice, action, complex emotions, and meaningful social interactions. A discussion of cortical structures and functions is essential for understanding how these relational processes develop out of the processing of sensory experience.

Information processing pathways

The cerebrum is divided from front to back by the longitudinal fissure, creating two cerebral hemispheres covered by the cortex (or neocortex). The cortex forms five lobes in each hemisphere: occipital, parietal, temporal, insular and frontal lobes. Figure 3.1 with anatomical directions provides a map of the cortex.

The insula lies hidden between the frontal, parietal, and temporal lobes shown in Figure 3.1, and the midbrain structures are located centrally between the right and left hemispheres. Higher to lower cortical functions are organized from front (anterior) to back (posterior) and from top (superior/dorsal) to bottom (inferior/ventral). Within these regions, neural pathways are organized structurally into different layers forming convolutions, which give the cortex its distinctive wrinkled appearance. These hills and valleys, respectively gyri and sulci, consist of gray matter forming the top of the gyri, which cover the underlying white matter (Berninger and Richards 2002). Deep sulci help identify boundaries between the five lobes, while sulci, in general, increase cortical surface area and vary somewhat from person to person. The cortex surrounds older, subcortical structures of the brain: brainstem areas responsible for involuntary or

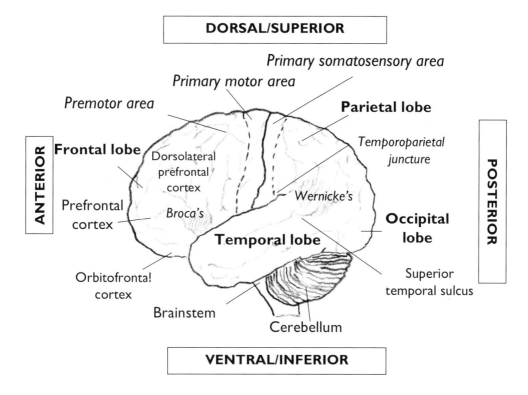

Figure 3.1 Lateral view of cortical lobes and specialized areas. Not indicated are the insula, which is hidden by the frontal, parietal, and temporal lobes, and medial locations located centrally between the right and left hemispheres.

automatic functions, and the limbic region responsible for autonomic, emotion, memory, motivation, and behavioral functions (Figure 3.2).

Limbic structures which include the caudate nucleus, thalamus, amygdala, and hippocampus connect to the cortex by projections of white matter fibers (Berninger and Richards 2002).

Cortical neuronal structure is characterized by gray and white matter. Gray matter consists of non-myelinated neuron bodies that process information while myelinated neuron axons appear white and serve to transfer information between neurons. Developmental maturation occurs as neurons myelinate, increasing the efficiency and synchronicity in the transmission of information between neural structures. Increased density of gray matter allows easier information processing through the formation of more pathways between neurons (Berninger and Richards 2002).

The white matter neural pathways form connections along bottom-up and top-down brain axes called projection pathways that link cortical and subcortical structures. Sensory receptors from each part of the body project through the brainstem and

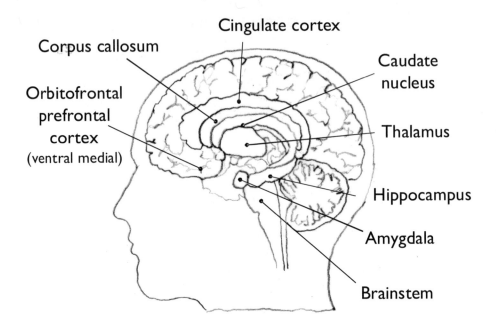

Figure 3.2 Medial view indicating locations of subcortical structures.

thalamus to a specific area of the cortex providing visceral information. Along a front-back axis, association fibers connect areas on the same side of the right or left cortical hemispheres (Berninger and Richards 2002).

A general processing principle is that vertical top/down processing associates with complex cognitive processes moderating sensory or emotional processes. Front/back or anterior/posterior processes associate with cognitive integration and regulation of sensory and emotional processes (Berninger and Richards 2002). Association pathways allow the sensory and motor cortices to connect so that what is sensed can be functionally integrated into decisions and action. These pathways contribute to the lobes' specific functions and support cross-hemispheric integration. Primary projection pathways transfer sensory information along sensory or afferent pathways from the lower brain structures and/or the body to the sensory or posterior portion of the cortex. The posterior regions of the cortex process sensory information first: visual information in the occipital lobe, auditory information in the temporal lobe, and sensory information from the body in the parietal lobe. Processed (bottom/up) information passes through the association areas to the frontal lobe, which plans for (top/down) movement and action. Projection pathways also send action messages from the frontal or motor portion of the cortex along motor or efferent pathways to lower brain centers and/or the body (Figure 3.3).

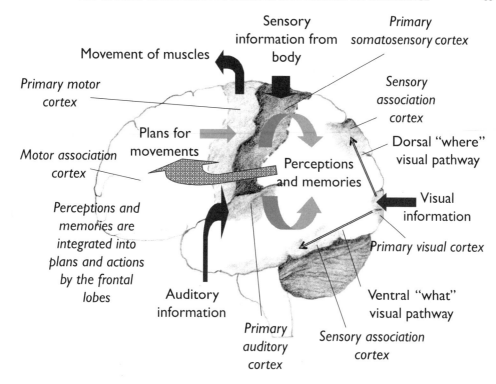

Figure 3.3 Projection pathways convey sensory information from lower regions to the posterior portion of the brain, and action messages from the frontal cortex to lower regions. Other pathways connect posterior and frontal cortices. Subcortical limbic processes (not shown) also contribute to cortical processing.

Most cortical areas contain third level or tertiary association areas that receive informa-tion from secondary association areas. These tertiary and secondary association pathways utilize more complex and abstract stimuli, which are less influenced by primary sensory input. Complex association contributes to higher-order thinking and computational skills (Berninger and Richards 2002).

Crossing the gap between the hemispheres, myelinated neuron bundles, called commissures, connect corresponding structures on each side of the brain. The corpus callosum (Figure 3.2) is the largest of these bi-lateral pathways (Berninger and Richards 2002). Bi-lateral integration of visual and tactile sensory systems, or bi-lateral linking of the hemispheres and their distinctive modes of processing sensory, emotional, or cognitive information, provides a means of coordinating a complex functional neural system fundamental to self-regulation and a sense of self (Siegel 1999).

The evidence for the lateralization of right and left hemisphere functions came from epilepsy patients who had had their corpus callosums severed during surgery. This splitting of the brain left each hemisphere's functioning isolated from the other (Berninger and Richards 2002). Split brain experiments identified left hemisphere specialization for language and functions requiring sequential processing and right hemisphere specialization for visual spatial skills and functions requiring simultaneous processing. Popularization of these concepts resulted erroneously in the belief that people were either right- or left-brained learners or thinkers. So-called visual learners and auditory learners further exemplified the oversimplification of complex processes involving numerous cortical structures and pathways. Functional processing and thinking requires integration of information utilizing vertical and lateral pathways throughout the brain.

Cortical structures and their functions provide redundancy so that if one cortical area fails, another can compensate for the missing function. Normal variations within genetic makeup and environmental experiences further vary the ways in which neural pathways develop. These normal variations provide a kind of fail-safe mechanism for survival—it is better to have several neural paths to solve a problem or achieve a goal than to depend upon one invariable neural pathway (Berninger and Richards 2002).

Neural pathways fire in parallel processes so that more than one brain task may be formulated at any one time. Functional systems work together to provide efficiency. Functionally, the cortex is associated with organizing sensory, motor, and conscious experiences; processing sensory perceptual information and voluntary movement; as well as executive-type functions, like reasoning, thought, and language. While brainstem structures and development largely reflect genetic determinants, cortical development is largely dependent on experience and learned interactions (Berninger and Richards 2002).

The occipital lobes and the association cortex

The visual system is an excellent example of how neural systems work together. The occipital lobe is the visual processing area of the cortex. Sensory stimulation of the retina is communicated through the thalamus to the occipital visual cortex, which continuously builds a kind of visual map of the world. The visual cortex maps low-level orientation, spatial frequency, motion, depth and distance, and color in small receptive fields. Information is transferred along the two pathways, the ventral and dorsal visual streams, to other visual processing areas in the occipital lobe and then to other cortical regions for further processing and integration (Berninger and Richards 2002).

The visual system utilizes two pathways for processing information (Figure 3.3). The ventral pathway, from occipital to temporal to frontal cortices, identifies objects, color, and fine details, while the dorsal pathway, from occipital to parietal to frontal cortices, processes motion and location in space. The occipital-parietal-temporal lobes form the association cortex which functions to forward information to the frontal lobes. The visual system forwards information to the association cortex in order for the frontal lobes to act upon visual information (Berninger and Richards 2002).

From a relational perspective, at about two months of age, the occipital visual function, especially the ventral stream to the temporal lobe, dramatically gains prominence by organizing non-verbal interactions between mother and child. The infant's gazing at the mother's face and emotional expressions, as well as his or her listening to mother's vocalizations, leads to infant and mother attachment interactions that develop affect regulation in the infant (Schore 2001).

Temporal lobes: emotional saliency and language

The temporal lobes receive visual information and utilize it to process interpersonally salient emotional stimuli, like faces (Schore 2001). The temporal lobes contain the primary auditory cortex involved in hearing. The left temporal lobe appears to be specialized for complex speech and language, naming, comprehension, and the identification of sound. Wernicke's area, unilaterally in the left temporal lobe, is associated with speech comprehension and syntax (Berninger and Richards 2002).

Broca's area in the left frontal lobe is associated with language production and comprehension. Along with Wernicke's, each area relates, respectively, to speech production and aural comprehension (Figure 3.1). Because Wernicke's myelinates by age two and Broca's myelinates around age four to six, children learn receptive language before they learn expressive language. Because the neural connection between the two areas myelinates slowly, development of the coordination of receptive and expressive language is slow (Berninger and Richards 2002).

Language incorporates complementary right/left processes (Beeman and Chiarello 1998). Left hemisphere functions include quickly processing and selecting categorical and plausible interpretations of language, while the right hemisphere contributes multiple meanings, attention to visual details in written words and acoustic features in spoken language, activation of multiple related concepts, metaphors, and activation of meaning outside the context of written or spoken language. These subtleties in lateralization once again evidence neural complexities (Berninger and Richards 2002).

The right temporal lobe also processes sound qualities like rhythm and melody in music. The temporal lobe encloses the hippocampus and amygdala, limbic structures important for memory and emotion. The medial temporal lobe appears to shape episodic/declarative memory. A particular area of the temporal lobe, the superior temporal sulcus (STS), and the temporoparietal junction (TPJ) are associated with emotional learning, knowing another's perspective, as well as knowing the other (Frith and Frith 1999).

Parietal lobes: visual spatial processing

Functionally, the parietal lobes integrate sensory information from the body (Figures 3.1 and 3.3), such as in visuospatial processing. They are important in orienting to spatial locations and in coordinating eye movements (Carter 1998) as well as shifting attention (Berninger and Richards 2002).

The somatosensory strip in the parietal lobe receives and processes information from all parts of the body. Precise locations in this area have been associated with specific body areas. A similar organization is reflected in the frontal motor cortex with precise locations identified as the source of impulses back to the body resulting in movement and action. The parietal lobes and the association cortex act in concert with the prefrontal lobe to better understand movement in the environment. Facilitating some of this integration are mirror neurons. Located in the brain where visual, motor, and emotional processing converge, mirror neurons respond to the observed actions and hand gestures of others. Evidence for mirror neuron networks in the parietal lobe, frontal premotor cortex, and the STS explain how we understand purposeful action through visual observation (Rizzolatti, Fogassi, and Gallese 2006). During observation and imitation, they provide for a learning experience. Mirror neurons also activate in anticipation of intended purposeful actions (Iacoboni *et al.* 2005). These findings also provide the hypothetical basis for how socially observed actions link with observed emotions, empathy, and how we experience others (Gallese 2003). Folk tales and images have reflected on this quality (Figure 3.4).

Insula cortex: bridging between body and cortex

Hidden within the frontal, parietal, and temporal lobes is the fifth cortical lobe, the insula or insular cortex (Dupont *et al.* 2003). It plays an integrative role between limbic structures and the frontal, parietal, and temporal lobes. It is organized somatotopically, like the motor and somatosensory cortex strips, which means that insular surface locations relate to specific body locations. The insula links the sense of self with self-control. It plays a role in mediating a range of emotions, awareness and expression of bodily states (our own and others'), extremes of emotion (from disgust to love), and behavior. Eye gaze and facial expressions such as fearful faces, expressions of disgust, and untrustworthiness activate this region and are involved in the assessment of threat and reward (Wicker *et al.* 2003). The ability to experience a somatic sense of self and to experience the pain of others, empathy, is related to activity in the insula (Cozolino 2006).

Prefrontal cortex: decisions, emotions and autobiographical memory

The prefrontal cortex (PFC) plays a significant role in executive planning, coordinating and controlling behavior as well as cognitive functions such as formulating language, impulse control, memory, socialization, and spontaneity (Banfield *et al.* 2004; Figure 3.5).

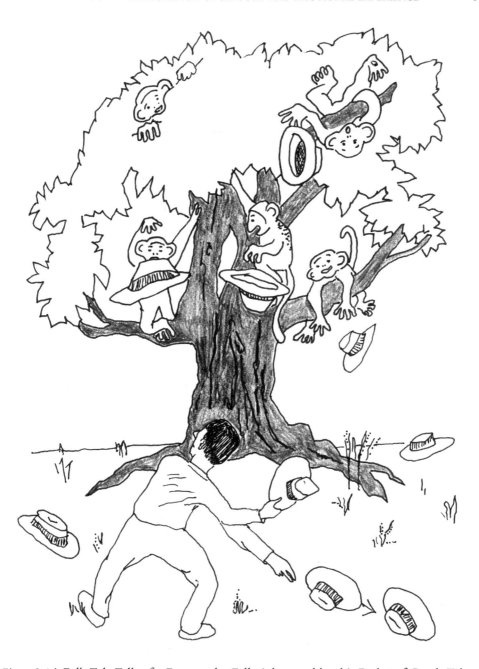

Figure 3.4 A Folk Tale Tells of a Farmer who Falls Asleep and has his Basket of Goods Taken Over by a Band of Monkeys. *When the farmer wakes he is taunted by the monkeys who are wearing his hats. The monkeys simply mimic his every movement—a case of mirror neurons in action. In vain the farmer chases the monkeys but finally decides to use his head (and his dorsolateral prefrontal cortex). The farmer throws his hat onto the ground and the monkeys follow suit. Art by Robin Vance.*

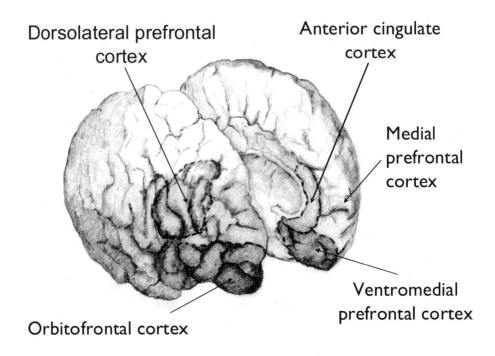

Dorsolateral prefrontal cortex

Anterior cingulate cortex

Medial prefrontal cortex

Ventromedial prefrontal cortex

Orbitofrontal cortex

Figure 3.5 Prefrontal cortex areas.

The PFC is considered the seat of consciousness and responsible for subjective reactions that shape personality. Through its control of lower order processes, it creates more self-regulation through the planning and execution of behavior. PFC executive functions include not only working memory, attention, memory, and choice, but also the control of emotion (i.e. affect, drive, and motivation).

The association and insular cortices process and forward internal and external information on to the prefrontal cortex for further processing and decision-making (Banfield *et al.* 2004). Frontal executive functions coordinate attention, emotions, cognition and actions integrating visceral, emotional, and behavioral information from other parts of the brain. It is in the prefrontal cortex that we develop ideas about others' beliefs, intentions, and perceptions, empathic thinking and the ability to regulate one's own emotions and impulses. Damage or dysfunction in the dorsal and orbital areas is associated with impairment in empathic behavior and antisocial behaviors.

The famous medical case of Phineas Gage, who survived massive prefrontal cortex damage in an 1848 railroad accident, provided evidence that the prefrontal cortex functions in personality expression and the delay of immediate gratification in behavioral choices (Damasio 1994). Gage's life became a tragedy as he exhibited bizarre behaviors and social interactions because he was unable to inhibit pleasurable, easy, and impulsive actions despite his awareness that these choices were self-defeating.

Strongly associated with frontal lobe structures are the functions of the anterior cingulate cortex (ACC). The ACC contributes to executive, evaluative, cognitive, and emotional functions through its connections with the prefrontal and parietal cortices, and the motor system (Carter 1998). It plays a role in attention, error detection, the monitoring of conflict, and reward-based processing and learning (Allman *et al.* 2001). The ACC receives input from the lateral prefrontal areas directing commands to motor areas and suppressing inappropriate motor responses (Turken and Swick 1999). In this way, the ACC modulates conflicting stimuli and activities by assigning priorities in order to achieve a desired goal.

The orbitofrontal cortex areas (OFC), behind and slightly above the orbits of the eyes, are biased toward right hemisphere executive functions. This region is also referred to as the ventral medial cortex. Its "hot" functions include the experience of reward and punishment, interpersonal social behavior, and the interpretation of complex emotions (Grafman and Litvan 1999). In contrast, the lateral or dorsolateral prefrontal cortex (DLPFC) provides functions biased toward left hemisphere functions. The "cold" functions of the DLPFC include mechanistic planning, verbal reasoning, and problem-solving. Both play a role in inhibition and control though their functions may differ, for example, the DLPFC may be involved in attentional decisions while the OFC will be involved in affective decisions (Schore 2001; Siegel 1999).

As part of the limbic system, the OFC connects to the ACC and the amygdala in a network that regulates and integrates emotions, motivation, and goal-directed behavior into experiences of attachment, fear, reward and punishment (Siegel 1999). If we have a good feeling about someone or act on attraction, it is probably this right hemisphere based, non-verbal, emotional appraisal system at work. This system helps us appraise faces that attract or repel, possible rewards or punishments (O'Doherty *et al.* 2001), and complex social situations. The appraisal process emerges from integrating social cognition (e.g. interpersonal social context, gaze, facial expression, non-verbal communication), awareness of body sensations and arousal, and input from the amygdala and hippocampus (Siegel 1999).

The OFC's integrative function includes the retrieval of autonoetic representations—autobiographical consciousness that provides a sense of self in the past, present, and future, as well as an ability to mediate perceptions of others. How social interactions are processed and assigned meaning affects action response flexibility and influences our ability to choose advantageous and adaptive behaviors in response to complex social situations. This self-reflective awareness appears to depend on emotionally meaningful interpersonal attachment experiences in early childhood. Emotional coherence and attunement in these experiences with caregivers facilitates the developing ability to regulate emotional arousal. Early experiences shape the OFC and its ability to regulate autonomic responses and emotions during social interactions that lead to empathy and collaborative social behaviors (Siegel 1999).

The lateral or dorsolateral prefrontal cortex (DLPFC), in conjunction with the hippocampus, has a major executive role in organizing working memory, focusing conscious attention, and integrating external and internal information in order to guide and inhibit behavior, manage conflict, set goals, plan, persevere, monitor, and self-regulate (Berninger and Richards 2002; Cozolino 2002; Siegel 1999). Developing procedural sequence learning skills reflects the DLPFC's ability to merge spatial information with working memory (Robertson *et al.* 2001). We may experience conscious awareness by linking diverse representations (i.e. external sensory stimuli, internally generated imagery from imagination or memory, and affective material) into a meaningful continuity through DLPFC functioning. An inability to integrate emotions through working memory may result in difficulty engaging in meaningful relationships, difficulty changing behavior, or difficulty in future planning resulting from a lack of awareness of one's own or others' emotions (Siegel 1999; Wood and Grafman 2003). Though these self-regulatory processes appear to be associated to particular cortical areas, such an approach is limited because of the complexity of interactions between brain areas that contribute to the cortex's integrative function (Banfield *et al.* 2004; Siegel 2006).

Emotional perception, the resulting emotional state and its behaviors, and the executive regulation of affective states and behaviors may be explained by two hypothesized emotional perception neural systems: one ventral and one dorsal (Phillips *et al.* 2003). The ventral emotional perception system is associated with the identification of emotional salience of a stimulus, the production of affective states, and the automatic (unconscious) mediation of automatic responses. The ventral emotional perception neural system includes the ventral areas of the prefrontal cortex, the OFC, the ventral anterior cingulate, insula, and amygdala. The dorsal emotional perception system provides effortful, executive control over the affective responses and behaviors. It includes the dorsal, lateral and medial areas of the prefrontal cortex, the dorsal anterior cingulate, and the hippocampus. These areas integrate cognitive and emotional processes utilizing selective attention, planning, and effort. Dysfunctions in these systems are implicated in disorders characterized by emotional and behavioral dysregulation like schizophrenia, bipolar disorder, and major depressive disorder (Phillips *et al.* 2003).

In summary, the PFC is responsible for the integration of internal subjective reactions to perceptions of the external world (Banfield *et al.* 2004). As such, it plays a vital role in the shaping of personality and interpersonal social functioning. Key to this integration is the subjective experience of others and the understanding of social experience.

Theory of mind, empathy and self-regulation

Theory of mind (ToM) is the ability to understand the mind, actions, and intentions of others (Frith and Frith 1999). Neurons found in the STS, inferior frontal regions, medial prefrontal regions, and ACC suggest that mindsight (Siegel 1999), essential to ToM, is a process that compares behavior we observe with our own experience that informs us about others' intentions. Mentalizing, which combines these aspects, depends upon autobiographical memory and activates the medial prefrontal regions (Frith and Frith 2003).

Mentalizing may be a component of language development and transmission of knowledge (Frith and Frith 2001). Language may have progressed from imitation and gesture, using mouth/facial and hand/arm actions, to vocalizations (Rizzolatti and Arbib 1998; Rizzolatti and Craighero 2004). This hypothesis gains support from a mirror neuron system for gestures located in Broca's area. Significant symptoms related to mirror neuron dysfunction include isolation, lack of empathy, an inability to mentalize and assess others' intentions, and socialization difficulties (Ramachandran and Oberman 2006).

Action goals also associate with mentalizing, abstract representations of goals, and mirror neurons in the STS (Frith and Frith 2001). The right STS is involved in the detection of motion. Implied motion, such as a photo of a running athlete, is perceived by the area that processes actual motion, the occipito-temporal junction (OTJ). Even sequential static images in different spatial locations, such as animation drawings, are perceived as motion by premotor and parietal cortices (Blakemore and Decety 2001). Other brain regions involved in mentalizing include the ACC, related to monitoring self mental states; the TPJ, related to reasoning about mental states (Saxe and Kanwisher 2003); the amygdala, related to emotional learning (Frith and Frith 2001); and the cerebellum, related to stored representations of our actions (Blakemore and Decety 2001). Frith and Frith (2001) hypothesize that the TPJ, located about halfway between two visual information processing streams, interfaces information processing about actions from one with information about objects and individuals from the other. The integrated information assists in the recognition of individuals or objects and their relationship to actions and intentions.

Understanding another's actions evokes cognitive, motor, and emotional functions underpinning comprehension (Gallese, Keysers, and Rizzolatti 2004). The processes are implicit, automatic, and unconscious. Hypothetically, the same process and neural systems facilitate the sensations and emotions that we call empathy: the ability to see oneself in another's position and to understand their emotional state (Gallese 2003).

Empathy has been conceptualized as "(1) an affective response to another person, which often but not always, entails sharing that person's emotional state, and (2) a cognitive capacity to take the perspective of the other person while keeping self and other differentiated" (Jackson, Meltzoff, and Decety 2005, p.771). This complex cognitive capacity allows an experience of self and other as connected yet differentiated.

Empathy involves bottom-up emotion sharing and top-down executive regulation of emotional experience. As such, empathy exemplifies the interface between "hot" emotional and "cold" rational functions in the PFC (Grafman and Litvan 1999).

When a person cannot remain differentiated from an event and begins to experience the painful situation as happening to them, personal distress increases. This experience of empathic failure and affect dysregulation utilizes the bottom-up processing that allows us to identify implicitly with another's experience but fails to recruit the top-down information processing necessary for emotional self-regulation. As affect regulation is disrupted, behavioral response flexibility is displaced by automatic responses. Emotional self-regulation accompanied by cognitive awareness of self and other is more apt to lead to both empathy and beneficial acts towards others (Decety and Lamm 2006).

Empathy is a complex interaction of multiple cortical and subcortical processes. These functions incorporate primitive emotional resonance or mirroring processes, attachment processes, and require higher cognitive processes involving mindsight, emotion identification, and perspective taking. Combined, these processes result in both cognitive and affective empathy (Watt 2005).

In conclusion, neuroscience provides insights into how the organization of neural networks develops in response to biological and environmental contingencies. Cortical functions develop in interpersonal contexts that provide models for integrating sensory, visceral, emotional, and cognitive functions. These processes bridge a subjective sense of self and others with the ability to self-regulate emotions and behaviors resulting from observed social interactions. Higher cognitive functioning depends on the ability to process and regulate somatic and emotional experiences.

References

Allman, J. M., Hakeem, A., Erwin, J. M., Nimchinsky, E., and Hof, P. (2001). The anterior cingulate cortex: The evolution of an interface between emotion and cognition. *Journal of Cognitive Neuroscience, 935,* 107–117.

Banfield, J. F., Wyland, C. L., Macrae, C. N., Münte, T. F., and Heatherton, T. F. (2004). The cognitive neuroscience of self-regulation. In R. F. Baumeister and K.D. Vohs (eds) *Handbook of Self-Regulation: Research, Theory, and Applications* (pp.62–83). New York: Guilford Press.

Beeman, M. J. and Chiarello, C. (1998). Complementary right-and left-hemisphere language comprehension. *Current Directions in Psychological Science, 7*(1), 2–8.

Berninger, V. W. and Richards, T. L. (2002). *Brain Literacy for Educators and Psychologists.* San Diego, CA: Academic Press/Elsevier Science.

Blakemore, S. J. and Decety, J. (2001). From the perception of action to the understanding of intention. *Nature Reviews, 2,* 561–567.

Carter, R. (1998). *Mapping the Mind.* Berkeley and Los Angeles, CA: University of California Press.

Cozolino, L. (2002). *The Neuroscience of Psychotherapy: Building and Rebuilding the Human Brain.* New York: W. W. Norton & Co.

Cozolino, L. (2006). *The Neuroscience of Human Relationships: Attachment and the Developing Social Brain.* New York: W. W. Norton & Co.

Damasio, A. R. (1994). *Descartes' Error.* New York: Avon Books.

Decety, J. and Lamm, C. (2006). Human empathy through the lens of social neuroscience. *The Scientific World Journal, 6,* 1146–1163.

DeVries, A. C., Glasper, E. R., and Detillion, C. E. (2003). Social modulation of stress responses. *Physiology & Behavior, 79*, 399–407.

Dupont, S., Bouilleret, V., Hasboun, D., Semah, F., and Baulac, M. (2003). Functional anatomy of the insula: New insights from imaging. *Surgery and Radiologic Anatomy, 25*, 113–119.

Frith, C. D. and Frith, U. (1999). Interacting minds: A biological basis. *Science, 286*, 1692–1695.

Frith, U. and Frith, C. (2001). The biological basis of social interaction. *Current Directions in Psychological Science, 10*(5), 151–155.

Frith, U. and Frith, C. D. (2003). Development and neurophysiology of mentalizing. *Philosophical Transactions of the Royal Society: Biological Science, 358*(1431), 459–473.

Gallese, V. (2003). The roots of empathy: The shared manifold hypothesis and the neural basis of intersubjectivity. *Psychopathology, 36*, 171–180.

Gallese, V., Keysers, C., and Rizzolatti, G. (2004). A unifying view of the basis of social cognition. *Trends in Cognitive Science, 8*(9), 396–403.

Grafman, J. and Litvan, I. (1999). Importance of deficits in executive functions. *Lancet, 354*, 1921–1923.

Greenspan, S. I. (1997). *Developmentally Based Psychotherapy*. Madison, CT: International Universities Press, Inc.

Iacoboni, M., Molnar-Szakacs, I., Gallesse, V., Buccino, G., Mazziotta, J. C., and Rizzolatti, G. (2005). Grasping the intentions of others with one's own mirror neuron system. *PLOS Biology, 3*(3), 529–535.

Jackson, P. L., Meltzoff, A. N., and Decety, J. (2005). How do we perceive the pain of others? A window into the neural processes involved in empathy. *Neuroimage, 24*(3), 771–779.

O'Doherty, J., Kringelbach, M. L., Rolls, E. T., Hornak, J., and Andrews, C. (2001). Abstract reward and punishment representations in the human orbitofrontal cortex. *Nature Neuroscience, 4*(1), 95–102.

Phillips, M. L., Drevets, W. C., Rauch, S. L., and Lane, R. (2003). Neurobiology of emotion perception: The neural basis of normal emotion perception. *Biological Psychiatry, 54*, 504–514.

Ramachandran, V. S. and Oberman, L. M. (2006). Broken mirrors: A theory of autism. *Scientific American, 295*(5), 62–69.

Rizzolatti, G. and Arbib, M. A. (1998). Language within our grasp. *Trends in Neurosciences, 21*(5), 188–194.

Rizzolatti, G. and Craighero, L. (2004). The mirror-neuron system. *Annual Review of Neuroscience, 27*, 169–192.

Rizzolatti, G., Fogassi, L., and Gallese, V. (2006). Mirrors in the mind. *Scientific American, 295*(5), 54–61.

Robertson, E. M., Tormos, J. M., Maeda, F., and Pascual-Leone, A. (2001). The role of the dorsolateral prefrontal cortex during sequence learning is specific for spatial information. *Cerebral Cortex, 11*, 628–635.

Saxe, R. and Kanwisher, N. (2003). People thinking about thinking people, The role of the temporo-parietal junction in "theory of mind." *Neuroimage, 19*, 1835–1842.

Schore, A. N. (2001). Effects of a secure attachment relationship on right brain development, affect regulation, and infant mental health. *Infant Mental Health Journal, 22*(1–2), 7–66.

Siegel, D. J. (1999). *The Developing Mind: Toward a Neurobiology of Interpersonal Experience*. New York: Guilford Press.

Siegel, D. J. (2006). An interpersonal neurobiology approach to psychotherapy: Awareness, mirror neurons, and neural plasticity in the development of well-being. *Psychiatric Annals, 36*(4), 248–256.

Turken, A. U. and Swick, D. (1999). Response selection in the human anterior cingulate cortex. *Nature Neuroscience, 2*(10), 920–924.

Watt, D. F. (2005). Social bonds and the nature of empathy. *Journal of Consciousness Studies, 12*(8–10), 185–209.

Wicker, B., Keysers, C., Plailly, J., Royet, J. P., Gallese, V., and Rizzolatti, G. (2003). Both of us disgusted in my insula: The common neural basis of seeing and feeling disgust. *Neuron, 40*, 655–664.

Wood, J. N. and Grafman, J. (2003). Human prefrontal cortex: Processing and representational perspectives. *Nature Reviews/Neuroscience, 4*, 139–147.

4

Neurotransmitters, Neuromodulators and Hormones: Putting It All Together

Richard Carr

With every second that passes, processes engaging our body's cellular communication alter our life experience quadrillions or more times. Miniscule changes stem from chemical messengers categorized as neurotransmitters, neuromodulators, and hormones. These protein-based messengers dynamically impact mood, memory, learning, cognition and body functions. They maintain and modify internal representations of self and other while shaping long-term health and personality. Knowing the effects that neurotransmitters, neuromodulators, and hormones create deepens one's appreciation of the intricacies of oneself and others. Chemically often more the same than different, how messengers reach their target, what they do and where they start are most significant.

Neurotransmitters excite or inhibit neurons that sequence together to reorganize mind-body processes. This sequencing of neurons forms neural networks that have specific functions like moving a muscle or stopping impulsive actions. The first and last cells in the network may be neurons or another kind of cell like a muscle cell or a pain receptor. Every cell in the network has receptors differentiated to receive specific neurotransmitter molecules like a key in a lock. To reach the receptors, neurotransmitters cross a space called a synapse that separates the neurotransmitter's originating neuron from a postsynaptic neuron. Postsynaptic neurons treat neurotransmitters as emissaries bearing important information (Castro *et al.* 2002). Branches on the postsynaptic neuron called dendrites contain specific receptors ready to receive the stimulation carried by the presynaptic neurotransmitter molecules. Thus, network communication travels from presynaptic to postsynaptic neurons. The process is illustrated and described further in Figure 4.1.

Presynaptic neurons manufacture and release, on average, three neurotransmitters (Howard 1994), along with other molecules to influence their message (Panksepp 1998). After delivering their exciting or inhibiting news, these messenger molecules are quickly demolished by synaptic enzymes or re-cycled back into the presynaptic neuron.

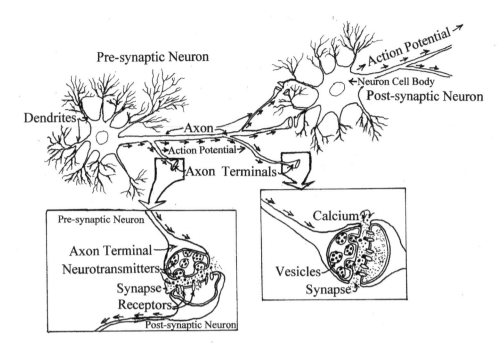

Figure 4.1 Neurons, synapses, and neurotransmitters. Information travels from pre- to post synapse in interconnected neurons. Stimulated postsynaptic dendrites excite the neuron cell body until an action potential (electrical impulse) is released and travels down the axon to an axon terminal, where neurotransmitters, neuromodulators, and/or neuropeptides release. These messengers cross the synapse (lower inserts) stimulating postsynaptic dendrites on the next neuron's cell body, which conveys its message in a like fashion to the next neuron in the sequence.

Over 100 billion neurons in the brain, utilizing 20 percent of the body's energy, create exceptionally quick reactions in this way. While hundreds of billions of neurotransmitter molecules are communicating critical information, each crosses only a single synapse to create rapid, brief responses. This differentiates them from hormones and neuromodulators.

Hormones produced by glands travel slower using fluid-based body systems, such as the vascular system. They help glands talk with other glands, diverse organs, tissues, cells, and/or neural networks. Using fewer energy resources than neurotransmitters, hormones circulate longer, slowly affecting receptors throughout the body. Thus, balancing hormonal effects are more difficult. Women, whose physiology is more impacted by hormones and stress than men, experience this complexity more often.

Hormonal systems require feedback loops to signal when to stop producing their hormones. Once a hormone's target is sufficiently stimulated, whether a gland or other structure, the target releases a related hormone into circulation that finds additional receptors on subsequent structures that continue, modify and/or end the function being performed. For example, the endocrine system stress response uses a feedback loop. Stimulated by stress, the hypothalamus secretes corticotropin-releasing hormone (CRH) into a tiny vascular system connecting to the master endocrine gland, the pituitary. The pituitary complies with adrenocorticotropic hormone (ACTH) secretions into the bloodstream leading to adrenal glands atop the kidneys. The adrenal gland's outer layer, the adrenal cortex, completes the loop by secreting cortisol into a vascular system leading back to the pituitary and hypothalamus. Cortisol finds every cortisol receptor along the way to aid and convey the body's preparation for stress. Hypothalamic and pituitary cortisol receptors convey that CRH and ACTH should be curtailed. When the stress/cortisol balance favors cortisol, feedback succeeds, the stress response tapers off, and relief follows. While slower than the nervous system, the endocrine system is more energy efficient and capable of widespread influence. However, neuromodulators bridge both neurotransmitter and hormone realms.

Neuromodulators influence message transfer in brain regions by impacting multiple synapses and their surrounding cells (Adelman and Smith 2004). They dampen or strengthen nerve signals that prompt action (Gill and Mizumori 2006). A wide range of neuroactive substances, from neuropeptides to steroids, is involved (von Bohlen und Halbach and Dermietzel 2006). In fact, some hypothalamic neuromodulators function as pituitary neurohormones that help link neural and hormonal effects to actions and environmental stimuli (Daruna 2004). Oxytocin, a hypothalamic neuropeptide, functions as both a neurotransmitter and a hormone. It influences affiliative bonding and breastfeeding experiences, decreases stress responses, and improves neural development. Certain emotional experiences stimulate oxytocin production as part of a feedback loop (Uvnäs Moberg 2003). For instance, a baby's cry may stimulate a mother's breast to weep.

Neuropeptides also function as neuromodulators, neurotransmitters, and hormones (Kaplan and Sadock 1995). Receptors for virtually every endocrine system peptide exist in neurons, effectively increasing endocrine/nervous system intercommunication. Many neuropeptides cross the blood brain barrier further linking brain activities to bodily functions. Feeling "sick" from anxiety can result from neuroimmune interactivity in the gut (von Bohlen und Halbach and Dermietzel 2006). In addition at least 40 small neuropeptides orchestrate specific emotional expressions by altering the intensity of neurotransmitter release (Panksepp 1998).

Learning (LTP), forgetting (LTD), and excitatory glutamate (Glu)

Processes of learning and forgetting exist on a neural basis to conserve energy and critically inform psychosocial functioning. Without learning, moment-to-moment stimulation of neurons would cause trial and error responses to environmental stimuli to exhaust the body's energy quickly. Even saying, "Hi, how are you?", for instance, requires learning-dependent memories that motivate rapid neuronal responses and habits that provide repetitive responses. Knowing and anticipating important cues facilitates energy conservation and the formation of purposeful patterns of action.

Activated neurons rely upon receiving glucose and oxygen from neighboring cells and blood vessels to survive. Throughout their lifespan, neural networks function based upon a use it or lose it principle. Neural dendrites extend rapidly and more frequently while seeking to strengthen links between neurons activated by related stimuli. Consequently, neural networks organize in accord with specific neurotransmitter functions, related influential neuromodulators and/or hormonal functions that encourage learning and integration. Network connections often form during critical and sensitive developmental stages, such as crawling, walking, and talking. When completed, learned or feed-forward linkages resist future change. As a counterpoint, feedback learning occurs when uncertainty of outcome persists. This results in synaptic plasticity (Ghosh 2002) that requires networks to reorganize and accommodate changing life needs. Impulses to act, react, or respond reflect different dynamic interplays between neuronal feed-forward (learned) and feedback (learning) processes that result in long-term potentiation (LTP) and long-term depression (LTD).

Long-term potentiation (LTP) or learning on a synaptic level strengthens and quickens specific stimulus-response links between nerve cells. Predictable neural network or feed-forward linkages result from LTP for hours to years. Brief high-frequency postsynaptic stimulation of LTP receptors shapes connections that provide long-lasting, enhanced, excitatory, synaptic strength (Shi 2001).

The interplay between two receptor types creates LTP. Both react to the brain's principal excitatory neurotransmitter glutamate (Glu) normally. One type responds in a typical stimulus-reaction sequence. The second type, an NMDA (N-Methyl D-Aspartic Acid) receptor, resists activation, like a child waiting to be coaxed. After enough repetitive and intense stimulation by Glu, NMDA receptors increase in number and reduce their activation thresholds, becoming very fast, reliable reactors. Dendrites with NMDA receptors escalate activity between neurons promoting networks that activate more easily, surpass previous reaction speeds and provide more reliability than the first type of glutamate receptors. Frequent stimulation of LTP increases network access to resources, ensuring its survival, and allowing refined behavior patterns to endure. Thus, over time art therapy clients might see art materials and feel an immediate LTP-based excitement about what and how to do art therapy.

Glutamate (Glu) projection circuits connect distant neocortex, limbic and brainstem areas (Letinic, Zoncu, and Rakic 2002) that are critical during development, cognition, memory, movement and sensing (Lipton and Rosenberg 1994). In order to facilitate limbic functions and motivate movement, Glu neurons connect the hippocampus, amygdala, and prefrontal cortex (PFC) to the nucleus accumbens, a pleasure center in the brain (Cauli and Morelli 2005). These structures critically mold learning experiences.

However, the response rapidity of NMDA receptors can pose significant dangers for a neuron. Prolonged Glu stimulation alters calcium and potassium concentrations inside and outside of the neuron, potentially causing neuronal damage or death from swelling and toxic conditions. This excitotoxicity becomes significant during strokes, hypoglycemia, trauma, amnesia, hyperalgesia, depression, anxiety, schizophrenia, epilepsy, Tourette's syndrome, Huntington's disease, Acquired Immune Deficiency Syndrome (AIDS), dementia, Lou Gehrig's disease, Parkinson's disease, and Alzheimer's disease (Gegelashvili and Schousboe 1997; Lipton and Rosenberg 1994; Meldrum

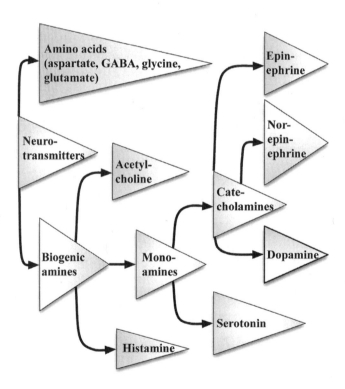

Figure 4.2 Chemical neurotransmitter relationships. Protein synthesis forms neurotransmitters. They differentiate into separate categories of specific molecules through step-wise chemical reactions (e.g. biogenic amines chemically change into monamines, which transform into different catecholamines called dopamine, norepinephrine, or epinephrine).

2000). To prevent excitotoxicity, fast and efficient reuptake of Glu is needed. Nearby support cells, called astrocytes or glial cells, in addition to providing glucose and oxygen (Swanson *et al.* 1997) accomplish this.

Long-term depression (LTD) is forgetting at a synaptic level. During LTD, actions normally excited by a neural network become inhibited. Learned or feed-forward responses become learning or feedback-based responses. In LTD neural responsiveness to specific stimuli can weaken from hours to years. Both LTP and LTD determine future responses differently in neurons utilizing NMDA receptors (Sheng and Kim 2002). Synaptic plasticity formed through LTD and LTP processes encode long-lasting inhibitory or excitatory memories in the brain (Sheng and Kim 2002) that are accessed through neurotransmitter release.

Over 50 different neurotransmitters are known. Like letters of the alphabet, they form an unlimited vocabulary that determines minute purposeful actions, shaping highly creative to extremely mundane to life-enhancing or life-threatening circumstances. Discussion of some chemically related neurotransmitters common in psychosocial responses follows (Figure 4.2).

Acetylcholine (ACh): neurotransmitter/neuromodulator

Acetylcholine (ACh) extensively adds to and alters arousal and attention processes in multiple anatomical regions supporting learning and memory (Gil, Connors, and Amitai 1997). Processing visual stimuli and concentration enhance and improve as a result (Atri *et al.* 2004; Levy *et al.* 2000; Raz 2004). In the dorsal visual stream, connecting the occipital to the parietal cortex (discussed in Chapter 5), ACh sharpens visuospatial attention and interrupts distractions from interfering with one's focus. Acetylcholine-impacted sensory networks more quickly and accurately lead to higher order cognitions and attention (Levy *et al.* 2000).

During learning, ACh hastily activates different neurotransmitter systems that help improve memory and comprehension (McIntyre, Marriott, and Gold 2003). Presynaptic ACh stimulates release of several neurotransmitters: norepinephrine, GABA (gamma-amino butynic acid) and serotonin, in the hippocampus (HC), a structure essential for explicit or consciously accessible memory functions. Hippocampal and parahippocampal regions become functionally enhanced through LTP. Thus, abundant ACh stimulation increases information access during problem-solving particularly when accompanied by high norepinephrine (NE), a neurotransmitter impacting vigilance and attention. Together they improve information recall (Panksepp 1998). Dopamine release stimulated by ACh motivates the striatum, a region contributing to recognition of stimulus salience and the nucleus accumbens, an area promoting reward, pleasure and addiction. Together, these improve regulation of normal memory functions: encoding, retention and retrieval (Atri *et al.* 2004). Overall, activating ACh hastens and enhances processes that involve sensory, especially visual, and memory components during problem-solving and learning contexts.

Art-making contexts involve novel sensory processing that would seem to activate the ACh system intrinsically. Arousal, attention, focus, visual processing and concentration engage synaptic plasticity, enhanced memory and learning functions. Art therapy media, setting, and processes would seem to stimulate ACh, thereby utilizing its contribution to emotion regulation, long-term memory, problem-solving and other overall cognitive changes found during successful art therapy endeavors. Because ACh is activated by visual and novel stimuli, this neurotransmitter may stimulate change processes operating during art therapy.

Dopamine (DA): neurotransmitter/neuromodulator

Dopamine function seems intrinsic to many of the activities and outcomes in art therapy as well. Feeling a sense of reward, pleasure, or thrill while achieving a predicted goal, like an art piece, is intrinsic to therapeutic art-making. Cognition conflicts, learning struggles, and anxiety-related difficulties that hinder attempts to physically shape goal-directed, reward-mediated, and motivation-dependent behaviors, stimulate what many art therapists consider an essential challenge within art therapy processes. Each context just mentioned also characterizes where researchers report that DA affects the arousal system (Raz 2004), higher brain functions, and action-oriented contexts (von Bohlen und Halbach and Dermietzel 2006).

Movement-related actions, basic emotions, visceral functions, reward-based learning and decision-making emerge from three DA pathways: the mesolimbic, the mesocortical and the nigrostriatal illustrated and discussed below (Figure 4.3).

For humans, these circuits involve processing diverse kinds of salient or rewarding stimuli, like those associated with cocaine, money, taste and beauty (Aron *et al.* 2004). Subcortical, mesolimbic DA pathway activation (evenly dashed line in Figure 4.3) helps motivate feelings and desires associated with gaining knowledge, like those found during positive therapeutic alliances. This mesolimbic pathway links with hippocampal activation to stimulate superior memory performance when available cues suggest significant rewards (Adcock *et al.* 2006). Pre-existing, long-term memories of related successes provided by hippocampal-activated DA circuits substitute until a new sense of reward can be achieved. Learning sensory cues that reliably precede rewarding events streamlines the mesolimbic system's participation in appropriately anticipating, preparing for, and pursuing experiences in a rewarding manner (Braver and Brown 2003). Outcomes based upon novelty, significance, emotional content, and feedback strengthen reward sensitivity during stimulus-driven or cause and effect-based learning (Adcock *et al.* 2006; Braver and Brown 2003; Seger and Cinotta 2005). Pre-existing memories of success (feed-forward) combine with outcome (feedback) experiences to reinforce pleasurable long-term memories that arise when anticipating accomplishment

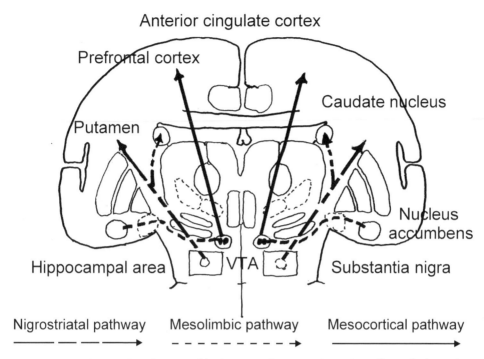

Figure 4.3 Dopamine circuits. This coronal brain section shows DA circuits in midbrain, limbic and cortical areas. Nigrostriatal pathway: substantia nigra, caudate, putamen, part of the striatum. Mesolimbic pathway: ventral tegmental area (VTA), nucleus accumbens, indirectly the hippocampus. Mesocortical pathway: ventral tegmental area, prefrontal cortex, indirectly the anterior cingulate. For a structure's functions see glossary or subsequent descriptions in text.

(new feed-forward linkages). Art-making and media manipulation provide clients with considerable stimulus-based feedback that link expressions of conscious and unconscious choices. Art-making affirms abilities used to express internal conditions, while reinforcing their presence, and increasing the client's confidence at predicting outcomes. Feelings that arise from sensing, desiring and accomplishing during art therapy seem to activate, rely upon and reshape brain functions utilizing this mesolimbic DA circuit. Perhaps future research will confirm when, how, and to what extent this circuit benefits art therapy processes and clients.

The mesocortical DA pathway or circuit (solid line in Figure 4.3) modulates higher order cognitive processes (Chavanon *et al.* 2007). This pathway helps assign positive and negative values to emotions, ideas and experiences (Dehaene, Kerszberg, and Changeux 1998) and aids stress adaptations by constraining activation in the hypothalamic-pituitary-adrenal (HPA) axis, the endocrine system's stress response (Sullivan and Dufresne 2006). The mesocortical pathway connects neocortical areas altering synaptic plasticity and cognitive and emotional processes to a subcortical area called the ventral tegmental area (VTA) that actively produces feelings of pleasure, reward, and addiction.

Mesocortical DA activity is also involved when something known is challenged. Resolution requires activation of the anterior cingulate cortex (ACC) and the lateral PFC, which holds information over time (Raz 2004). The ACC involved with cognitive control and volition activates when tasks that require people to respond to strong, compelling or conflictual stimuli occur. For example, a client may be simultaneously drawn to and repelled by characteristics of clay, which, while easily manipulated, could seem messy and reminiscent of forbidding memories. Detection of this conflict preceding the attempted resolution activates the medial PFC (Raz 2004). While making selections, experiencing conflict, supervising, or during focused and metacognitive attention processes mesocortical DA arousal in the ACC, the basal ganglia, and the PFC blend (Raz 2004). The mesocortical DA circuit's involvement with executive functions may highlight important aspects of meta-cognitive changes taking place during art therapy.

Functionally disrupted DA circuits were correlated with neuropsychiatric disorders (Wang *et al.* 2003). Having too little DA has been associated with feelings of meaninglessness, lethargy, social withdrawal, lack of attention and concentration, deficit motivation-dependent behavior and imbalanced emotional perception. Excesses of DA have been correlated with hallucinations and paranoia, uncontrolled speech and movement (Tourette's syndrome), agitation and repetitive action, and exaggerated convictions of "meaningfulness" (von Bohlen und Halbach and Dermietzel 2006). Dopamine dysfunctions have been found to alter normal associative processes, contributing to schizophrenia, depression, anhedonia, and anxiety disorders (von Bohlen und Halbach and Dermietzel 2006).

Subcortical, nigrostriatal pathway neurons (unevenly dashed line in Figure 4.3) note errors while a person is predicting rewards. Error detection promotes assessing how to alter goal-oriented behavior (Aron *et al.* 2004) such as making abstract designs and patterns fit. Executive decision-making arouses mesocortical and nigrostriatal pathways along with DA receptors in the ACC, which enable cognitive control and volition (Raz 2004). Responding to salient or rewarding events stirs all three DA circuits (Aron *et al.* 2004). Over the course of art therapy, all of the above functions engage and seem to affect change. These midbrain, limbic and prefrontal circuits primarily target the brain's reward circuitry (ventral striatum, orbitofrontal and medial prefrontal cortex) to motivate and create change (Aron *et al.* 2004)

Epinephrine/adrenaline (E): neurotransmitter/neuromodulator

Most people have experienced a rush of adrenaline. Adrenaline, also called epinephrine (E), is part of the sympathetic nervous system's mobilization of a flight or fight response to threat or stress. It enables body reactions to speed up and survival motivations to take priority over other functions, like eating or healing. While initiating flight or fight responses, the amygdala engages the sympathetic nervous system to activate E release from the adrenal medulla atop the kidneys (Liang 2001). In response to signals of danger, E release viscerally primes memory (Knox, Sarter, and Berntson 2004) and enhances learning and memory retention, especially during inhibitory or active avoidant tasks (Liang 2001). The cessation of E activation corresponds with the end of danger.

Emotional reactions to evocative imagery and novel media stimulate amygdala activation and E release below the awareness threshold, during which time, rapid and visible body changes occur, such as sweating, change in pupil size, dry mouth, or cold clammy hands. These heightened physiological reactions signal stress that could motivate the client to approach issues previously avoided, and the therapist's need to monitor the client's increasing overwhelm. Successful art therapy interventions help over time to de-sensitize reactions to such images. When achieved, these kinds of images stir memories devoid of significant E activation probably due to LTD.

Norepinephrine/Noradrenaline (NE): neurotransmitter/neuromodulator

Norepinephrine and E are released into the body from the adrenal medulla in reaction to fear, anxiety or stress. The release of NE/E is critical to sympathetic nervous system alterations of behavior. In the brain, NE comes primarily from the midbrain's locus coeruleus (LC), which innervates over 70 percent of the forebrain's cortical and limbic structures along with the lower cerebellum, medulla, and spinal cord in the body (Ressler and Nemeroff 2000). The LC-NE system is the central component in the sympathetic adrenal stress system (De Bellis 2002).

Norepinephrine activation impacts and controls more comprehensive brain events related to sensory arousal than discrete behavioral processes (Panksepp 1998). For example, new information acquisition, working memory and the attentional aspects of memory storage are all modulated by NE (Vermetten and Bremner 2002). Activating the LC-NE circuitry to the right parietal and frontal cortices causes general attention to become alert, aroused, or vigilant (Raz 2004). This heightened attention initiates multidimensional psychological processes that interact closely with one another to create multiple behavioral and physiological changes.

Decision-making requires sensing task-relevant stimuli, identifying them and then joining them with an appropriate response within hundreds of milliseconds before the decision is enacted. NE enables this complex sequence. Motivationally significant events stimulate the LC-NE system to heighten attention and prepare for action (Nieuwenhuis, Aston-Jones, and Cohen 2005). Social-emotional interactions stimulate LC-NE activation specifically to alter self-perception and social motivation (Bond 2001). Too little NE in the PFC causes decreases in alerting and attention functions associated with Attention Deficit/Hyperactivity Disorder where cues from the parietal cortex interrupt and re-orient attention, distracting any previous focus (Beane and Marrocco 2004).

Norepinephrine significantly shapes depression and other forms of psycho-pathology (Ressler and Nemeroff 2000; Sapolsky 2004). Elevated NE levels in depressed, pregnant mothers have been correlated with premature birth, low birthweight and seemingly depressive behaviors in newborn infants (Field, Diego, and Hernandez-Reif 2006). Postnatally, infants, like their mothers that show increased NE and cortisol and decreased DA (Field *et al.* 2004), demonstrate higher risks for later psychopathology. These infants often go on to develop attention, learning and memory dysfunctions (Huizink, Mulder, and Buitelaar 2004). Similar increases in NE and depression are found in children and adolescents suffering significant early maternal separations, trauma, and abuse (De Bellis 2002). Early, tactile mother-infant experiences, such as skin-to-skin holding, touching and massaging, stimulate neuropeptides, cholecystokinin (CCK) and endogenous opioids that can reverse stress effects from LC-NE elevations (Meaney, Brake and Gratton 2002; Weller and Feldman 2003).

Serotonin (5-HT): neurotransmitter/neuromodulator

The 5-HT system and the LC-NE system functionally counterbalance each other. While the LC-NE system orients towards attention and the environment, the 5-HT system prioritizes homeostasis and restores internal functioning and calm.

Serotonin neurons "project from the brainstem extensively throughout the cortical and subcortical structures" (Ressler and Nemeroff 2000, p.3). Well known for involvement in mood and anxiety disorders, 5-HT is sometimes referred to as the nervous system's brake (Ressler and Nemeroff 2000). For instance, behavioral inhibition, freezing rather than flight or fight, increases when certain 5-HT receptors activate (Panksepp 1998). A temperament dimension called Harm Avoidance, personality characteristics of self-directedness and to a lesser extent cooperativeness, and increased social skills all correlated with 5-HT activation (Bond 2001). Amygdala inhibition, neurogenesis and hippocampal resilience all depend upon 5-HT activation. Low 5-HT levels and/or prenatal stress (Huizink, Mulder and Buitelaar 2004) were also associated with aggression, impulsive behavior, and disrupted sleep. Dreaming similarly reflected decreased 5-HT inhibition of brainstem stimulation promoting internal sensory awareness in the visual cortex (Ressler and Nemeroff 2000). Underactivation of serotonin accompanied by complex NE dysregulation, primarily overactivation, is thought to occur during depressive disorders.

Serotonin neurons respond only modestly to environmental stimuli until intensified stress increases their activation. At that point, the higher levels of 5-HT diminish motivation and emotional behaviors (Panksepp 1998). High 5-HT facilitates increased tolerance and decreased memory of aversive contexts—the opposite of the LC-NE system stress activation. Repetitive behaviors and thoughts common in anxiety disorders like OCD (obsessive compulsive disorder) raise stress to a level that finally stimulates 5-HT systems to decrease amygdala-based anxiety and fear responses and aversive memory formation. When 5-HT is hyporesponsive, stress reactivity increases and aversive memories form (Ressler and Nemeroff 2000).

Panic disorders and borderline personality disorders have also demonstrated dysregulation of 5-HT functioning (Grosjean and Tsai 2007; Maron *et al.* 2004). During therapy, clients shift between outward and inward attention-based processes, suggesting balances or imbalances in LC/NE and 5-HT systems. Understanding of 5-HT functions advantages therapeutic choices, which facilitate or interfere with outward and inward attention-based shifts.

Gamma-amino butyric acid (GABA): neurotransmitter

Gamma-amino butyric acid (GABA) is the brain's major inhibitory neurotransmitter. Organs outside the central nervous system, like the ovaries, testes and the gastrointestinal tract, exhibit abundant GABA receptors (Schousboe and Waagepetersen 2004). It occurs in 30 to 40 percent of all synapses, second only to glutamate, the brain's major excitatory neurotransmitter. GABA's concentration in the brain is one to two thousand times greater than ACh or other monoamines (Figure 4.2). Prenatally, GABA is excitatory, helping form primitive patterns of activity similar to those postnatal glutamate creates while facilitating NMDA connections. Maternal oxytocin inhibits fetal neurons that switch GABA from an excitatory prenatal neurotransmitter to an inhibitory postnatal one. This switch in GABA function quiets neuronal activation, reduces stress effects and increases resistance to insults during delivery (Tyzio *et al.* 2006). Postnatally, GABA activates inhibitory dendritic receptors that block excitatory receptors from responding thus diminishing a network's activity. The brain's overall level of inhibition reflects GABA activation of its receptors, the number of GABA synapses, and the strength of these inhibitory synapses (Kandler 2004). In the neocortex, GABA inhibits local circuitry rather than projection circuits covering larger distances (Letinic *et al.* 2002). Local circuit synapses affect recombining of cortical information (Gil *et al.* 1997) rather than corticolimbic information or vice versa.

Emotional conflict resolution and moment-to-moment integration of negative and positive emotions into aspects of creating art may facilitate shifting and improving functional inhibitory networks. During negative affect processing, GABA decreases orbitofrontal cortex (OFC) regulation of emotion from the amygdala, which itself is plentiful with GABA receptors. GABA increases processing in the medial PFC, a site that detects emotional conflict (Northoff *et al.* 2002) and self-referential activity (Szpunar, Watson, and McDermott 2007). Positive emotions reverse these patterns of GABA induced responses increasing OFC regulation of the amygdala and decreasing processing in the medial PFC. Both the OFC and the amygdala utilize GABA in regulating psychogenic stress responses. The amygdala uses GABA in the way a double negative functions in grammar—inhibiting inhibitory synapses, which enhances hypothalamic hormone secretion. The OFC inhibits ACTH production through GABA use. Inhibiting ACTH production can cause functional imbalances in GABA and glutamate neurons. GABA/glutamate imbalances play a major role in HPA dysregulation contributing to aging and disease (Herman, Mueller, and Figueiredo 2004).

Activity-dependent synaptic reorganization is crucial in establishing functional inhibitory networks. Elimination or strengthening of GABA synapses helps organize local networks more precisely:

> Deeper insight into the principles of how inhibitory circuits become organized and functionally fine-tuned can shed some much-needed light on the biological basis of psychiatric diseases such as epilepsy, anxiety disorders, depression, and schizophrenia, many of which are associated with specific changes in distinct GABAergic circuits rather than changes in the overall level of inhibition. (Kandler 2004, p.101)

Learning how to inhibit neurochemical imbalances is crucial in treating psycho-pathology. Art therapy's role in inhibition learning remains a dynamic question for future research.

Summary

Human nature, behavior, feelings, emotions, thoughts, and decision-making emerge from neuromodulator, neurotransmitter, and hormone systems that fine-tune interactions within complex systems that define organ, tissue, and cellular functioning. Our beliefs, motivations, actions and dysfunctions reflect and alter the influences of these interactions. Dynamically balanced and blended hormones, neurotransmitters and neuromodulators shape learning and memory during psychotherapy in substantial and reliable ways that change a person's self and worldview. Psychotherapy processes and psychopharmacology alter neurotransmitter, neuromodulator and hormone balances in an effort to change psychopathology and improve health. Understanding the contributions to internal communication processes that these messengers create makes a person's inner life more accessible.

This chapter broadly bridged neurotransmitter, neuromodulator and hormonal functioning reported in neuroscience research with ideas about art therapy. Sensory and especially visual processes, novel stimuli, active feedback, pragmatic problem-solving, emotion, expressivity, and the contextual ability to address and reduce stress and threat—all characteristic of art therapy contexts—were discussed as evocators of neurotransmitters.

From a neurotransmitter point of view, art therapy may be especially advantaged by the ACh system. This interesting system responds exceptionally well to visual and novel stimuli; promotes faster cognitive and emotional processing; facilitates learning and memory while lessening distractibility; and recruits other neurotransmitter systems to combine their functioning synergistically while stimulating brain functions. The DA system motivates; provides a sense of pleasure and reward; facilitates improved problem-solving, helps overcome mistakes and achieve goals; and emboldens self-esteem and self-confidence. Glutamate, the brain's major excitatory neurotransmitter, excites arousal and memory processes while facilitating long-term learning and memory (LTP/LTD). Glutamate's counterpart GABA, the brain's major inhibitory neurotransmitter, helps shape focused and/or considered processing of cortical information, regulation of psychogenic stress responses, and emotional awareness. Generally, negative emotions signal that something needs changing, while positive emotions enhance quality of life issues. GABA increases conflict detection and self-referential activity while helping the amygdala increase awareness of negative emotions and secrete hormones in preparation for challenging contexts. For positive emotions, GABA decreases amygdala functioning and increases emotion-based executive functions. Adrenaline promotes physiological expressions to stress and improves emotional memory, especially of adverse moments. Norepinephrine elevates attention processes to a higher level and increases memory of stressful moments. Serotonin puts the brakes on arousal and juxtaposes NE effects by promoting homeostasis and deterring stress responses in order to create a calming effect. NE also initiates multidimensional psychological processing of sensory arousal that impacts and controls broad ranging psychological events, self-perception and social motivation.

By engaging intrinsic communication processes facilitated by neurotransmitters and hormones, art therapy seems poised to enable positive therapeutic changes while possibly enhancing synaptic plasticity and creating multi-tiered psychological outcomes.

References

Adcock, R. A., Thangavel, A., Whitfield-Gabrieli, S., Knutson, B., and Gabrieli, J. D. E. (2006). Reward-motivated learning: Mesolimbic activation precedes memory formation. *Neuron, 50*, 507–517.

Adelman, G. and Smith, B. H. (2004). *Encyclopedia of Neuroscience* (3rd edition). New York: Elsevier B. V.

Aron, A. R., Shohamy, D., Clark, J., Myers, C., Gluck, M. A., and Poldrack, R. A. (2004). Human midbrain sensitivity to cognitive feedback and uncertainty during classification learning. *Journal of Neurophysiology, 92*, 1144–1152.

Atri, A., Sherman, S., Norman, K. A., Kirchhoff, B. A., Nicolas, M. M., Greicius, M. D., *et al.* (2004). Blockade of central cholinergic receptors impairs new learning and increases proactive interference in a word paired-associate memory task. *Behavioral Neuroscience, 118*, 223–236.

Beane, M. and Marrocco, R. T. (2004). Norepinephrine and acetylcholine mediation of the components of reflexive attention: Implications for attention deficit disorders. *Progress in Neurobiology, 74*, 167–181.

Bond, A. J. (2001). Neurotransmitters, temperament and social functioning (review article). *European Neuropsychopharmacology, 11*, 261–274.

Braver, T. S. and Brown, J. W. (2003). Principles of pleasure prediction: Specifying the neural dynamics of human reward learning. *Neuron, 38*, 150–152.

Castro, A. J., Merchut, M. P., Neafsey, E. J., and Wurster, R. D. (2002). *Neuroscience: An Outline Approach.* St. Louis, MO: Mosby.

Cauli, O. and Morelli, M. (2005). Caffeine and the dopaminergic system. *Behavioral Pharmacology, 16*, 63–77.

Chavanon, M.-L., Wacker, J., Leue, A., and Stemmler, G. (2007). Evidence for a dopaminergic link between working memory and agentic extraversion: An analysis of load-related changes in EEG alpha 1 activity. *Biological Psychology, 74*, 46–59.

Daruna, J. H. (2004). *Introduction to Psychoneuroimmunology.* San Diego, CA: Elsevier Academic Press.

De Bellis, M. (2002). Developmental traumatology: A contributory mechanism for alcohol and substance use disorders. *Psychoneuroendocrinology, 27,* 155–170.

Dehaene, S., Kerszberg, M., and Changeux, J. P. (1998). A neuronal model of a global workspace in effortful cognitive tasks. *Proceedings of the National Academy of Sciences—Neurobiology, 95,* 14529–14534.

Field, T., Diego, M., Dieter, J., Hernandez-Reif, M., Schanberg, S., Kuhn, C., *et al.* (2004). Prenatal depression effects on the fetus and the newborn. *Infant Behavior & Development, 27,* 216–229.

Field, T., Diego, M., and Hernandez-Reif, M. (2006). Prenatal effects on the fetus and newborn: A review. *Infant Behavior & Development, 29,* 445–455.

Gegelashvili, G. and Schousboe, A. (1997). High affinity glutamate transporters: Regulation of expression and activity. *Molecular Pharmacology, 52,* 6–15.

Gil, Z., Connors, B. W., and Amitai, Y. (1997). Differential regulation of neocortical synapses by neuromodulators and activity. *Neuron, 19,* 679–686.

Gill, K. M. and Mizumori, S. J. Y. (2006). Context-dependent modulation by D1 receptors: Differential effects in hippocampus and striatum. *Behavioral Neuroscience, 120*(2), 377–392.

Ghosh, A. (2002). Learning more about NMDA receptor regulation. *Science, 295,* 449–450.

Grosjean, B. and Tsai, G. E. (2007). NMDA neurotransmission as a critical mediator of borderline personality disorder. *Journal of Psychiatry & Neuroscience, 32,* 103–115.

Herman, J. P., Mueller, N. K., and Figueiredo, H. (2004). Role of GABA and glutamate circuitry in hypothalamo-pituitary-adrenocortical stress integration. *Annals of the New York Academy of Sciences, 1018,* 35–45.

Howard, P. J. (1994). *The Owner's Manual for the Brain, Everyday Applications from Mind-Brain Research.* Austin, TX: Bard Press.

Huizink, A. C., Mulder, E. J. H., and Buitelaar, J. K. (2004). Prenatal stress and risk for psychopathology: Specific effects or induction of general susceptibility? *Psychological Bulletin, 130,* 115–142.

Kandler, K. (2004). Activity-dependent organization of inhibitory circuits: Lessons from the auditory system. *Current Opinion in Neurobiology, 14,* 96–104.

Kaplan, H. I. and Sadock, B. J. (1995). *Comprehensive Textbook of Psychiatry* (6th ed., Vol. 1&2). Baltimore, MD: Williams & Wilkins.

Knox, D., Sarter, M., and Berntson, G. G. (2004). Visceral afferent bias on cortical processing: Role of adrenergic afferents to the basal forebrain cholinergic system. *Behavioral Neuroscience, 118*(6), 1455–1459.

Letinic, K., Zoncu, R., and Rakic, P. (2002). Origin of GABAergic neurons in the human neocortex. *Nature, 417,* 645–649.

Levy, J. A., Parasuraman, R., Greenwood, P. M., Dukoff, R., and Sunderland, T. (2000). Acetylcholine affects the spatial scale of attention: Evidence from Alzheimer's disease. *Neuropsychology, 14,* 288–298.

Liang, K. C. (2001). Chapter 9: Epinephrine modulation of memory, amygdala activation and regulation of long-term memory storage. In P. E. Gold and W. T. Greenough (eds) *Memory Consolidation: Essays in Honor of James L. McGaugh* (pp.165–183). Washington, DC: APA Books.

Lipton, S. A. and Rosenberg, P. A. (1994). Excitatory amino acids as a final common pathway for neurologic disorders. *The New England Journal of Medicine, 330,* 613–622.

Maron, E., Kuikka, J. T., Shlik, J., Vasar, V., Vanninen, E., and Tiihonen, J. (2004). Reduced brain serotonin transporter binding in patients with panic disorder. *Psychiatry Research: Neuroimaging 132,* 173–181.

McIntyre, C. K., Marriott, L. K., and Gold, P. E. (2003). Cooperation between memory systems: Acetylcholine release in the amygdala correlates positively with performance on a hippocampus-dependent task. *Behavioral Neuroscience, 117,* 320–326.

Meaney, M. J., Brake, W., and Gratton, A. (2002). Environmental regulation of the development of mesolimbic dopamine systems: A neurobiological mechanism for vulnerability to drug use? *Psychoneuroendocrinology, 27,* 127–138.

Meldrum, B. S. (2000). Glutamate as a neurotransmitter in the brain: Review of physiology and pathology. *Journal of Nutrition, 130,* 1007S–1015S.

Nieuwenhuis, S., Aston-Jones, G., and Cohen, J. D. (2005). Decision-making, the P3, and the locus coeruleus-norepinephrine system. *Psychological Bulletin, 131*(4), 510–532.

Northoff, G., Witzel, T., Richter, A., Gessner, M., Schlagenhauf, F., Fell, J., *et al.* (2002). GABA-ergic modulation of prefrontal spatio-temporal activation pattern during emotional processing: A combined fMRI/MEG study with placebo and Lorazepam. *Journal of Cognitive Neuroscience, 14,* 348–370.

Panksepp, J. (1998). *Affective Neuroscience: The Foundations of Human and Animal Emotions.* New York: Oxford University Press.

Raz, A. (2004). Anatomy of attentional networks. *The Anatomical Record (Part B: New Anatomist), 281B*, 21–36.

Ressler, K. J. and Nemeroff, C. B. (2000). Role of serotonergic and noradrenergic systems in the pathophysiology of depression and anxiety disorders. *Depression and Anxiety, 12*(supplement 1), 2–19.

Sapolsky, R. M. (2004). *Why Zebras Don't Get Ulcers: An Updated Guide to Stress, Stress-related Diseases, and Coping* (3rd edition). New York: W. H. Freeman and Company.

Schousboe, A. and Waagepetersen, H. S. (2004). Gamma-amino butyric acid (GABA). In G. Adelman and B. H. Smith (ed.) *Encyclopedia of Neuroscience* (3rd edition). New York: Elsevier.

Seger, C. A. and Cinotta, C. M. (2005). The roles of the caudate nucleus in human classification learning. *The Journal of Neuroscience, 25*(11), 2942–2951.

Sheng, M. and Kim, M. J. (2002). Postsynaptic signaling and plasticity mechanisms. *Science, 298*, 776–780.

Shi, S.-H. (2001). AMPA receptor dynamics and synaptic plasticity. *Science, 294*, 1851–1852.

Sullivan, R. M. and Dufresne, M. M. (2006). Mesocortical dopamine and HPA axis regulation: Role of laterality and early environment. *Brain Research, 1076*, 49–59.

Swanson, R. A., Liu, J., Miller, J. W., Rothstein, J. D., Farrell, K., Stein, B. A., *et al.* (1997). Neuronal regulation of glutamate transporter subtype expression in astrocytes. *The Journal of Neuroscience, 17*(3), 932–940.

Szpunar, K. K., Watson, J. M., and McDermott, K. B. (2007). Neural substrates of envisioning the future. *Proceedings of the National Academy of Sciences of the United States of America, 104*, 642–647.

Tyzio, R., Cossart, R., Khalilov, I., Minlebaev, M., Hübner, C. A., Represa, A., *et al.* (2006). Maternal oxytocin triggers a transient inhibitory switch in GABA signaling in the fetal brain during delivery. *Science, 314*, 1788–1792.

Uvnäs Moberg, K. (2003). *The Oxytocin Factor, Tapping the Hormone of Calm, Love and Healing*, Cambridge, MA: Da Capo Press.

Vermetten, E. and Bremner, J. D. (2002). Circuits and systems in stress. I. Preclinical studies. *Depression and Anxiety, 15*, 126–147.

von Bohlen und Halbach, O. and Dermietzel, R. (2006). *Neurotransmitters and Neuromodulators* (2nd edition). Wienheim: Wiley-VCH.

Wang, X., Zhong, P., Gu, Z. and Yan, Z. (2003). Regulation of NMDA receptors by dopamine D4 signaling in prefrontal cortex. *The Journal of Neuroscience, 23*(30), 9852–9861.

Weller, A. and Feldman, R. (2003). Emotion regulation and touch in infants: The role of cholecystokinin and opioids. *Peptides, 24*, 779–788.

5

Visual System in Action

Noah Hass-Cohen and Nicole Loya

Art therapy practices are routinely informed by visual stimuli and mental imagery. Visual integration is influenced by intrapersonal affects, interpersonal demands, and relational support. The amazing ability of humans to uniquely process, organize, and express retinal signals highlights the distinctiveness of each individual's mental imagery and the artwork they produce. For instance, people with right hemispheric brain lesions do not draw on the left side of the page, while artists with left hemispheric damage often simplify their art, changing its style (Wald 1999). The choices of shapes, color palettes, and imagery locations on the page tell the brain's story (Lezak, Howieson and Loring 2004; Zaidel 2005) and help regulate affect.

Making artwork is exciting and may arouse media safety issues related to the feelings that the materials bring up. Understanding how the visual system pathways function assists in increasing a felt sense of safety: collage images with or without implied movement can enhance clients' feelings of mastery and safety while mediating stress responses aroused by novel stimuli. Conversely, utilizing photographs of images of familiar faces may evoke stronger emotional reactions than would utilizing other images.

Recognizing that the processing of mental imagery and visual stimuli share most neural pathways (Kosslyn, Thompson, and Ganis 2006) provides further clues about art therapy's advantages. While guided imagery approaches and verbal therapy approaches are inclusive of mental imagery, art therapy practices actively seek to integrate sensory experiences probably contributing to neural integration, strengthening mental imagery and as Riley (1999) often pointed out, providing concrete and therapeutic visual feedback. As most people do, the authors in this chapter use mental imagery as synonymous with visual imagery, even though what constitutes mental imagery continues to be a very interesting debate (Kosslyn *et al.* 2006).

The meaning of visual inputs is determined by non-linear flows of information between subcortical sensory and emotional processing, and cortical perceptions and cognitions. The left hemisphere processes visual information from the right half of each eye's visual field; the right hemisphere processes from the left half. The brain's association of visual information endows human activities with meaning. Visual stimuli perceived in the retina travel along the optic track to the thalamus and then to the occipital lobe. The occipital lobe is the primary visual cortex from which visual processing regions and pathways extend to the higher cortex. Partnered with the parietal and temporal lobes, as well as the motor system, the visual cortex translates visual stimuli into pictures that are progressively associated into the forebrain. Visual signals are also fed back to the thalamus, and then transmitted directly to the prefrontal cortex. Figure 5.1 shows many of the thalamic pathways (Kalat 2004).

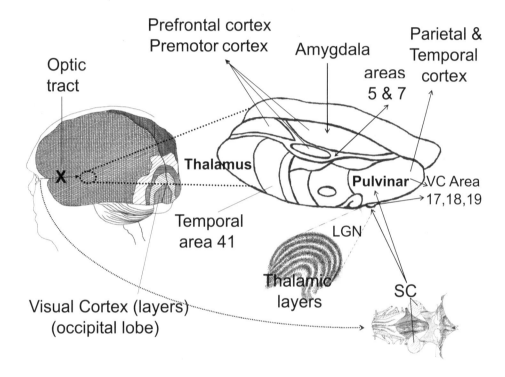

Figure 5.1 The visual system with enlarged view of the thalamus. Retina, optic tract, thalamus, thalamic lateral geniculate nuclei (LGN), thalamic pulvinar nucleus, superior colliculus (SC), visual cortex (VC areas 1–19) and parietal and temporal lobe pathways. The SC connects to the pulvinar nucleus. Arrows indicate direction of information flow.

The thalamus receives all sensory information except for olfactory, smell. The thalamus also receives mental images generated by the frontal lobe and retrieved from memory (Ganis, Thompson and Kosslyn 2004). However, these mental images are weaker impulses when compared to the impulses generated by sensory information. This explains why it is easier to generate mental imagery from sensory stimuli. Thalamic-cortical connections differ from individual to individual, changing how each person sees and reacts to the world (Bjartmar *et al.* 2006; Shatz 1996). From a developmental perspective the maturation of visual subcortical areas is experience-dependent and is linked with the development of cortical connectivity and the emergence of the visual system (Horng and Sur 2006; Sur, Angelucci, and Sharma 1999). Contributions from subcortical thalamic processing to cortical consciousness and awareness underscore the psychological value of art therapy sensory inputs and mental imagery. Within the thalamus, the lateral geniculate nucleus (LGN) and the pulvinar nuclei engage in complex visual processing (Kaas 2005; Michael and Buron 2005; Figure 5.1). The LGN screens and relays visual stimuli and the pulvinar acts as a stimuli processor. The LGN closely connects with vigilance and attention and is the first site where what we see is influenced by how we feel (Kastner and Pinsk 2004; O'Connor *et al.* 2002). The LGN's neuronal makeup directly contributes to this function. The layers of large magnocellular cells illustrated in Figure 5.2 respond quickly to visual stimuli, whereas smaller parvocellular cells are involved in meaning-making.

1. Two layers of magnocellular (M) ganglion cells are larger and mediate light and dark. The heavily myelinated M cells take less time to process information, but do not process information with much detail.

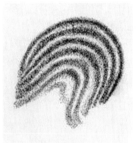

2. Two layers of parvocellular (P) ganglion cells are smaller and mediate color. Less well myelinated P cells take longer to process incoming information in detail.

3. In between layers consist of smaller koniocellular, non-M/non-P cells. K cells may play a role in color perception, however their role is less clear. K cells project to LGN and to the SC.

Figure 5.2 LGN six layers of quick and slow processing.

Large magnocellular processing integrated with small parvocellular processing characterizes most visual system functioning. Therefore, it is likely that therapeutic shifts between quick processing of images and slower content exploration and meaning-making are hard-wired. Depending on the clinical need, clients may react quickly to the visuals or feel safe enough to take the time to process the art. The visual system is exquisitely sensitive to detecting danger and its function is dedicated to the self's survival.

Thalamic orchestration of wordless information also involves survival-oriented responses in the superior colliculus (SC; Figure 5.1). The SC, a subcortical structure, receives information directly from the optic tract, the thalamus and the primary visual cortex. The SC is pivotal in detecting danger through its sensitivity to auditory input, peripheral vision, light and motion stimuli (Colonius and Diedrich 2004). It directly contributes to primary visual cortex processing of potentially dangerous motion signals.

Recognition helps determine the need for a fast reaction and the primary visual cortex (V1-V3) acts as a buffer that assists in recognizing visual stimuli (Kosslyn *et al.* 2006). From the primary visual cortex, processing disperses to more than 30 areas (Van Essen 1995) in dorsal (upper) and ventral (lower) pathways. The dorsal stream, called the *where-how* stream, and the ventral stream, called the *what* stream, are pathways through the association cortex where visual stimuli integrate into a full picture (Ungerleider and Haxby 1994). The detailed information on the dorsal and ventral pathways processing in Figure 5.3 provides a point of reference for the upcoming discussion.

The dorsal stream: where is the danger?

The visual system quickly adapts to a rapidly changing environment. The dorsal *where-how* system is the visual system's functional gatekeeper, and primarily processes spatial properties. Tracking and scanning peripheral movement that occurs outside the very center of gaze *where-how* is an unconscious, early warning system attuned to identifying simple novel forms (Cromwell and Buhman-Wiggs 2005).

The ability to locate movement that is outside of the direct line of vision is helped by the SC, which helps the dorsal stream scan and detect objects and their spatial location (Li and Basso 2005). The SC is like a reflex center; for example, it reacts to a flash of peripheral light, causing the eyes and head to move in that direction. Subcortically the intermediate, deeper layers of the SC integrate visual, somatosensory, and auditory inputs. The SC structure increases the accuracy of the dorsal-parietal association of spatial processing. As we notice a moving object, an area in the posterior parietal lobe detects and analyzes other-and-self movements while supplementary cortical areas integrate the visual and somatosensory information (Bear, Connors, and Paradiso 2006). Complex visual spatial information carried by the dorsal system projects back to the lateral geniculate nucleus (LGN), forming corrective feedback loops between the LGN, visual cortex and the prefrontal lobe (Casagrande, Royal, and Sary 2005).

When clients first orient to the art psychotherapy environment, dorsal *where-how* reactions most likely activate. They are sensitive to any changes in the art therapist's office and to any unexpected movements on her part. A consistent, organized studio space can mitigate the effects of introducing novel media and dynamic interventions and help avoid unintentionally jump-starting this stream in a fearful individual.

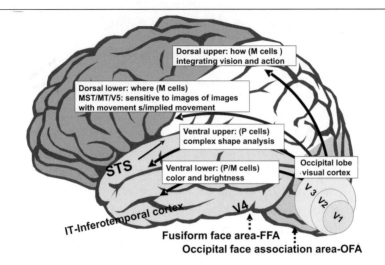

Purposes of the dorsal *where-how* stream

1. The dorsal stream is sensitive to motion in space.
2. Quick reactions are facilitated mostly by large M cells (magnocellular) with well-myelinated axons.
3. The upper *how* sub-stream quickly integrates vision with action.
4. The lower *where* sub-stream detects movement and location. Medial temporal/medial superior temporal cortical areas (MT/MST/V5) sense movement and images with implied movement.

Purposes of the ventral *what* stream

1. The ventral stream processes shape, color and meaning.
2. Associates object information with the temporal lobe functions of emotion, recognition and memory.
3. The upper sub-stream engages complex shape analysis. It has slower acting neurons, P cells.
4. The lower sub-stream is sensitive to color and brightness. It has both M and P cells.

How visual association pathways work

The occipital lobe forwards information to the parietal lobe. The parietal lobe, association cortex, forwards information to the prefrontal cortices so that it can be diminished, enhanced and/or enacted.

- The primary and secondary visual areas (V1; V2) are surrounded by tertiary (V3) and extrastriate-associative visual areas (V4, V5-MT).
- Areas V1 to V3 differentiate visual stimuli into dots, straight lines and diagonal lines.
- Areas V2 and V3 select for orientation. V3 is sensitive to color and movement. V4 receptive fields are sensitive to color, shapes and orientation and contribute to ventral and dorsal processing. V4 connects to the inferotemporal cortex (IT) that responds to a wide range of colors and simple geometric shapes. IT cells play a role in visual memory.
- Extrastriate regions outside of the visual cortex (V1 to V3) have larger receptive fields. At least 30 extrastriate areas progressively associate other sensory signals with visuals creating integrated, multisensory representations.

Facial processing areas

Face and color tasks activate the fusiform face area (FFA) in the IT; the occipital face association area OFA in the occipital lobe; and the STS—superior temporal sulcus.

Figure 5.3 Visual information processing.

Otherwise, unfamiliar conditions that do not match the client's first impressions of the art therapy office can activate dorsal warnings.

The *where-how* stream likely activates during media manipulation; it guides clients as they reach out to pick up the art media and products. Dorsal scanning of size, position and spatial orientation helps exercise visual-motor control over objects (Cromwell and Buhman-Wiggs 2005; Faw 2003; Gazzaniga 2004; Kalat 2004; Kourtzi and Kanwisher 2000).

Neuroimaging showed the dorsal stream to be less reactive to redundant, repetitive, or continuous stimuli presentations (Cromwell and Buhman-Wiggs 2005). It is informed by habituation to stimuli. We believe that, over time, the dorsal stream habituates and gets used to the novelty of art therapy set-up and practices. A neutral familiar baseline for therapeutic change is established as *where-how* becomes less reactive to novelty and non-repetitive motions aroused by the art-making. As a result, clients and therapists can increase references to safety, mastery and control while using the media, static imagery and the art space. Conversely, when clients seem stuck in therapy, novel interventions, such as suggesting a new media and/or changing whether the client sits or stands up while making the art, excite the dorsal stream and re-engage therapeutic attention. The dorsal stream's lack of habituation to new media or new directives provides an additional window of therapeutic opportunity.

In addition to possible outcomes from repetitive or novel art activities, spatial processing is exquisitely sensitive to images that imply motion, even when encoded in static photographs (Kourtzi and Kanwisher 2000). The extended dorsal substream projects to temporal and occipital lobe regions, sensitive to human parts and biological movement (V5-MT, Figure 5.3; Downing *et al.* 2001; Peuskens *et al.* 2005). For example, a picture of hands that were implying the action of gripping increased corticospinal excitability when compared with images of rested hands or hands indicating completed motions (Urgesi *et al.* 2006). When first making collages, clients often choose beautiful, glossy and serene images with no human or animal movement. Previously, Noah Hass-Cohen considered this tendency a form of psychological defense. However, the research (Kourtzi and Kanwisher 2000) suggests that pictures without implied motion calm the dorsal stream. Offering clients landscape collages may help them settle into therapeutic art-making.

Matching pictures with the client's previous mental imagery helps them translate implicit meanings. For example, people generally find beautiful landscape or glossy symmetrical facial images attractive (Zaidel and Cohen 2005) and become frustrated when drawn images do not turn out as beautiful. Most likely, this attraction activates the brain's dopaminergic reward circuitry, the orbital medial prefrontal cortex, the ventral striatum, and the nucleus accumbens (Aron *et al.* 2005). Art therapy relational neuroscience (ATR-N) principles (Hass-Cohen 2008) underscore the value of using attractive collage images without implied movement to help clients increase mastery and control and to stimulate pleasurable experiences.

Ventral stream: what we see is influenced by what we remember and feel

Recognizing what we see is important to the ventral stream. The ventral visual stream is the temporal lobe (Kalat 2004). Ventral pathways link fine details with visual salience resulting in reward-seeking behaviors and/or in sophisticated and planned, skilled escape sequences (Bullier 2001). The slower *what* stream builds consciously formed representations that identify objects (Cromwell and Buhman-Wiggs 2005). Ventral object processing is important to attention, working memory, and identifying stimulus salience. Once an object is recognized, its image projects to the amygdalar-thalamic-hippocampal complex and is processed for danger, threat, and emotional relevance. Basal amygdalar neurons direct attention by projecting directly to the visual cortex (Adolphs 2004) and enhancing recognition. The amygdala and the prefrontal cortex help determine any fit between tangible properties such as color, texture, shape, and their emotional associations (Shaw *et al.* 2005). Asking clients to describe what they are seeing most likely engages the ventral stream's deliberate processing, and helps the person slow down and assign meaning to the event depicted.

Emotional connections between what is seen and what is recognized are driven by memory. In Capgras's syndrome, amygdala connections are severed and people cannot make affective sense of what they see. Ramachandran (1994) described a case of a young man who recognized his mother's face but did not feel the affect associated with her. The discrepancy caused him to assume that an alien had taken over his mother. Emotion and memory systems link and continually update a sense of self in relationship to others.

Looking further into connections between the visual system, memory, and emotion, we see that mental imagery and external visuals often coincide. For example, while experiencing intense emotions, such as those stirred during a horror movie, limbic processing does not differentiate between external and internal images (Kuhtz-Buschbeck *et al.* 2003). When we imagine, the visual cortex activates overlapping visual perception and mental imagery neural substrates (Carli *et al.* 2006; Ganis *et al.* 2004; Slotnick, Thompson and Kosslyn 2005). Furthermore, the amygdala appraises both visual inputs produced by the art and internal imagery generated by the frontal cortex. As appraising fear comes before conscious evaluation, it can cause quick non-verbal responses affecting decision-making and actions. Clients' imaginary anticipatory reactions can initiate a stress response and the body may experience the chemical changes that would normally occur only if one were actually in danger.

Understanding visual stream functions suggests updating traditional art therapy media continuum (Malchiodi 1998; Virshup, Riley and Shepherd 1992). Traditionally, this continuum has focused on the degree of fluidity versus structure and crumbliness of media (paint versus clay for example). Safety in this continuum was associated with increased structure. Based on the neuroscience, we suggest that it is likely that the firmer the media, the safer the assessment given by the amygdala. To further associate safety with dorsal/ventral visual stream functioning, we suggest including media location and implied movement along with novelty shape, color, and meaning as illustrated in Table 5.1.

Ventral bias for facial recognition and expression: an art therapy palette

The preference for seeing familiar faces and objects shapes the self throughout the lifespan (Schore 2000) and contributes to non-verbal modes of client-therapist exchanges. How we feel about faces and what we do with them propels visual processing (Gauthier et al. 1999). Social-emotional identification and interpretation of faces and facial expressions involves a wide network of overlapping subcortical and cortical visual networks (Ishai, Schmidt and Boesiger 2005; Vuilleumier and Pourtois 2007).

From the beginning of life, the ventral stream tunes to familiar objects, faces and human gazes (Taylor, Batty and Itier 2004). As early as eight weeks old, an infant's visual system links to right hemispheric processing resulting in a socially attuned brain (Schore 2000). The right hemisphere's ventral stream specializes in analyzing low frequency auditory tones expressing the emotional intonation of caregivers' language and low frequency visual perceptions such as the soft, shadowy patterns of a mother's face (Ungerleider and Haxby 1994). Babies are exquisitely attuned to their mothers' faces (Cleveland, Kobiella and Striano 2006; Crandell, Patrick and Hobson 2003; Tronick and Cohn 1989). Infants find their mother's soft-edged face to be a pleasurable and significant visual stimulus (Schore 2000). Gazing at the faces of significant others helps shape the baby's developing brain (Schore 1996) and toddlers continue to participate in a mutual coordinated dance of eye contact and smiles with their mother. Facial expressions and gestures communicate a sense of safety and play that results in social and emotional growth. Over time, reassuring body language communications are utilized from a distance, allowing the child to explore the world safely. Mutual eye contact continues to be a most significant human experience throughout the lifespan, developing into a life-long preference and longing for faces and familiar object forms.

Automatic responses to facial expressions are universal reactions critical to our species survival (Nomura et al. 2004; Whalen et al. 1998). Visual processing is initially unconscious and very quick, happening in 110 milliseconds (ms) in the occipital lobe and 165 ms in the fusiform area (Halgren et al. 2000). Bottom-up integration of subcortical facial networks and cortical neural networks contribute to the recognition of familiar, non-familiar and self-faces (Platek et al. 2006; Sugiura et al. 2005.) Face-sensitive visual networks include the fusiform face area (FFA), the occipital face association area (OFA) (Kanwisher, McDermott and Chun 1997; Kanwisher and Yovel 2006, review), and the superior temporal sulcus (STS) that delineates the temporal and the parietal lobes (see Figure 5.3 for their location). The STS involves emotional visual

Table 5.1 Updated art media psychological continuum of safety and mastery.

Media placement adds to a sense of safety. From a dorsal perspective, media placed peripherally may be more threatening than media placed directly in front. From a ventral perspective, novel unfamiliar messages may be more threatening when in direct view. *Objects, faces or landscapes.

| Media | Less safety movement—dorsal safety | | | | Meaning—ventral novel and less safe (N) familiar and safer (F) | | |
	No implied movement	Implied movement	Undefined shapes	Human movement	Shapes (N/F)	Color (N/F)	Texture (N/F)	Content (N/F)*
Pencils								
Color pencils								
Collage full journals								
Precut collage images								
Felt pens								
Oil pastels								
Plasticine (oily clay)								
Chalk pastels								
Paint								
Watercolors								
Clay								

processing, the OFA responds to physically isolated, inverted, or upright facial parts and the FFA perceives face configuration similarities and upright facial presentations (Kanwisher and Yovel 2006, review). Processing of familiar faces activates emotional-cognitive areas, insula, middle temporal, inferior parietal, and medial frontal lobe, whereas self-face processing involves increased activation of cognitive areas, the right superior frontal gyrus, medial frontal and inferior parietal lobes, and left middle temporal gyrus (Platek *et al.* 2006; Sugiura *et al.* 2005; Table 5.2).

Table 5.2 Non-familiar, familiar and self-face processing advantages.

Unfamiliar faces	Familiar faces	Self-faces
Perceptual-emotional processing	Emotional-cognitive processing	Increased cortical-cognitive processing

We hypothesize that drawing self-portraits involves a considerable amount of cognitive effort compared to drawing familiar faces. Asking for a self-portrait may therefore be contraindicated while clients are experiencing many other demands. Instead, therapists may consider working with less familiar facial images that enhance perceptual processing and contribute to feelings of control. From our experience, we know that familiar faces bring affect to the table. Clients often actively seek images of faces that they love, know, and recognize. Nicole's drawing illustrates this inclination as her mother's familiar face emerges from the white pages (Figure 5.4).

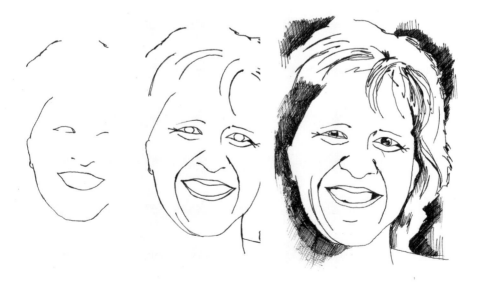

Figure 5.4 My Mom *by Nicole Loya.*

The visual network is capable of sorting individual faces, and differentiating the familiar face (Gauthier *et al.* 1999; Rossion, Schiltz and Crommelinck 2003). People's extensive expertise seeing and identifying faces throughout the lifespan may be one factor leading to the development of preferential responses to familiar faces (Gauthier *et al.* 1999; Kanwisher and Yovel 2006, review) and to familiar objects. The ventral fusiform gyrus has a generalized bias towards familiarity. According to the expertise approach, participants who developed familiarity at viewing funny-looking novel three-dimensional objects called "Greebles" showed more FFA activation than baseline or in comparison to the control participants (Gauthier and Tarr 1997; Gauthier *et al.* 1999; Figure 5.5).

A simple directive common in initial art therapy sessions capitalizes on the brain's love of familiarity: "Choose some collage images that you like and tell me about them." The directive invites clients to engage the temporal lobe by bringing familiar images and dopaminergic rewards into the studio and/or therapy room. Clients' interpretation of visual marks as positive and familiar may indicate right hemisphere dopaminergic activation (Louilot and Besson 2000). The study suggested that attraction or aversion

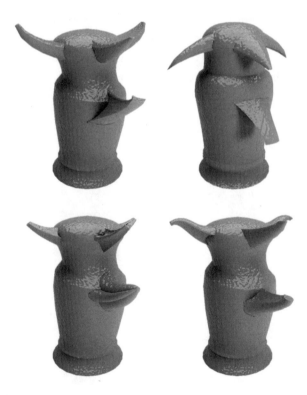

Figure 5.5 The Greebles *were created for researchers Michael J. Tarr and Isabel Gauthier. There are two different genders, which according to the research are easy to discriminate. Reprinted with permission (http://www.tarrlab.org/stimuli/novel-objects).*

toward a stimulus correlate with dopamine variations in the nucleus accumbens, and that the basolateral amygdala controls affective behavioral responses.

Targeted use of collage facial images can excite or calm. To invite relational affects, family art therapists may want to engage clients with familiar family and home pictures. The fusiform face area (FFA) responds more strongly to viewing intact front-view faces rather than to scrambled faces, front-view photos of houses, and three-quarter-view face photos with hair concealed (Kanwisher et al. 1997). Thus, the regulation of relational emotions may be assisted by pictorial choices. The "Greebles" study (Gauthier et al. 1999) suggests repetition and expertise with easy-to-make stick figures or abstract marks endow them with affect. In other words, clients can develop ventral expertise with individualized stylistic marks representing family members.

The fusiform face area generalizes responses for a variety of face types as it perceives and identifies non-familiar human faces, cat faces and cartoon faces (Kanwisher, Tong and Nakayama 1998; Tong et al. 2000). Using highly stylized and non-familiar facial images may arouse less emotion and is a good approach to the beginning stages of therapy and/or a way to lead clients gently towards becoming more involved in processing familiar facial images and/or marks that may represent emotionally charged relationships.

The brain networks that are most associated with processing emotional facial expressions are in the right cortical regions (Adolphs et al. 1996). The right hemisphere is also better at perceiving upright faces and transfers this information to the left hemisphere (McCarthy et al. 1999). Art therapists wanting to recruit a client's left hemispheric function should consider presenting inverted faces, as the left hemisphere was found to be better at perceiving inverted faces and transmitting information to the right hemisphere (McCarthy et al. 1999). Therefore, the literature about recruiting the right hemisphere by drawing an upside down picture (Edwards 1999) is most likely not supported. Moreover, it is difficult to apply some of these findings outside of a lab environment, as most clients will most often look at images with both their eyes engaging both hemispheres. Additional research is needed in order to determine how to present facial images spatially in therapy.

Art therapists wanting to support integrated right-left processing may want to include collage images of printed letters. While faces trigger a strong EEG (electroencephalogram) response (N170) in the right hemisphere (Yovel et al. 2003), printed letters trigger an equally strong response in the left hemisphere. Including images of faces and printed words in the collage box can potentially stimulate right and left hemispheres and perhaps contribute to integrating right and left hemispheric function.

Hemispheric lateralization helps discern between neutral, happy and sad facial expressions (Jansari, Tranel and Adolphs 2000). Normal participants were better at discriminating happy from neutral faces when the happy face was to the viewer's right of the neutral face (presenting the visual stimuli to the client's left hemisphere). Conversely, discriminating sad from neutral faces was better when the sad face was to the left. The art therapist may sit to the client's left and/or present positive facial images to the client's left to facilitate moments of faster, more accurate processing of information about positive possibilities. Clients with left and/or right brain injury may need the art therapist to reverse his/her seating approach. Research participants with damage on the right performed less well in discerning sad faces shown on the left, whereas research participants with either left or right damage actually performed better when discriminating happy faces shown on the left. The research concluded that perception of negative valence relies preferentially on the right hemisphere, whereas perception of positive valence relies on both left and right hemispheres (Adolphs, Jansari and Tranel 2001; Jansari *et al.* 2000; Table 5.3).

Table 5.3 How to present faces.

Therapist		
Sad	Neutral	Happy
RH processing		LH processing and RH processing
Client		

The research on FFA-OFA ventral processing of faces also suggests that art therapists be mindful of the kind of face images presented to and/or created by their clients. Face-dependent EEG measures (N170) present when both high (crisp) and low (blurry) spatial frequencies are present in the facial images (Goffaux, Gauthier and Rossion 2003). When only high spatial frequencies were presented, like smiley cartoon faces, the typical N170 inversion characteristics were missing (Goffaux *et al.* 2003; Sagiv and Bentin 2001). N170 facial characteristics are dependent on low spatial frequency information, the same sort of visual information seen by infants with undeveloped eyesight (Goffaux *et al.* 2003), and which babies associate with close relationships. Adolescents may often draw schematic sharp faces that include shading and high spatial frequencies, like a cartoon smiley face (Gardner 1980; Lowenfeld and Brittain 1987). Helping adolescents incorporate naturalistic face characteristics (soft, blurry, low spatial features) may assist in the exploration of intimacy and connectedness. Clinical observation of how the eyes are drawn may be helpful: fear associates with eyes surrounded by the whites of the eye (Whalen *et al.* 2004), and inquiring about the feelings stimulated by cartoon-like eyes may help mitigate some fears. Crosshatch shading in drawn faces may be indicative of self-doubt and anxiety (Hammer 1997). The literature on infant gazing and the ventral system preference for faces raises relational questions. Could shading reflect doubt in the relationship? Could introducing soft blurry spatial qualities invite intimacy and closeness into the room?

A face can make more than ten thousand expressions (Ekman 2003). Therefore, art therapy facial images may stimulate more than ten thousand emotion-based interpretations. Relational communication depends upon our expertise in interpreting these facial expressions. Facial expressions generate feelings within us, affect the feelings of others around us and enhance ventral meaning-making. Possibly, we automatically estimate someone's approximate age, gender, mood, and assign emotional meanings and stories to facial expressions. These reactions are probably mediated by the STS (Kanwisher and Yovel 2006, review; Figure 5.3). We notice where people focus their attention, how attentive they are, as well as whether or not we find them attractive.

Facial expression research using photographs (Ekman 2003) suggests the likelihood that for children and adults, collage and drawn facial expressions arouse similar reactions as facial expressions in real life. Emotional facial expressions within face-sensitive brain networks activate the anterior cingulate, the insula, the thalamus and primarily the amygdala (Whalen et al. 1998). The amygdala automatically deciphers trustworthiness or approachability in other people based upon their facial presentation (Adolphs 1999). The thalamus communicating with right somatosensory strip generates internal empathic representations of how the other person might feel (Adolphs et al. 2000). While still being studied, facial recognition tasks suggest these areas operate in concert with the bilateral fusiform gyrus, the medial temporal lobe, the right parietal lobe, and the prefrontal cortex (Iidaka et al. 2001). Cortical activation helps translate emotional information into action. This social brain network is bi-lateral with a right hemispheric bias (Allison et al. 1999; McCarthy et al. 1997; Rossion et al. 2003a, 2003b). Right hemispheric empathic responses are essential for adaptive communication. The left amygdala is also involved in processing new faces for positive and negative values (Baas, Aleman and Kahn 2004, review). Sometimes, one may encounter problems reading facial expressions if amygdala deficits exist (Whalen et al. 2004). As most facial expression processing converges on prefrontal areas (Bar et al. 2006; Sprengelmeyer et al. 1998), art therapy interventions may strengthen transmission of information that engages conscious prefrontal-organized discussions (Figure 5.6).

Reactions to angry facial expressions may involve the stress response, which alters heart rate, blood flow, and skin temperature (Ekman 2003). After immediately activating the amygdala, the hippocampus and the prefrontal cortex response follows, allowing long-term autobiographical memory to instill a calming response. However, reactions to facial expressions are context-driven. A daughter seeing the image of her father's angry face may feel safety and calm instead of fear, as long-term memories of his protective qualities are remembered. The emotional reaction primarily depends upon whose face it is, rather than an identification of facial expression. When visual information is ambiguous or insufficient, the orbitofrontal cortex (OFC) activates and utilizes potential reward value responses derived from the familiar, rather than allowing ambiguity to continue (Kosslyn et al. 2006).

Some clients have difficulty engaging in eye contact and interpreting social facial expressions associated with amygdala function deficits (Glascher et al. 2004). Collages have the advantage of being one step removed from the intensity involved in real-life gaze. Therefore, art images of faces and facial expressions afford clients opportunities to

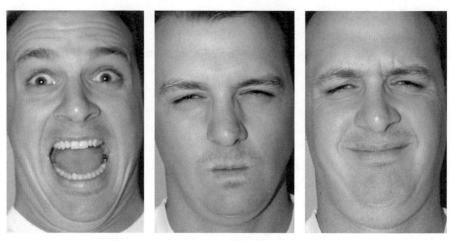

Fearful (on left): amygdala, right fusiform gyrus, left dorsolateral frontal cortex.

Angry (middle): posterior right cingulate gyrus, left medial temporal gyrus, amygdala.

Disgust (right): right putamen, left insula cortex, inferior left frontal cortex.

Figure 5.6 Separate and convergent neurocorrelates of fearful, angry and disgusted facial expressions. All three visual outputs converge on the inferior left frontal cortex for processing.

practice interpreting human expressions, control and master therapeutic communication, and enhance affective attunement.

Summary

Historically, research on vision has been limited to the investigation of the basic mechanics of the projection of visual information onto the visual cortex. We have expanded the investigation to show how the interface between quick/slow and detailed/broad cortical pathways constitutes a relational visual system. Art therapy clinical micro-skills include shifting between *where-how* and *what* systems, as well as engaging higher cortical functions triggered by drawing and observing self-portraits. In looking at and making images, concurrent visual streams engage. Dynamic association of top-down mental imagery and bottom-up visual stimuli allow clients to execute novel pieces of art masterfully, and imbue them with familiar meaning. The ability to manipulate visual media and make meaningful images helps regulate unsettling yet meaningful emotions. It also opens the door to dramatic memories.

On a first order of change, there is a sense of empowerment: *I made something in the moment and it is mine.* A sense of accomplishment activates as ventral neurochemical reward circuits engage and expertise, familiarity with self-generated objects, feelings of ownership and degrees of mastery and control develop. On a second order of change, there are more enduring meta-meanings of mastery and control—going back and forth between internal and external images—and balancing familiar and novel stimuli. Clients use the art to move volitionally to slower explorations of meaning and familiarity. As ventral pathways engage, clients' memories trigger, stabilize, and/or change during therapeutic interplays of external and internal visual stimuli processing. Autobiographical meaning-making is mediated by visual processing, suggesting that what I see is coherent with who my memories tell me that I am. This second order of change contributes to an updated coherent sense of self. Visual information processing not only answers, "What and who is it?"; it also answers, "How do I feel about what I see and what do I do about it? How will what I do reward me, and will I want to do more?"

References

Adolphs, R. (1999). Social cognition and the human brain. *Trends in Cognitive Sciences, 3*(12), 469–479.

Adolphs, R. (2004). Emotional vision. *Nature Neuroscience, 7*(11), 1167–1168.

Adolphs, R., Damasio, H., Tranel, D., and Damasio, A. R. (1996). Cortical systems for the recognition of emotion in facial expressions. *The Journal of Neuroscience, 16*(23), 7678–7687.

Adolphs, R., Damasio, H., Tranel, D., Cooper, G., and Damasio, A. R. (2000). A role for somatosensory cortices in the visual recognition of emotion as revealed by three-dimensional lesion mapping. *Journal of Neuroscience, 20*, 2683–2690.

Adolphs, R., Jansari, A., and Tranel, D. (2001). Hemispheric perception of emotional valence from facial expressions. *Neuropsychology, 15*(4), 516–524.

Allison, T., Puce, A., Spencer, D. D., and McCarthy, G. (1999). Electrophysiological studies of human face perception. I: Potentials generated in occipitotemporal cortex by face and non-face stimuli. *Cerebral Cortex, 9*, 415–430.

Aron, A., Fisher, H., Mashek, D. J., Strong, G., Li, H., and Brown, L. L. (2005). Reward, motivation, and emotion systems associated with early-stage intense romantic love. *Journal of Neurophysiology, 94*, 327–337.

Baas, D., Aleman, A., and Kahn, R. S. (2004). Lateralization of amygdala activation: A systematic review of functional neuroimaging studies. *Brain Research. Brain Research Reviews, 45*(2), 96–103.

Bar, M., Kassam, K. S., Ghuman, A. S., Boshyan, J., Schmid, A. M., Dale, A. M., *et al.* (2006). Top-down facilitation of visual recognition. *Proceedings of the National Academy of Sciences of the United States of America, 103*(2), 449–454.

Bear, M. F., Connors, B., and Paradiso, M. (2006). *Neuroscience: Exploring the Brain* (3rd edition). Baltimore, PA: Lippincott, Williams and Wilkins.

Bjartmar, L., Humberman, A. D., Ullian, E. M., Renteria, R. C., Liu, X., Xu, W. *et al.* (2006). Neuronal pentraxins mediate synaptic refinement in the developing visual system. *The Journal of Neuroscience, 26*(23), 6269–6281.

Bullier, J. (2001). Integrated model of visual processing. *Brain Research Reviews, 36*, 96–107.

Carli, G., Rendo, C., Sebastiani, L., and Santarcangelo, E. L. (2006). Suggestions of altered balance: Possible equivalence of imagery and perception. *The International Journal of Clinical and Experimental Hypnosis, 54*(2), 206–223.

Casagrande, V. A., Royal, D. W., and Sary, G. (2005). Extraretinal inputs and feedback mechanisms to the lateral geniculate nucleus (LGN). In J. Kremers (ed.) *The Primate Visual System: A Comparative Approach* (pp.191–211). Chichester: John Wiley & Sons.

Cleveland, A., Kobiella, A., and Striano, T. (2006). Intention or expression? Four-month-olds' reactions to a sudden still-face. *Infant Behavior and Development, 29*(3), 299–307.

Colonius, H. and Diedrich, A. (2004). Multisensory interaction in saccadic reaction time: A time-window-of-integration model. *Journal of Cognitive Neuroscience, 16*(6), 1000–1009.

Crandell, L. E., Patrick, M. P., and Hobson, R. P. (2003). "Still-face" interactions between mothers with borderline personality disorder and their 2-month-old infants. *The British Journal of Psychiatry: The Journal of Mental Science, 183*, 239–247.

Cromwell, H. C. and Buhman-Wiggs, A. (2005). Commentary on Joel Norman: Early and late constructive features in two visual systems. Retrieved 2/16/06 from http://www.bbsonline.org/Preprints/Norman/cromwell.html.

Downing, P. E, Jiang, Y., Shuman, M., and Kanwisher, N. (2001). A cortical area selective for visual processing of the human body. *Science, 293*(5539), 2470–2473.

Edwards, B. (1999). *The New Drawing on the Right Side of the Brain.* New York: Jeremy P. Tarcher/Putnam.

Ekman, P. (2003). *Emotions Revealed: Recognizing Faces and Feelings to Improve Communication and Emotional Life.* New York: Times Books.

Faw, B. (2003). Pre-frontal executive committee for perception, working memory, attention, long-term memory, motor control, and thinking: A tutorial review. *Consciousness and Cognition, 12*(1), 83–139.

Ganis, G., Thompson, W. L., and Kosslyn, S. M. (2004). Brain areas underlying visual mental imagery and visual perception: An fMRI study. *Brain Research. Cognitive Brain Research, 20*(2), 226–241.

Gardner, H. E. (1980). *Artful Scribbles: The Significance of Children's Drawings.* New York: Basic Books, Inc.

Gauthier, I. and Tarr, M. J. (1997). Becoming a "Greeble" expert: Exploring mechanisms for face recognition. *Vision Research, 37*(12), 1673–1682.

Gauthier, I., Tarr, M. J., Anderson, A. W., Skudlarski, P., and Gore, J. C. (1999). Activation of the middle fusiform "face area" increases with expertise in recognizing novel objects. *Nature Neuroscience, 2*(6), 568–573.

Gazzaniga, M. S. (ed.) (2004). *The Cognitive Neurosciences.* Cambridge, MA: MIT Press.

Glascher, J., Tuscher, O., Weiller, C., and Buchel, C. (2004). Elevated responses to constant facial emotions in different faces in the human amygdala: An fMRI study of facial identity and expression. *BMC Neuroscience, 5*(1), 45.

Goffaux, V., Gauthier, I., and Rossion, B. (2003). Spatial scale contribution to early visual differences between face and object processing. *Brain Research. Cognitive Brain Research, 16*(3), 416–424.

Halgren, E., Raij, T., Marinkovic, K., Jousmaki, V., and Hari, R. (2000). Cognitive response profile of the human fusiform face area as determined by MEG. *Cerebral Cortex, 10*(1), 69–81.

Hass-Cohen, N. (2008). *CREATE*: Art therapy relational neurobiology principles (ATR-N). In N. Hass-Cohen and R. Carr (eds) *Art Therapy and Clinical Neuroscience.* London and Philadelphia, PA: Jessica Kingsley Publishers.

Hammer, E. F. (ed) (1997). *Advances in Projective Drawing Interpretation.* Springfield, IL: Charles C. Thomas Pub Ltd.

Horng, S. H. and Sur, M. (2006). Visual activity and cortical rewiring: Activity-dependent plasticity of cortical networks. *Progress in Brain Research, 157,* 3–11.

Iidaka, T., Omori, M., Murata, T., Kosaka, H., Yonekura, Y., Okada, T., *et al.* (2001). Neural interaction of the amygdala with the prefrontal and temporal cortices in the processing of facial expressions as revealed by fMRI. *Journal of Cognitive Neuroscience, 13*(8), 1035–1047.

Ishai, A., Schmidt, C. F., and Boesiger, P. (2005). Face perception is mediated by a distributed cortical network. *Brain Research Bulletin, 67,* 87–93.

Jansari, A., Tranel, D., and Adolphs, R. (2000). A valence-specific lateral bias for discriminating emotional facial expressions in free field. *Cognition and Emotion, 14*(3), 341–353.

Kaas, J. H. (2005). The evolution of visual cortex in primates. In J. Kremers (ed.) *The Primate Visual System: A Comparative Approach* (pp.267–283). Chichester: John Wiley & Sons.

Kalat, J. W. (2004). *Biological Psychology* (8th edition). Belmont, CA: Thomson/Wadsworth.

Kanwisher, N., McDermott, J., and Chun, M. M. (1997). The fusiform face area: A module in human extrastriate cortex specialized for face perception. *The Journal of Neuroscience, 17*(11), 4302–4311.

Kanwisher, N., Tong, F., and Nakayama, K. (1998). The effect of face inversion on the human fusiform face area. *Cognition, 68,* B1–B11.

Kanwisher, N. and Yovel, G. (2006). The fusiform face area: a cortical region specialized for the perception of faces. *Philosophical Transactions of the Royal Society of London. Series B, Biological Sciences, 361*(1476), 2109–2128.

Kastner, S. and Pinsk, M. A. (2004). Visual attention as a multilevel selection process. *Cognitive, Affective, and Behavioral Neuroscience, 4*(4), 483–500.

Kosslyn, S. M., Thompson, W. L., and Ganis, G. (2006). *The Case for Mental Imagery.* Oxford, New York: Oxford University Press.

Kourtzi, Z. and Kanwisher, N. (2000). Activation in human MT/MST by static images with implied motion. *Journal of Cognitive Neuroscience, 12*(1), 48–55.

Kuhtz-Buschbeck, J. P., Mahnkopf, C., Holzknecht, C., Siebner, H., Ulmer, S., and Jansen, O. (2003). Effector-independent representations of simple and complex imagined finger movements: A combined fMRI and TMS study. *The European Journal of Neuroscience, 18*(12), 3375–3387.

Lezak, M. D., Howieson, D. B., and Loring, D. W. (2004). *Neuropsychological Assessment* (4th edition). New York: Oxford University Press.

Li, X. and Basso, M. A. (2005). Competitive stimulus interactions within single response fields of superior colliculus neurons. *The Journal of Neuroscience, 25*(49), 11357–11373.

Lowenfeld, V. and Brittain, W. L. (1987). *Creative and Mental Growth* (8th edition). New York: Macmillan.

Louilot, A. and Besson, C. (2000). Specificity of amygdalostriatal interactions in the involvement of mesencephalic dopaminergic neurons in affective perception. *Neuroscience, 96*(1), 73–82.

Malchiodi, C. A. (1998). *The Art Therapy Sourcebook*. Los Angeles, CA: Lowell House.

McCarthy, G., Puce, A., Belger, A., and Allison, T. (1999). Electrophysiological studies of human face perception. II: Response properties of face-specific potentials generated in occipitotemporal cortex. *Cerebral Cortex, 9*, 431–444.

McCarthy, G., Puce, A., Gore, J. C., and Allison, T. (1997). Face-specific processing in the human fusiform gyrus. *Journal of Cognitive Neuroscience, 9*(5), 605–610.

Michael, G. A. and Buron, V. (2005). The human pulvinar and stimulus-driven attentional control. *Behavioral Neuroscience, 119*(5), 1353–1367.

Nomura, M., Ohira, H., Haneda, K., Iidaka, T., Sadato, N., Okada, T., *et al.* (2004). Functional association of the amygdala and ventral prefrontal cortex during cognitive evaluation of facial expressions primed by masked angry faces: An event-related fMRI study. *NeuroImage, 21*(1), 352–363.

O'Connor, D. H., Fukui, M. M., Pinsk, M. A., and Kastner, S. (2002). Attention modulates responses in the human lateral geniculate nucleus. *Nature Neuroscience, 5*(11), 1203–1209.

Peuskens, H., Vanrie, J., Verfaillie, K., and Orban, G. A. (2005). Specificity of regions processing biological motion. *European Journal of Neuroscience, 21*, 2864–2875.

Platek, S. M., Loughead, J. W., Gur, R. C., Busch, S., Ruparel, K., Phend, N., *et al.* (2006). Neural substrates for functionally discriminating self-face from personally familiar faces. *Human Brain Mapping 27*, 91–98.

Ramachandran, V. S. (1994). *Encyclopedia of Human Behavior*. San Diego, CA: Academic Press.

Riley, S. (1999). *Contemporary Art Therapy with Adolescents*. London: Jessica Kingsley Publishers.

Rossion, B., Caldara, R., Seghier, M., Schuller, A.-M., Lazeyras, F., and Mayer, E. (2003a). A network of occipito-temporal face-sensitive areas besides the right middle fusiform gyrus is necessary for normal face processing. *Brain, 126*, 2381–2395.

Rossion, B., Joyce, C. A., Cottrell, G. W., and Tarr, M. J. (2003b). Early lateralization and orientation tuning for face, word, and object processing in the visual cortex. *NeuroImage, 20*, 1609–1624.

Rossion, B., Schiltz, C., and Crommelinck, M. (2003). The functionally defined right occipital and fusiform "face areas" discriminate novel from visually familiar faces. *NeuroImage, 19*, 877–883.

Sagiv, N. and Bentin, S. (2001). Structural encoding of human and schematic faces: Holistic and part-based processes. *Journal of Cognitive Neuroscience, 13*(7), 937–951.

Schore, A. N. (1996). The experience-dependent maturation of a regulatory system in the orbital prefrontal cortex and the origin of developmental psychopathology. *Development and Psychopathology, 8*, 54–87.

Schore, A. N. (2000). Attachment and the regulation of the right brain. *Attachment and Human Development, 2*(1), 23–47.

Shatz, C. J. (1996). Emergence of order in visual system development. *Proceedings of the National Academy of Sciences of the United States of America, 93*(2), 602–608.

Slotnick, S. D., Thompson, W. L. and Kosslyn, S. M. (2005). Visual mental imagery induces retinotopically organized activation of early visual areas. *Cerebral Cortex, 15*(10), 1570–1583.

Shaw, P., Bramham, J., Lawrence, E. J., Morris, R., Baron-Cohen, S., and David, A. S. (2005). Differential effects of lesions of the amygdala and prefrontal cortex on recognizing facial expressions of complex emotions. *Journal of Cognitive Neuroscience, 17*(9), 1410–1419.

Sprengelmeyer, R., Rausch, M., Eysel, U. T., and Przuntek, H. (1998). Neural structures associated with recognition of facial expressions of basic emotions. *Proceedings. Biological Sciences/The Royal Society, 265*(1409), 1927–1931.

Sugiura, M., Watanabe, J., Maeda, Y., Matsue, Y., Fukuda, H., and Kawashima, R. (2005). Cortical mechanisms of visual self-recognition. *NeuroImage, 24*(1), 143–149.

Sur, M., Angelucci, A., and Sharma, J. (1999). Rewiring cortex: The role of patterned activity in development and plasticity of neocortical circuits. *Journal of Neurobiology, 41*(1), 33–43.

Taylor, M. J., Batty, M., and Itier, R. J. (2004). The faces of development: A review of early face processing over childhood. *Journal of Cognitive Neuroscience, 16*(8), 1426–1442.

Tong, F., Nakayama, K., Moscovitch, M., Weinrib, O., and Kanwisher, N. (2000). Response properties of the human fusiform face area. *Cognitive Neuropsychology, 17*, 257–279.

Tronick, E. Z. and Cohn, J. F. (1989). Infant-mother face-to-face interaction: Age and gender differences in coordination and the occurrence of miscoordination. *Child Development, 60*(1), 85–92.

Ungerleider, L. G. and Haxby, J. V. (1994). "What" and "where" in the human brain. *Current Opinion in Neurobiology, 4,* 157–165.

Urgesi, C., Moro, V., Candidi, M., and Aglioti, S. M. (2006). Mapping implied body actions in the human motor system. *The Journal of Neuroscience, 26,* 7942–7949.

Van Essen, D. C. (1995). Behind the optic nerve: An inside view of the primate visual system. *Transactions of the American Opthalmological Society, 93,* 123–133.

Virshup, E., Riley, S., and Shepherd, D. (1992). *The Art of Healing Trauma: Media, Techniques, and Insights.* Sunland, CA: Southern California Art Therapy Association.

Vuilleumier, P. and Pourtois, G. (2007). Distributed and interactive brain mechanisms during emotion face perception: Evidence from functional neuroimaging. *Neuropsychologia, 45*(1), 174–194.

Wald, J. (1999). The role of art therapy in post-stroke rehabilitation. In C. Malchiodi (ed.) *Medical Art Therapy with Adults* (pp.25–42). London: Jessica Kingsley Publishers.

Whalen, P. J., Kagan, J., Cook, R. G., Davis, F. C., Kim, H., Polis, S. *et al.* (2004). Human amygdala responsivity to masked fearful eye whites. *Science, 306*(5704), 2061.

Whalen, P. J., Rauch, S. L., Etcoff, N. L., McInerney, S. C., Lee, M. B., and Jenike, M. A. (1998). Masked presentations of emotional facial expressions modulate amygdala activity without explicit knowledge. *The Journal of Neuroscience: The Official Journal of the Society for Neuroscience, 18*(1), 411–418.

Yovel, G., Levy, J., Grabowecky, M., and Paller, K. A. (2003). Neural correlates of the left-visual-field superiority in face perception appear at multiple stages of face processing. *Journal of Cognitive Neuroscience, 15*(3), 462–474.

Zaidel, D. W. (2005). *Neuropsychology of Art: Neurological, Cognitive, and Evolutionary Perspectives.* New York: Psychology Press.

Zaidel, D. W. and Cohen, J. A. (2005). The face, beauty, and symmetry: perceiving asymmetry in beautiful faces. *The International Journal of Neuroscience, 115*(8), 1165–1173.

6

The Stress Response and Adaptation Theory

Kathy Kravits

Understanding the role of relationships in mitigating and modifying stress responses, stress' impact upon learning, the influence of image making upon stress response regulation and conditions associated with prolonged or exaggerated stress responses are part of the therapist's skill set. Stress is often thought of in negative terms as something to overcome, manage, and minimize. Clinical neuroscience and attachment theory provide a conceptual framework for understanding how relationships and social engagement modulate stress and promote adaptive coping responses. Interfacing art therapy, attachment theory and neuroscience creates a rich common language useful in describing an integrated therapeutic model of survival, growth, adaptation and social interaction extending and promoting mastery.

Stress response

Consider our human ancestors stepping onto the savannah in small family bands, large predators hunting them, and other humans competing with them for food. Survival demanded a rapid and effective response to danger. Protection lay not in sharp claws or venomous bites, but in their ability to identify, anticipate and respond to threats. Today's stress response is our ancestors' evolutionary legacy. The heightened arousal state that occurs during the perception of a threat or stressor results from the interaction of complex systems of biological, psychological and social processes (Christopher 2004). The purpose of this stress response is to mitigate the threat allowing an individual to regain allostatic balance (Sapolsky 1998). For example, a patient receiving his first chemotherapy treatment experiences significant distress. However, with time and relational support the rhythms and routines of the experience become familiar, reducing anxiety and distress. This familiarity forms a new allostatic state replacing the distress. Allostasis results in adaptive, stress-reducing behaviors that can be repeated with minimal attention during similar life contexts. The allostatic-orchestrated pattern of functioning promotes a rapid pathway to reducing stress as the body shifts from one activity context to another. Once successful, allostatic balance is memorialized as the allostatic state needed to resolve or avoid a specific type of stressor in the future (McEwen and Wingfield 2003; Table 6.1).

Table 6.1 Allostatic levels.

Adaptation to stress	Description
Allostasis	Adaptation processes balancing and stabilizing basic physiological life functions during changing environmental and developmental contexts.
Allostatic state	Patterned allostatic adaptation to environmental and/or life stage contexts requiring altered functioning, like a bear's hibernation.
Allostatic load	Cumulative distortions in body functioning as allostatic shifts encounter unpredictable environmental influences.
Allostatic overload	When energy demands exceeding combined energy income and stored accessible resources cause serious pathophysiology.

Stressors that we experience as threatening or novel initiate stress responses, engaging needs for new allostatic solutions. These stressors may be external circumstances and/or internal processes activating memories of unpleasant, unknown, or threatening events. As an oncology nurse, this author often works with chemotherapy patients. It is not unusual to hear that certain smells immediately produce episodes of nausea and vomiting even in the absence of the chemotherapy. The smells in question are ones noticed during treatment as the patients experienced episodes of nausea and vomiting. The initial episode of nausea and vomiting occurs as an effect of the administration of chemotherapy on the central nervous system. Chemotherapy is an external stressor producing nausea, vomiting and an associated stress response. The smells present during the administration of the chemotherapy are associated with the negative experience of throwing up, which becomes stored as part of that memory. Exposure to those smells in the future, without the presence of chemotherapy, subsequently triggers other episodes of nausea, vomiting and stress responses. This conditioned response becomes an allostatic state displaying significant allostatic load.

Patients occasionally report that just the thought of chemotherapy can trigger stress, nausea and vomiting. Anticipatory thoughts and imagery activate internal stressors, stimulating unpleasant memories of vomiting that manifest as anxiety and fear (Murray and Richmond 2001). Exaggerated and prolonged stress responses found in generalized anxiety disorder and post-traumatic stress disorder exemplify allostatic overload.

Direct and indirect pathways of stress responses: central nervous system processing

Stress responses initiate when input from sensory neurons in the periphery provide challenging data to the central nervous system. Sensory information including visual, auditory, tactile, proprioceptive, nociceptive, gustatory, vestibular, and olfactory is first sent to the thalamus where it is routed to appropriate brain areas for processing. These brain areas are delineated below (LeDoux and Muller 1997; Figure 6.1).

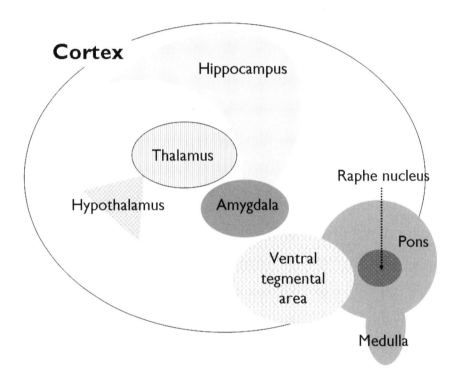

Figure 6.1 Limbic related structures. Subcortical structures transmit impulses in a coordinated manner so that an organized response to danger is achieved. The hippocampus is associated with memory formation, the amygdala with fear, the hypothalamus with the stress response and hormonal urges, the thalamus with sensory processing, the ventral tegmental area with reward or pleasure, the raphe nucleus with serotonin production, the pons with arousal and sensory relay between the cerebellum and cerebrum, and the medulla with autonomic life functions.

The stress response is partially an automatic response influenced by rapid transmission of impulses from the sensory to the limbic system. A quick, *direct path* (LeDoux and Muller 1997) forwards sensory impulses from the thalamus directly to the amygdala in the limbic system. The amygdala processes them, relays the impulses to the hypothalamus, and then along multiple pathways resulting in complex responses, including flight, fight, freeze and social engagement (Porges 2001). This quick, direct response for accessing the limbic system involves fewer neuronal pathways.

While impulses race along the *direct path* to the lateral amygdala, and on to sympathetic nerve fibers, they also connect from the thalamus to the amygdala along an *indirect path* (LeDoux and Muller 1997). The *indirect path* leaves the thalamus, travels to the primary sensory cortex, the entorhinal cortex, the orbitofrontal cortex, the hippocampus and finally to the lateral amygdala. The *indirect path* engages cortical areas where analysis and judgment involve many more neurons and responding occurs more slowly (LeDoux and Muller 1997; Figure 6.2).

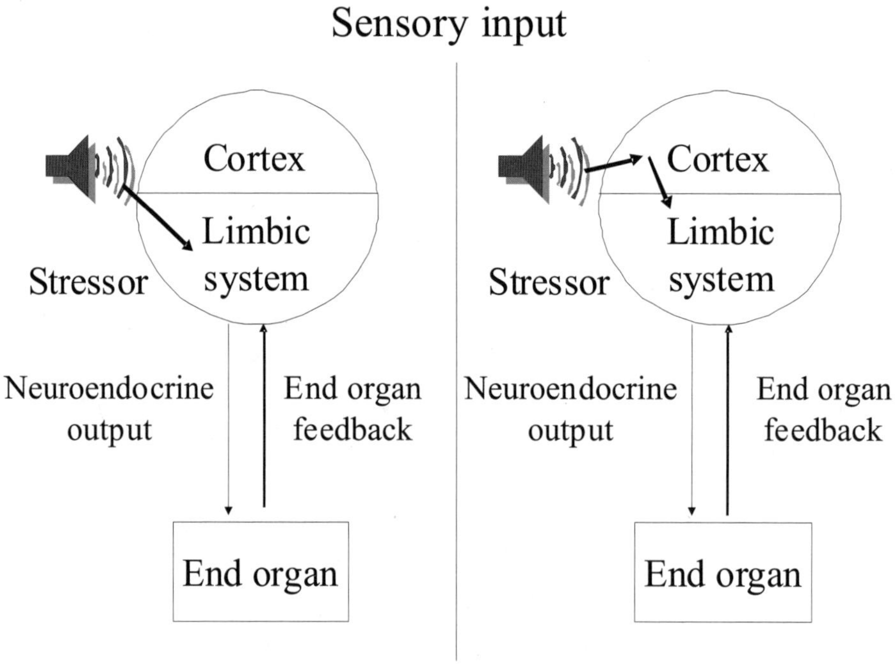

Figure 6.2 Direct and indirect pathways. Direct path: Sensory input transmitted to the limbic system results in neuroendocrine stimulation of essential organs such as the heart, lungs, and so forth. Subsequent changes in metabolic status relay back to the brain creating a negative feedback loop. Indirect path: Sensory input transmitted to the cortex allows time for evaluating the data. Impulses then relay to the limbic system and on to the body as illustrated. The indirect path requires more time for information to be communicated to the cortex where judgment modifies the response.

The *direct path*, triggered by unconscious stimuli that were perhaps in the past dangerous, but that in the moment are not necessarily threats, reacts quickly. Implicit or automatic memories regulated by the amygdala correspond to a set of circumstances close enough to match a past threatening experience and, before the conscious mind can interfere, a stress response occurs. Clinical conditions, like anxiety disorders, phobias and post-traumatic stress disorder, can manifest as a result of this mechanism.

The direct response is modified by processing in the primary sensory cortex, the entorhinal cortex, and the hippocampus. Relevant implicit and explicit memories are now routed to appropriate systems for action (LeDoux and Muller 1997).

It is not unusual for patients to have completed their chemotherapy and continue to have a *direct* stress response rooted in their chemotherapy experience. A patient reported vomiting at the sight of her physician's office for many months after completing treatment. She avoided traveling near his office due to her anxiety about this response. Her response, generated by the sight of the office, stimulated an implicit, unconscious, memory (vomiting at the time of treatment) relayed to the amygdala that stimulated the nerve paths producing emesis (Murray and Richmond 2001). This example shows how cognitive awareness cannot take place before the response generated via the *direct path* is already under way. Therefore, experience and judgment cannot mitigate, modify or otherwise influence the initial response (LeDoux and Muller 1997).

Relaxation techniques can assist in interrupting this cycle. Therapeutic interruption of *direct path* activation allows processes resulting from *indirect path* stimulation (analysis and judgment) to modulate perceived threats reducing anxiety and vomiting. Therapeutic art interventions can activate relaxation, a parasympathetic response. The parasympathetic system is essentially the brake for the alarm-sympathetic system (Porges 2001). Sympathetic tone is constant and in the absence of stress, the parasympathetic system dampens sympathetic tone in order to maintain the basic level of arousal necessary to carry out normal day-to-day functions. Parasympathetic stimulation reduces sympathetic influence: heart rate and respiratory rate slow, intestinal blood flow increases, and blood flow to major muscle groups decreases (Figure 6.3).

Guided imagery has been shown to effectively recruit parasympathetic responses that may be less available through conscious retrieval and naming (Avrahami 2005; Redd, Montogomery, and DuHamel 2001). Stimulating relaxation responses and using therapeutic suggestion promotes focused attention and facilitates the alteration of implicit/automatic memories underpinning the experience of nausea and vomiting (Redd *et al.* 2001). *Indirect path* interventions slow the immediacy of *direct path* controlled responses and can be achieved through a conscious activation of deep breathing, image-making, and discussion. Activation of the *indirect path* allows an opportunity for the threats to be redefined, new learning to occur, new behaviors to be adopted and memories to be modified.

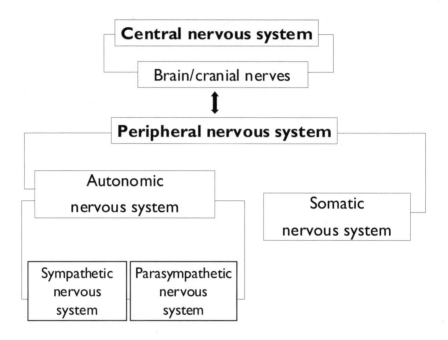

Figure 6.3 Divisions of the nervous system. The central nervous system consists of the brain, spinal cord, and cranial nerves. The peripheral nervous system contains the autonomic and somatic nervous systems. The autonomic nervous system divides further into sympathetic and parasympathetic nervous systems.

Short- and long-term stress responses: sympathetic adrenal medulla (SAM), peripheral nervous system, and hypothalamus-pituitary-adrenal (HPA) contributions

The *sympathetic adrenal medulla* (SAM) axis response is responsible for what is generally thought of as the flight or fight response. Triggered by the amygdala and the hypothalamus, sympathetic nervous system stimulation generates metabolic resources (glucose and oxygen), so that the body may act swiftly to protect itself immediately. The sympathetic nerves utilize norepinephrine (NE) as the primary neurotransmitter. NE is a catecholamine produced by the adrenal medulla, a gland on top of the kidney. The end organs receiving stimulation from the sympathetic fibers respond to its release. The results include increased respiratory rates, heart rates, and blood flow to major muscle groups in the arms and legs, along with decreased blood flow to the intestinal tract, and slowing of peristalsis, and stimulation of glycogen release in the liver, which is then rapidly metabolized into glucose for feeding the muscles and the brain. Endogenous opiates or endorphins are also produced by the adrenal medulla during this period. These opiates create a type of anesthesia decreasing awareness of injury and pain. The SAM response readies the brain to think faster and the muscles to perform (Figure 6.4).

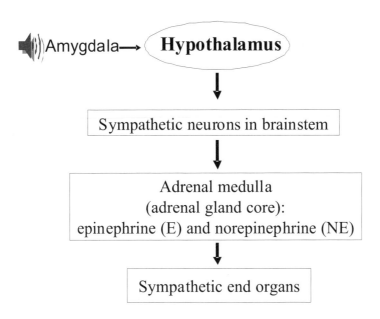

Figure 6.4 Primary structures activated during a response of the SAM axis. The SAM response occurs as a result of activation by the hypothalamus of the central nervous system, the sympathetic ganglions located in the brainstem and adrenal medulla. Catecholamines, epinephrine and norepinephrine circulate through the vascular system stimulating selected target organs. The central nervous system detects circulating catecholamine levels, which results in dampening of the SAM response via a negative feedback loop.

A quick and immediate SAM response has been conceptualized as functionally signaling a person's attempts to be in control and/or striving for control (Henry and Wang 1999). This functional description allows art therapists to understand the SAM response as an adaptive response. For example, patients who research all cancer treatment options and have consultations with many doctors are exhibiting striving for control responses. In art therapy sessions, hurried marks on the page, which illustrate this process, portray visual imprints of an adaptive response.

The hypothalamus-pituitary-adrenal (HPA) stress response is a long-term stress response. Psychologically, it occurs with a sense of a loss of control, and represents an adaptation to chronic states of arousal (Henry and Wang 1999). A prolonged SAM response leads to fatigue and exhaustion while helplessness is associated with arousal of the HPA axis. The hypothalamus is pivotal in activating both autonomic nervous system and endocrine system responses associated with stress. The hypothalamus intimately linked with the structures forming the limbic system lies adjacent to and directly above the pituitary gland. Exposed to a threat, the hypothalamus releases CRH (corticotropin-releasing hormone) into the bloodstream. Within seconds, the anterior pituitary produces ACTH (adrenocorticotropic hormone). ACTH travels via circulation to the adrenal glands (small glands that rest atop each kidney) and stimulates the glucocorticoid release from the adrenal cortex. Glucocorticoids circulate and stimulate the glucose release by the liver, suppress inflammation and halt the formation of new lymphocytes by the thymus. When glucose levels rise sufficiently in the blood, the hypothalamus is stimulated to stop the CRH release (a negative feedback loop), reducing ACTH and glucocorticoid production (Figure 6.5).

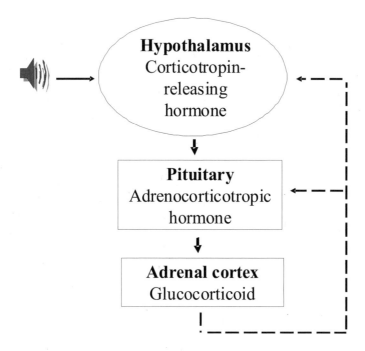

Figure 6.5 Hypothalamus-pituitary-adrenal axis. Serious and/or chronic stimulation of the stress response results in the activation of the hypothalamus-pituitary-adrenal axis. Corticotropin-releasing hormone (CRH) emitted by the hypothalamus stimulates the pituitary to produce adrenocorticotropic hormone (ACTH). ACTH is carried in the circulation to the adrenal gland where it acts on the adrenal cortex to produce glucocorticoids or cortisol.

In the short term, an HPA response is adaptive. It allows grief to take its course. The body shuts down long-term projects and shifts from active coping to "a passive non-aggressive coping style. The emphasis is now on 'self preservation'" (Henry and Wang 1999, p.866).

Cortisol, a glucocorticoid, affects the immune system by reducing cytokine production and suppressing the ability of lymphocytes to respond to threat (Figure 6.6).

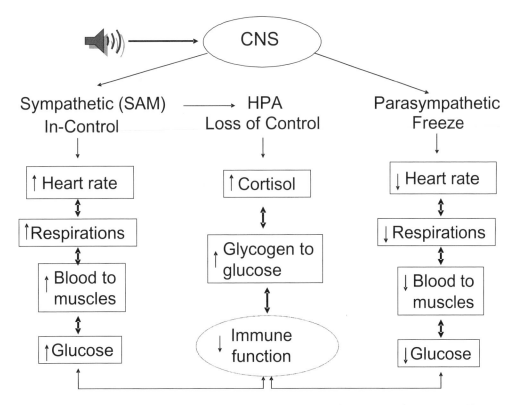

Figure 6.6. Impact of the stress response on the body. Increased sympathetic tone results in increased heart rate, respiration, blood flow to the muscles and increased circulating glucose. Activation of the HPA axis stimulates the adrenal cortex to produce glucocorticoids. When the threat reaches lethal levels, parasympathetic tone predominates with decreases in heart rate, respiratory rate, blood flow to muscles and circulating glucose.

Cytokines are protein compounds produced within the body that turn on the immune system. They facilitate maturation and proliferation of lymphocytes, which are the primary cells that fight infection. Lymphocytes divide into groups. T cells, once produced, migrate to the thymus where they reside until cytokine stimulation promotes their maturation and release. B cells mature in the bone marrow and then circulate within the vascular system. Some are held within the spleen. Again, cytokines activate their response to foreign protein-like bacteria. Cortisol suppresses cytokine production, which can reduce the inflammatory response often seen in reaction to trauma. Cortisol production also liberates glucose, which is required to feed the brain.

Prolonged elevation of cortisol levels creates very negative consequences for the body. For example, cortisol can suppress and kill lymphocytes, the primary infection fighting cells. Cortisol can also destroy hippocampal neurons resulting in impaired memory function. In the short term, cortisol keeps the brain fed by releasing glucose. During heightened or sustained long-term use, negative effects overcome the positive.

The Polyvagal Theory: social engagement and the sympathetic nervous system

Polyvagal Theory describes the neurobiological mechanisms that promote social engagement and their interaction with the stress response. Looking and listening link with variations in heart rate to regulate behavioral states and promote prosocial encounters. Safe and unsafe situations are associated with affective experience, emotional expression, facial gestures, vocal communication, and behavioral responses that promote survival responses (Porges 2001; Figure 6.7).

The vagus is the longest nerve in the body and a critical component of the parasympathetic nervous system. An important cranial nerve innervating many visceral organs, the vagus complements functional nerve fibers in the sympathetic nervous system by creating a mutual, dynamic system of stimulation and relaxation.

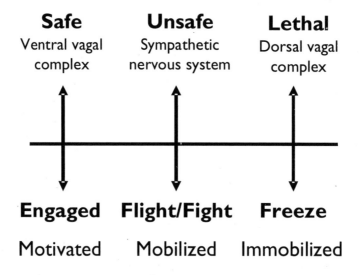

Figure 6.7 Social engagement. This continuum displays in a linear fashion the relationship between appraisal of the degree of threat and type of interactions. Environments assessed as unsafe do not support proactive social interactions.

In human beings, the vagus has evolved to have two parts, the dorsal vagal complex (DVC) and ventral vagal complex (VVC). The DVC is phylogenetically the older component that humans share with most vertebrates. The DVC is composed of unmyelinated, slower responding, nerve fibers that leave the central nervous system and travel to several end organs in the body, including the stomach, intestines, and lungs. Stimulation of the DVC is essentially automatic and unaffected by cortical control. The function of the DVC is to conserve bodily resources through behavioral strategies such as immobilization and avoidance (Porges 2001). Immobilization is protective and shared by insects, animals and humans. It is the activation of the DVC immobilizing freeze response that is associated with Voodoo, heart-stopping deaths (Cannon 1942). Similar to the direct path, the DVC reaction is a crisis response to threat.

The VVC is a system of discrete myelinated nerve fibers that include segments of cranial nerves V, VII, IX and XI and the myelinated division of the vagus. Myelinated vagal fibers communicate with the cortex by the corticobulbar pathway. Phylogenetically, it is the newest vagal pathway. The stimulation of the VVC is thought to promote social interaction as result of its influence on heart rate, facial expression, breathing, listening and vocalization (Porges 1998). The Polyvagal Theory postulates that the VVC regulates lifting of the eyelids and tensing of middle ear muscles involved in linking the person we are looking at with listening to her voice. Stimulation of the VVC also allows for rapid adjustments in heart rate from fast to slow. Slowing the heart rate creates perceptions of calm, enhancing the possibility of positive social interaction (Porges 2001; Figure 6.8).

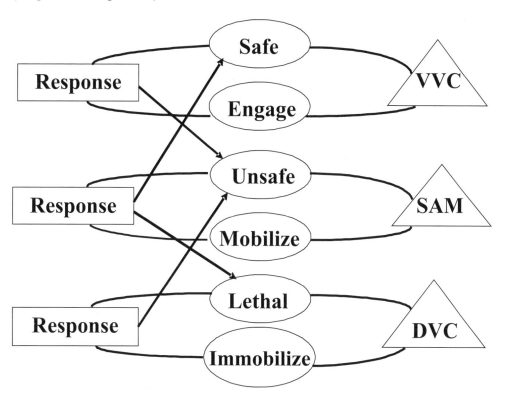

Figure 6.8 Polyvagal system and stress response. The stress response is dynamic—changing as the level of threat and degree of mastery or control changes. Safe environments promote stimulation of the ventral vagal complex (VVC). VVC activation results in rapid shifts in heart rate with slowing predominating. Slow heart rate helps create an environment supporting social interaction. Unsafe environments promote sympathetic nervous system stimulation as well as HPA axis activation. Striving for mastery and control is supported. Lethal stressors activate the dorsal vagal complex (DVC) and generate freeze behaviors. Control is lost.

Attachment and the stress response

Individuals who have experienced secure attachment with a primary caregiver experience less stress and show more resilience when exposed to stressors (van Bakel and Riksen-Walraven 2004). Human development has evolved to include a prolonged period of dependence in infancy and early childhood. This period of vulnerability demands that a caretaker be able to attend and attune to the child appropriately in order for him or her to develop, mature and survive. The anatomical structures and physiologic processes of the central nervous system, peripheral nervous system, and endocrine system are exquisitely sensitive to attachment interactions between caretaker and child. They shape allostatic states that continue throughout life supporting relationships with others.

> In recent reviews on the role of stress in human attachment, it has been discussed
> that stressors can trigger a search for pleasure, proximity and closeness (i.e. attach-
> ment behaviors), thereby promoting the re-balancing of altered physiological and
> psychological states. (Esch and Stefano 2005, p.177; Figure 6.9)

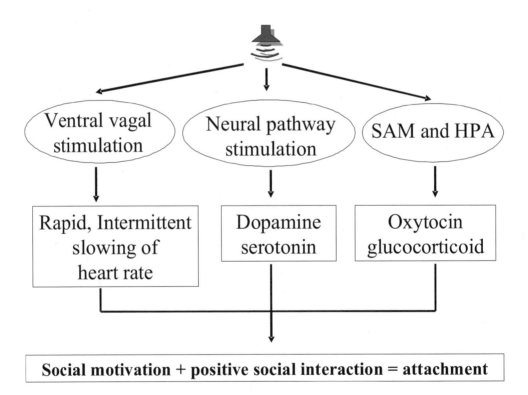

Figure 6.9 Stress and attachment. Three neurobiological systems supporting social motivation and proactive social contact result in attachment: the SAM, motivation pathway, and ventral vagal complex.

Seeking social support has been identified as one of the most important emotional coping strategies. Hormone-like substances play a role in creating an internal environment that is ready for social interaction, like oxytocin. Oxytocin is released by the posterior pituitary and is chemically related to the hormone vasopressin. It plays a role in promoting uterine contractions during childbirth, lactation, the development of maternal nurturing behaviors and human proximity seeking.

Oxytocin influences the transmission of impulses by the dorsal motor nucleus of the vagus, which is part of the DVC mentioned previously. When feedback returns from the viscera, oxytocin alters thresholds for action that effectively maintain homeostasis (Porges 2001). Oxytocin reduces sympathetic tone and restrains the release of glucocorticoids, which are so damaging to the body (Esch and Stefano 2005). In other words, oxytocin supports internal states that are resistant to the flight or fight response associated with stress.

Oxytocin was implicated as an element in the response to positive touch that promotes emotional regulation. Research suggests that physical contact associated with oxytocin release from the hypothalamus promotes (1) increased endogenous opioid activity and (2) stimulation of dopamine receptors (Esch and Stefano 2005). Oxytocin is associated with feelings of pleasure and well-being. However, it is unclear if this effect is generalizable to all relationships. It may only be seen in the context of relationships infused with specific levels of positive or neutral regard. A therapeutic relationship might qualify as such a relationship. Future research also needs to explore the impact of touching, comforting media on well-being and oxytocin release.

Vasopressin, a neuropeptide chemically very similar to oxytocin, is manufactured and released by the same structures as oxytocin. Vasopressin also plays a role in promoting relationships. Simultaneous release of oxytocin and vasopressin may produce both a parasympathetic and sympathetic response resulting in a state of arousal as well as a sense of well-being. The release may be the physiologic state that supports intimacy between individuals.

Social interaction, including attachment, occurs through a combination of effects created by the stimulating cranial nerves, sensory input and motor responses to shift gaze, turn the head, and smile. Sympathetic and parasympathetic body tone is poised to mobilize or connect as well as regulate end organ responses effecting fast or slow heart rate and agitated or calm mood. Finally, we cortically process safe or unsafe contexts as neuropeptides create a sense of well-being and pleasure. Without these structures and processes in place, humans would not have the mechanisms necessary to engage in proactive positive contact (Porges 2001).

Motivation is the intention or desire to seek pleasure and avoid pain (Esch and Stefano 2005), which is involved in positive social contact. Structures involved in the motivation system include the prefrontal cortex, the amygdala, the hippocampus, the hypothalamus, the locus coeruleus, the dorsal raphe nucleus, and the nucleus accumbens. The neurotransmitters serotonin and dopamine also play significant roles in motivation processes.

Primary motivational systems in the brain involve the cortex, ventral striatum and motor structures. Dopamine is associated with the primary motivational system influencing the translation of desires into action and the learning of new behaviors (Chambers, Taylor, and Potenza 2003). Serotonin, operating in concert with the structures of the secondary motivational system (hippocampus, amygdala, hypothalamus, and septal nuclei), facilitates the delivery of contextual data, i.e. memories to the primary circuitry influencing resulting behaviors (Chambers *et al.* 2003). Eating, sex, nurturing, even playing are a result of the motivational system effects. Without it, social relationships and their salutary effects on the stress response would not exist.

Attention originating in the RAS, the reticular activating system, allows individuals to control the sensory information to which the most attention is paid. The RAS, located at the top of the brainstem, regulates arousal and focus. It serves as a gatekeeper for the limbic system, by regulating attended sensory stimuli passed on for processing (Lyons 1999; Figure 6.10).

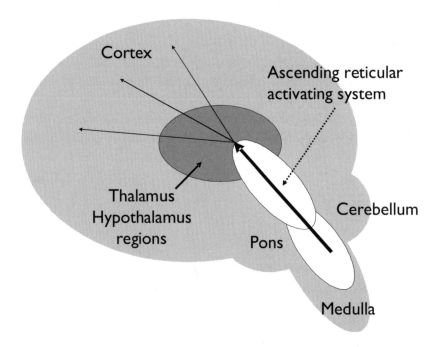

Figure 6.10 Reticular activating system (RAS). The RAS functions promote focused attention that is critical to the successful modulation of the stress response.

Attention, directed by the individual, modulates the stress response by directing the focus to specific aspects of experience. Obsession exemplifies a heightened state of directed attention.

Reception and integration of sensory information allows sensory input to be processed and organized in a manner facilitating analysis and the creation of coherent meaning systems. Meaning-making assists the individual to incorporate new information and life experiences into his or her worldview. Internal maps of the self and the world include an understanding of personal worth. Circumstances identified as very threatening and/or non-negotiable often trigger the creation of new meaning systems as a way to reduce stress and promote growth.

The following case illustrates meaning-making as a strategy for managing stress. A 49-year-old patient with relapsed leukemia decided to pursue a bone marrow transplant as a last option for cure. He knew his situation was very critical, and that a high probability existed that he could not be cured. After talking to his nurse and psychologist about his situation, he felt that although God did not cause his cancer, God gave him this opportunity to face this challenge and deepen his faith. He felt that his faith had become an example to his family and friends, and in particular to people who were not believers and that perhaps his ordeal and strong faith might be inspirational, causing others to believe. The new worldview allowed him to define his life as valuable regardless of the outcome of treatment. It reduced the negative impact of disease-related stress on his neurochemistry.

The stress response is impacted by thought, analysis, and judgment (Folkman and Greer 2000). Temperament, especially a bias towards a positive affect, promotes a more tolerant appraisal of threat, whereas a bias towards negative affect promotes assessing a greater degree of threat (Rosenkranz *et al.* 2003; van Bakel and Riksen-Walraven 2004). Cognitive competence allows a complex analysis of the degree of threat, generating a more accurate understanding of the risk (van Bakel and Riksen-Walraven 2004). Memories create a context for understanding a stimulus as a threat or not. Taken together, these qualities contribute to creating an appraisal of threat that supports the most effective response.

Summary

Consider the stress response and attachment-based movements towards relationships as dynamic, interconnected systems of behavior that promote human survival and mental and physical health. It is not useful to try to define stress as good or bad (Christopher 2004). Clients need to be educated that stress can have long lasting negative or positive effects (McEwen 1998, 2002; Sapolsky 1998). It is important, therefore, to note that a stress response facilitates restoration of allostatic balance, which results in decreasing circulating glucocorticoids as soon as possible. A benign stress response can be facilitated in a safe environment by engaging others. In an unsafe environment, SAM and

HPA responses stimulate fleeing and fighting. In a lethal environment, freezing, a polyvagal response, may occur. Emotional expression, facial gestures, vocal communication and social behavior are contingent with the polyvagal system function. Safety is best attained through promoting and understanding the benefits of interacting with others. Unsafe contexts leading to intense or prolonged flight or fight response or freeze reaction motivate an individual towards predisposed survival responses and away from social solutions. It is problematic when psychosocial stressors, rather than physical environmental constraints, create the stress response. Education and successful social experience-building solutions reduce chronic stress, preserve optimal attachment functioning and encourage the longevity of health and increased quality of life.

It is useful to reframe the concept of stress as a transformative experience. Regardless of the nature of the change, we are altered at every level by the experience (Christopher 2004). Clients' assessment of an experience as safe/unsafe, threatening/exciting and controllable/uncontrollable influences the activation of the physiological processes associated with the stress response as well as the coping mechanisms chosen to mitigate the challenge (Folkman and Moskowitz 2000). An art therapist's reframing of stress facilitates the client's growth and minimizes the negative physical consequences. Modulating the stress response by reframing experience in positive terms and providing pleasurable art activities can minimize the exposure to chronic stressors and cultivates a relaxation response. Encouraging positive affect promotes restoring allostatic balance with minimum load and overload consequences (Folkman and Moskowitz 2000). Relationship building and creating meaning-making through the art offer some powerful strategies for mitigating the negative consequences of the stress response and promoting growth.

References

Avrahami, D. (2005). Visual art therapy's unique contribution in the treatment of post-traumatic stress disorders. *Journal of Trauma & Dissociation, 6*(4), 5–38.

Cannon, W. B. (1942). "Voodoo" death. *American Anthropology, 44,* 169–181.

Chambers, R. A., Taylor, J. R., and Potenza, M. N. (2003). Developmental neurocircuitry of motivation in adolescence: A critical period of addiction vulnerability. *American Journal of Psychiatry, 160*(6), 1041–1052.

Christopher, M. (2004). A broader view of trauma: A biopsychosocial-evolutionary view of the role of the traumatic stress response in the emergence of pathology and/or growth. *Clinical Psychology Review, 24,* 75–98.

Esch, T. and Stefano, G. B. (2005). The neurobiology of love. *Neuroendocrinology Letters, 3*(26), 175–192.

Folkman, S. and Greer, S. (2000). Promoting psychological well-being in the face of serious illness: When theory, research and practice inform each other. *Psycho-oncology, 9,* 11–19.

Folkman, S. and Moskowitz, J. T. (2000). Positive affect and the other side of coping. *American Psychologist, 55*(6), 647–654.

Henry, J. P. and Wang, S. (1999). Effects of early stress on adult affiliative behavior. *Psycho-neuroendocrinology, 23*(8), 863–875.

LeDoux, J. E. and Muller, J. (1997). Emotional memory and psychopathology. *Philosophical Transactions of the Royal Society of London, 352,* 1719–1726.

Lyons, C. A. (1999). Emotions, cognition and becoming a reader: A message to teachers of struggling learners. *Literacy, Teaching and Learning, 4*(1), 67–87.

McEwen, B. (1998). Protective and damaging effects of stress mediators. *The New England Journal of Medicine, 338*, 171–179.

McEwen, B. (2002). The neurobiology and neuroendocrinology of stress: Implications for post-traumatic stress disorder for a basic science perspective. *Psychiatric Clinics of North America, 25*, 469–494.

McEwen, B. S. and Wingfield, J. C. (2003). The concept of allostasis in biology and biomedicine. *Hormones and Behavior, 43*, 2–15.

Murray, E. A. and Richmond, B. J. (2001). Role of perirhinal cortex in object perception, memory, and associations. *Current Opinion in Neurobiology, 11*, 188–193.

Porges, S. W. (1998). Love: An emergent property of the mammalian autonomic nervous system. *Psychoneuroimmunology, 23*(8), 837–861.

Porges, S. W. (2001). The polyvagal theory: Phylogenetic substrates of a social nervous system. *International Journal of Psychophysiology, 42*, 123–146.

Redd, W. H., Montogomery, G. H., and DuHamel, K. N. (2001). Behavioral intervention for cancer treatment side effects, a review. *Journal of the National Cancer Institute, 93*(11), 810–823.

Rosenkranz, M. A., Jackson, D. C., Dalton, K. M., Dolski, I., Ryff, C. D., Singer, B. H., *et al.* (2003). Affective style and in vivo immune response: Neurobehavioral mechanisms. *Proceedings of the National Academy of Sciences of the United States of America, 100*(19), 11148–11152.

Sapolsky, R. (1998). *Why Zebras Don't Get Ulcers.* New York: W. H. Freeman and Company.

van Bakel, H. J. A. and Riksen-Walraven, J. M. (2004). Stress reactivity in 15-month-old infants: Links with infant temperament, cognitive competence, and attachment security. *Developmental Psychobiology, 44*, 157–167.

Part II

The Ideas

7

The Neurobiology of Relatedness: Attachment

Kathy Kravits

Emotional resonance

Successful development occurs as the result of an exquisite interaction between the genetic makeup of the individual and the environment. A significant environmental factor critical to adaptive development appears to be the quality of the relationship between the infant and the caregiver (De Wolff and van Ijzendoorn 1997; Smyke *et al.* 2007). An internally stable caregiver is able to provide the developing fetus and infant sufficient opportunities for comfort and stimulation, promoting the development of a healthy central nervous system (Schore 2002). Brain organization, synaptic development, neurochemical thresholds and stress responses are influenced by pro-social attachments, whether secure or insecure, and by any loss of stable caregiver relationship (Nickerson 2006; Smyke *et al.* 2007). Insecure attachment can result in neurological changes that include reductions in the number and type of synapses, reduction in growth hormones, and elevated cortisol levels (Weiss and Bellinger 2006).

A lost generation

Under the government of President Nicolai Ceausescu, Romanians in the 1960s, 1970s and 1980s were encouraged to have a minimum of five children regardless of whether or not they could feed them. Parents who found themselves unable to care for their children were encouraged to place them in state-sponsored institutions. The decision to place children in these institutions voluntarily was characterized and promoted by Romanian authorities as a responsible choice, not as abandonment. Thus began the deprivation and the loss of a generation of Romanian youth (McGeown 2005).

For the children, many of whom were not orphans, the care they received met their needs for cleanliness, food, and shelter. However, their needs for human contact and emotional comfort were not met, as evidenced by the use of emotionally uninvolved caregivers, multiple caregivers, and prolonged periods without caregiver interaction (Gloviczki 2004). The consequences of such treatment included stunted physical growth, impaired cognition and profoundly restricted affective development (Nickerson 2006). Research examining the impact of institutional care as compared to family care of young children suggested that the presence of attuned and emotionally resonant individualized care, which is more possible in family settings, significantly improved developmental outcomes (De Wolff and van Ijzendoorn 1997; Smyke *et al.* 2007).

Attachment sensitive developmental events

Essential to human development, the neurobiological mechanisms and consequences of attachment allow for the regulation of negative affective states, resilient negotiation of stressful experiences, enhanced capacity for joy and excitement, and positive social interactions (Schore 1997). Secure attachment promotes resilience. Resilience states are internal working models that are biased towards positive responses to novel experiences. Insecure attachment leads to the storage of negative affect laden memories that contribute to the creation of negatively biased internal working models. Insecure attachment impairs resilience.

A genetically dictated timeline orders the specific development of brain structures that later result in attachment behaviors. An infant must be in a relationship with a primary caregiver capable of interacting in an emotionally resonant manner on a consistent basis in order for secure attachment to result and for proper neurodevelopment to occur (Perry 2001). Attuned interaction between the emotionally involved and available primary caregiver promotes the most adaptive expression of genetic material. However, the primary caregiver does not need to be perfectly attuned to the infant at all times. In fact, attunement, followed by mis-attunement, which is then repaired, resulting in re-attunement, promotes the development of resiliency (Schore 2002). This interactive process begins before birth.

Conception to birth

The fetus in the womb needs affectively positive maternal anticipation to support brain development. An expectant mother who experiences life and the pregnancy as positive generates more oxytocin and vasopressin, two neuropeptides, that promote the development of the social bond and that help regulate the hypothalamus-pituitary-adrenal (HPA) axis (Carter 2005). The mother's hormones regulate the expression of the baby's genes and provide a mechanism through which the mother structurally and functionally influences the organization of the baby's brain (Burrow, Fisher and Larsen 1994; Mirescu and Gould 2006; Mirescu, Peters and Gould 2004; O'Connor *et al.* 2002).

An expectant mother embroiled in stressful life circumstances has an internal physical environment saturated with cortisol and catecholamines, fundamental biochemical mediators of the stress response. Maternal cortisol acts on the placenta to stimulate the production of adrenocorticotropic hormone (ACTH), which produces increased fetal cortisol levels. Prenatal cortisol exposure alters the corpus callosum, a bridge between the right and left cerebral hemispheres, which facilitates bi-lateral hemispheric integration. In males, the size of the corpus callosum is increased by exposure to cortisol, and in females, the size is decreased (Coe, Lulbach, and Schneider 2001). Stress also impairs prenatal hippocampal neurogenesis, resulting in learning and memory deficits after birth (Glover and O'Connor 2002). Amygdala enlargement is associated with maternal prenatal stress and increased newborn irritability (Salm *et al.* 2004). A hypersensitive HPA axis in the infant has also been associated with maternal antenatal stress and infant irritability (Davis and Sandman 2006; Fowden and Forhead 2004; Kapoor *et al.* 2006; Talge, Neal, and Glover 2007). In summary, the mother's responses to a stressful environment and/or to negative affectively charged internal representations of the attachment relationship generate biochemicals that may alter the fetal brain development in undesirable ways (De Graaf-Peters and Hadders-Algra 2006; Table 7.1).

The internal working model (IWM) of maternal attachment is often a legacy of the primary attachment experience as well as subsequent attachment opportunities across the life span. Anticipation of the birth of a child is the product of a complex set of maternal experiences that may result in the formation of an IWM of a flawed mother/infant relationship (Spangler and Zimmermann 1999). Dysregulated negative emotions associated with the activation of maternal negative IWM generate elevated stress hormones (cortisol and catecholamines) shared with the developing fetus (O'Connor *et al.* 2002). Postnatally, the maternal IWM further reinforces the child's neurological organization molded in utero (Perry 1999) and can lead to mis-attunements, neglect and hostility.

From birth to two months

At birth, the infant's brain weighs approximately 400 grams. It nearly triples in weight during the first 12 months of life, through the addition of new dendrites, myelinated axons, and synaptic connections that accompany maturation of established structures (Schore 2002). Brain maturation is genetically pre-programmed and experience-dependent (Schore 2000). The right cerebral hemisphere, the limbic structures and the HPA axis predominate functionally after birth. These affectively biased structures facilitate the management of non-verbal information. Maturing motor and sensory capacities, especially smell, taste, and touch, provide primary access to sensory data from the environment. During this postnatal period, sympathetic and subcortical systems regulate states of pleasure and displeasure (Schore 2000).

Due to the predominance of sympathetic and subcortical systems, the young baby has difficulty filtering the internal and external world, and can be perceived as a screaming machine. She is able to take in and experience sensory data in a limited fashion shaped during the prenatal experience, and is learning to process other meanings of that data as functioning in key brain structures matures. The primary caregiver protects, nourishes and provides external regulation for the unfettered

Table 7.1 Attachment developmental milestones.

The evolution of attachment corresponds to the neurobiological maturation of the child. Maturation is associated with myelination of the neurons. Critical to the evolution of stable attachment patterns is the myelination of the limbic structures and the associated cortical structures. Pro-social interactions with the primary caregiver promote the expression of the genetic tendencies that result in a secure attachment and resilience.

Age	Developmentally dominant structures / Maturational process	Pro-social interactions	Attachment achievement
Antenatal	Maternal hormones regulate expression of fetal genes (i.e. cortisol, thyroxine, etc.)	Positive maternal anticipation of relationship to newborn	The mother bonds with fetus in manner predisposing her towards pro-social interactions with newborn
	Brain growth spurts initiate in third trimester	Fetus discerns and responds to sounds and other environmental stimuli and to mother's physiology and moods	Noticing and incorporating fetal responsiveness to stimuli, whether foods, moods, external or internal
	Maternal/infant relationship rooted in maternal internal working model of attachment		
Birth to 2 months	Right cerebral hemisphere, structures of limbic system, autonomic nervous system, and the HPA axis are functional	Infant explores environment with limited sensory-motor capabilities	Organizes more complex emergent functions: processing of emotion, new learning, and adaptation to environment
	Sympathetic subcortical systems predominate fueling excitatory states of pleasure and displeasure	Caregiver responds to the infant by engaging in physical contact, meeting physical needs and providing comfort	
	Maturing amygdala, motor and sensory capacities of smell, taste and touch		
2 months	Right cerebral hemisphere, structures of limbic system, autonomic nervous system, and the HPA axis are functional	Intense periods of mutual gaze	Early communication leading to mutually attuned interactions, "moment to moment state sharing" (Schore 1997)
	Primary visual cortex and occipital cortex mature	Infant's large pupils capture caregiver attention	Emerging self
		Infant and mother synchronize affect in order to regulate the intensity of interactions	

Age	Developmentally dominant structures *Maturational process*	Pro-social interactions	Attachment achievement
2–7 months	Primary visual cortex and occipital cortex has matured Brain to brain interactions in the context of positive affect relationship required for growth and development Patterns of response in anterior cingulate and insula coordinate	Interactive attunement and co-regulation Successful infant regulation by mother promotes successful negotiation of stressful state transitions Interactive amplification of positive affect states through play	Regulates negative affective states in partnership with the primary caregiver and then on own Amplification of positive affect promotes positively charged curiosity and exploration Core self, attachment style emerge and stabilize
7–36 months	Right orbitofrontal cortex and parasympathetic cortical inhibitory systems mature Myelination supports maturation Limbic and right cerebral hemisphere functional Right orbitofrontal cortex monitors and regulates duration, intensity and frequency of positive and negative affective states Maturation of parasympathetic cortical inhibitory systems promotes regulation Myelination of corpus callosum speeds communication between right and left cerebral hemispheres	Nurturance must happen in order for the limbic nuclei to develop appropriately Interactive attunement Interactive amplification of positive affect states through play	Sense of self and self with other (internal working models) develops (subjective self) Shared attention, intention and emotion between caregiver/child Established attachment patterns Shared words with caregiver and emergence of verbal self Autobiographical narrative defines self resulting in narrative self

responses of the sympathetic and subcortical systems during this time. The caregiver loans the child her own ability to regulate emotion. The caregiver's comforting touch, soft voice, and gaze communicate to the child that everything is all right. The caregiver's reassurance facilitates the child's return to a state of calm and begins the process of developing resilience within the child.

I see you (two to seven months)

Critical episodes of brain development occur at two months with the maturation of the primary visual cortex (Yamada *et al.* 2000). Synapses in the occipital cortex are modified by visual experience. Behaviorally, exchanges of intense gaze between caregiver and infant begin to occur. The mother's face becomes a rich and engaging visual stimulus for the child. The infant's large-pupiled eyes provide positive re-enforcement to the mother's connected gaze. This mutual face-to-face examination by mother and child is a dynamic, fluid system of communication. Mutual gazing creates positive feedback loops that generate new social-emotional pathways of neural activation within the infant brain (Schore 2002).

This experience of mutual gaze can be emotionally intense. The caregiver and infant synchronize affective states while learning to regulate intensity (Figure 7.1).

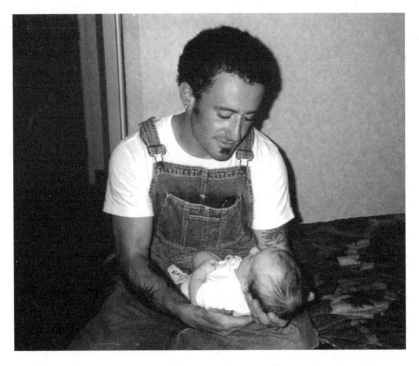

Figure 7.1 "I see you." The caregiver, Daddy or Mommy, in collaboration with the infant creates an emotion regulating system by their use of gaze. Eye contact and, when signaled by the infant, eye aversion promotes emotion management. Photo by Kathy Kravits.

When an infant averts his eyes for periods of time, he is signaling over-stimulation and is attempting to quiet his internal environment (Tronick, Cohn and Shea 1986). Caregivers who fail to allow this period of withdrawal by continuing to pursue interaction and eye contact contribute to an escalating, intense, affective experience while negatively re-enforcing previous mutual sharing. Mis-attunement expressed by continued caregiver eye contact contributes to the dysregulation of the infant's internal emotional environment (Figure 7.2).

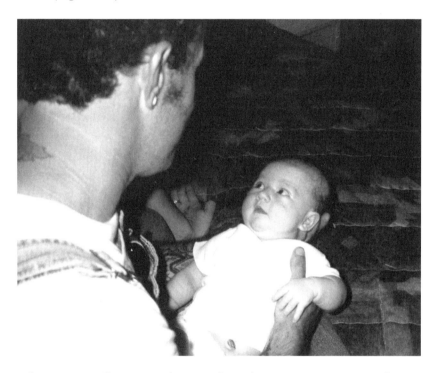

Figure 7.2 "I see you, too." *Eye contact between infant and caregiver creates a reciprocal communication process promoting transitions between different internal states. Photo by Kathy Kravits.*

Stability (7 to 36 months)

The child develops a stable attachment style with the caregiver by approximately seven months of age (Schore 2002). In most cases, caregiver and child express predictable patterns of emotional resonance, demonstrating established affect regulation and state transitions. Curiosity and exploration assume an important role supported by amplification of positive affect during play between the caregiver and the child (Figure 7.3).

Before the first year ends, the primary inter-subjectivity established during mutual gazes transitions into secondary inter-subjectivity: sharing mental states through common interests and purposes. Interesting objects entice caregiver and infant to include a mutual focus on a third element to develop. The mutual excitement and sharing

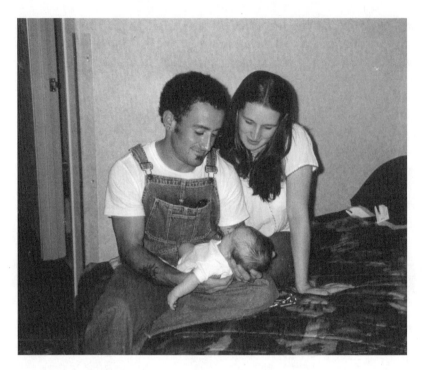

Figure 7.3 Mutual engagement of attachment dynamics. While the primary caregiver is often assumed to be the mother, the influence of both primary caregivers must be considered when understanding the attachment dynamics of a family unit.

created by this new form of interaction helps the infant's vocal and gestural "comments" integrate into the caregiver's and the infant's mutual meaning-making (Trevarthen 2001). This is a sensitive period for the development of limbic structures and cortical associations. The maturation of inhibitory systems, supported in the right orbitofrontal cortex and parasympathetic nervous system by myelination, allows more sophisticated monitoring and regulation of affective states by the child. However, nurturance and affective regulation provided by the caregiver continues to be critical to the successful development of these structures, especially the limbic nuclei (Schore 2000).

Up until this time, the sympathetic nervous system and associated structures have predominated, but maturation of the inhibitory capacities of the orbitofrontal cortex and parasympathetic nervous system creates brakes for output from the sympathetic system. The infant, no longer a screaming machine, forms tools necessary for self-regulation of affective states.

Bilateral attachment: hemispheric communication (36 months)

The right cerebral hemisphere is dominant for the first three years of the child's life. Its maturational schedule and linkages to limbic and other subcortical structures support its role in early development of emotions and attachment. However, things begin to change between ages two and three years with the myelination of the corpus callosum. By three years of age, it is fully myelinated. Communication between the hemispheres occurs at a more rapid rate. The left hemisphere participates more actively in regulating affective states and in creating verbally symbolic, conscious internal working models of the world.

Ruptures and repairs: successful state transitions as road to resilience

Resilience is the ability to respond optimistically on a consistent basis and adapt to changing circumstances. It is a dynamic, functional state dependent upon the evolving neurobiology and social interactions of the self across the lifespan (Cicchetti and Rogosch 1997) that ensure survival benefits. Resilience is created by individual qualities, interpersonal relationships (Siegel 2001), and secure attachments (Schore 2002). It can be characterized by cognitive integration of new experiences into the meaning system, successful affect regulation strategies, and the ability to sustain relationships with peers and parents (Siegel 2001). Impaired resilience is the consequence of insecure attachment.

Joy and play: key features of successful attachment

Emotionally resonant attunement is vital to the development of secure attachment and ultimately a coherent sense of self. However, it is not enough for the caregiver to participate interactively with the infant in regulating emotion. In order for curiosity, exploration and just plain joy to manifest, the brain must activate the neural pleasure pathways. Play may do this by promoting genetic activation of substances within the brain that promote neuronal growth and therefore brain development (Gordon *et al.* 2003). Play is a powerful stimulant for organizing a brain that fosters the creation of joy, curiosity, and exploration.

Vulnerability

Considerable evidence suggests that insecure attachments support vulnerability in individuals because they promote the development of inauthentic and/or fragmented self-states (Siegel 1999). Insecure attachment is associated with a variety of different presentations, all demonstrating a fundamental malfunction in appraisal and coping systems (Spangler and Zimmermann 1999). Dysfunctions in appraisal and coping produce a mismatch between reality and subjective reality. Affective regulation in such situations can only be effective to a limited degree (Spangler and Zimmermann 1999).

Infant and child attachment styles

Between the ages of 7 and 18 months, the child develops a stable attachment style with predictable behavior patterns. Secure attachment promotes the development of a firm sense of self and other, use of pro-social interactions, ability to regulate emotions, express curiosity and a desire to explore the environment (Siegel 2001).

Insecure attachments distort internal models of self and other and result in impaired ability to regulate emotions successfully. These attachments lead to inaccurate appraisals of the environment and increase the infant/child's vulnerability (Siegel 2001). Avoidant insecure attachment is characterized by an avoidance of seeking comfort from the primary caregiver. Ambivalent/resistant insecure attachment is characterized by an infant/child who is preoccupied with the primary caregiver and yet is unable to be comforted by the caregiver (Spangler and Zimmermann 1999). A disorganized/disoriented attachment style presents when an infant/child who would otherwise be identified as secure, avoidant or ambivalent/resistant displays disorganized behaviors, including dissociation, when under stress in the presence of the caregiver. This attachment style occurs when an infant/child has been exposed to patterns of frightening behaviors from the primary caregiver (Hesse and Main 2000; Table 7.2).

Attachment across the lifespan

Attachment is a dyadic, emotion regulating system that contributes to the development of internal representations of the self and the world. Infant attachment status frequently corresponds to adult attachment status (Ogawa *et al.* 1997). Attachment theory provides a useful model for understanding adolescent and adult behavior.

Secure attachment provides the individual with sufficient resources to be able to experience and explore both the internal and external world congruently. It provides the internal structure for the development of psychological resilience (Spangler and Zimmermann 1999). Adolescents with secure attachment styles demonstrate better relationships with peers, less internalization and fewer acting-out behaviors that would bring them into conflict with the legal system (Allen *et al.* 1998). Adults demonstrating secure attachment styles are able to engage successfully in dynamic relationships in a manner that preserves autonomy for the self and the other (Caspers *et al.* 2006). However, adults with continuous secure attachment and earned secure attachment do present different psychological profiles: adults with earned attachment show higher rates of mood disturbances than do adults with continuous secure attachment (Caspers *et al.* 2006).

Adolescent preoccupied attachment styles are associated with more acting-out and conduct disturbances (Allen *et al.* 2002). Preoccupied adolescents who are in relationships with highly autonomous and directing mothers are at increased risk for severe problems with conduct, including vulnerability to substance abuse (Allen *et al.* 2002).

Autonomy is threatening to the preoccupied adolescent (Waldinger *et al.* 2003). Female adolescents with a preoccupied attachment style present with increased

Table 7.2 Infant/child attachment styles.*

Attachment styles	Caregiver and infant mental organization	Infant behavior
Secure	Caregiver: Maternal sensitivity is highly correlated with secure infant attachment	Engages in active exploration of familiar and novel environments. Indicates distress when separated from parent. Eagerly reunites with the parent and returns to play
	Infant: Expected cortisol levels and patterns of synchronized emotional regulation between infant and caregiver predominate	
Avoidant (insecure)	Caregiver: Unstable and/or changing family circumstances, primary caregiver sensitivity and childrearing arrangements are correlated with insecure and disorganized attachment patterns	Fails to cry on separation from parent. Actively avoids and ignores parent on reunion. Little or no proximity seeking, no distress, no anger
	Infant: Elevation of cortisol levels confirms ongoing mis-attunement and sub-optimal emotional regulation	
Ambivalent resistant (insecure)	Caregiver: Unstable and/or changing family circumstances, primary caregiver sensitivity and childrearing arrangements are correlated with insecure and disorganized attachment patterns	May be wary and/or distressed when exposed to novel environments. Preoccupied with parent and may seem angry or passive. Fails to settle and be comforted by parent after a separation. Fails to return to exploration after reunion
	Infant: Elevation of cortisol levels confirms ongoing mis-attunement and sub-optimal emotional regulation	
Disorganized disoriented	Caregiver: Unstable and/or changing family circumstances, impaired primary caregiver sensitivity and chaotic childrearing arrangements are correlated with insecure attachment patterns that contain episodes of disorganized behavior	Displays disorganized and/or disoriented behaviors in the parent's presence that are dominated by episodes of dissociation
	Infant: Elevation of cortisol levels confirms ongoing mis-attunement and sub-optimal emotional regulation	

* Compiled from De Wolff and van Ijzendoorn 1997, Siegel 1999, Spangler and Zimmermann 1999.

symptoms of internalization. Males with this attachment style demonstrate a tendency toward externalizing behaviors or acting-out (Allen *et al.* 2002). Adults with a preoccupied attachment style often engage in anxious interpersonal relationships and experience increased levels of negative emotions. They are vulnerable to substance abuse and other deviant behaviors (Caspers *et al.* 2006). On the positive side, the preoccupied type adolescent as well as the earned secure adult are more likely to participate in treatment, psychotherapy and/or medication than those with the dismissing attachment style (Caspers *et al.* 2006).

A dismissing attachment style is characterized by behaviors that minimize the experience of negative circumstances and internal states. Adolescents with this style demonstrate higher levels of substance abuse than the secure attachment styles (Rosenstein and Horowitz 1996; Caspers *et al.* 2005). Adults and adolescents with a dismissing attachment style display emotional distancing and rely on the self rather than others (Caspers *et al.* 2006).

Disorganized attachment styles are associated with severe disturbances in the ability to regulate emotions, cope effectively and relate to others (Siegel 2001). Prone to dissociation, adults with this attachment style often feel a loss of a coherent experience of self and other (Carlson 1998). While disorganized attachment may occur in the context of frightening maternal behaviors, there is also evidence that certain infants may be predisposed to developing this attachment style due to a genetic polymorphism in the dopamine D4 receptor (Lakatos *et al.* 2000). Genetic expressions and genetic predisposition may interact with and be influenced by experience.

Children presenting with disorganized attachment can exhibit role-reversal in relationship to the caregiver, elevated levels of anxiety and/or continued episodes of dissociation (Hesse and Main 2000). Adolescents with disorganized attachments often go on to develop aggressive behaviors. Adults demonstrate profound disruptions in thought and narrative in discussions of loss and/or abuse. They constitute a significant number of the hospitalized psychiatric and criminal population (Hesse and Main 2000; Table 7.3).

Roadmap for the caregiver

Resilience is beneficial for survival; adaptation is contingent upon it. Consequently, it is possible to earn a secure attachment later in life. This concept is the basis underlying therapy with individuals who have insecure attachment styles. The qualities of a therapeutic relationship that promote the development of earned security include those behaviors demonstrated by an appropriately attuned caregiver and infant dyad. Reciprocal nonverbal as well as verbal communication is one therapeutic strategy useful in facilitating the development of trust. Creating shared meaning systems by using coherent narratives and emotionally rich dialogue facilitates the repair of ruptured attachments and promotes development of earned secure attachment status (Siegel 2001).

Table 7.3 Adult attachment styles.[*]

Attachment style	Mental organization	Behaviors
Secure	Affective systems for appraisal and coping; organized and adaptable behavioral regulation	Freely perceive and experience as well as communicate positive and negative feelings; unrestricted emotional expression accurately reflecting circumstances; coherence between internal and external experience communicated without restriction or impairment
Dismissing	Impaired affective systems for appraisal; instead idealization and avoidance	Decreased ability to experience and communicate negative feelings; restricted emotional expression that reflects in a limited manner, negative circumstances; lack of coherence between internal and external experience that is communicated with minimization of negative circumstances
Preoccupied	Impaired use of affective systems for appraisal; negative feeling states dominate; inappropriate appraisal and ineffective coping	Communication of negative or ambivalent feelings predominates; restricted emotional expression that reflects in a limited manner negative circumstances; lack of coherence between internal and external experience that is communicated with minimization of negative circumstances
Disorganized	Lack of affective systems for appraisal; inability to regulate emotionally when confronted with traumatic experiences and/or triggers	Presence of verbal and/or mental incoherence or irrational thinking as evidenced by apprehension, confusion, contradiction, and/or dissociation

[*] Compiled from De Wolff and van Ijzendoorn 1997, Siegel 1999, Spangler and Zimmermann 1999.

Return to the Romanian orphans

Longitudinal studies of the effects of institutionalization on the abandoned Romanian children have demonstrated that no matter how wonderful the institution, a family-focused setting with a consistent caregiver is more beneficial to the development of children (Smyke *et al.* 2007). Children raised in institutions show deficits in emotional, social and cognitive development (MacLean 2003). What is missing from institutional care? What is missing are consistent caregivers engaged enough to create mutually reciprocal communication systems for the purpose of regulating emotion and promoting exploration of the environment (Siegel 2001).

What has happened to the orphans of Romania? As of 2006, approximately 30,000 Romanian orphans remain institutionalized and 8000 continue to be abandoned each year despite aggressive efforts to curtail the circumstances leading to institutionalization (Nelson 2007). Many of the abandoned children have grown up and left the orphanages. It is remarkably difficult to identify where they are and who they are. Save the Children tried to compile a database of the institutionalized children and was not able to finish the task. Upon leaving the orphanages, these children had become largely untraceable. At age 18, they were released into society, abandoned once again (McGeown 2005).

The fortunate children were those who found homes through adoption or fostering (Nelson 2007) before the age of two years old. One such child was Mimi. Abandoned at birth, she spent the first 18 months in an institution. Mutually engaged interactions with a consistent caregiver and play were missing from those first 18 months of life. She showed the effects of such deprivation. She was listless, undersized, unable to feed herself, unable to walk, and unable to talk. She was then fostered with a family. After four years in a family home, Mimi's IQ has entered the normal range. She smiled and liked animals (Nickerson 2006).

The significant factor in saving Mimi was a consistent, attuned relationship that stimulated and soothed her. In the context of that kind of nurturance and an enriched psychosocial environment, the brain can mature and synaptic connections can be created. Memories of care and comfort can be stored and hope can be reborn. The power of attachment forms and is re-formed during relatedness—a lesson we should not forget.

References

Allen, J. P., Marsh, P., McFarland, C., McElhaney, K. B., Land, D. J., Jodl, K. M., *et al.* (2002). Attachment and autonomy as predictors of the development of social skills and delinquency during mid-adolescence. *Journal of Consulting Clinical Psychology, 70*(1), 56–66.

Allen, J. P., Moore, C., Kuperminc, G., and Bell, K. (1998). Attachment and adolescent psychosocial functioning. *Child Development, 69*(5), 1406–1419.

Burrow, G. N., Fisher, D. A., and Larsen, P. R. (1994). Maternal and fetal thyroid function. *The New England Journal of Medicine, 331*, 1072–1078.

Carlson, E. A. (1998). A prospective longitudinal study of disorganized/disoriented attachment. *Child Development, 69,* 1107–1128.

Carter, C. S. (2005). The chemistry of child neglect: Do oxytocin and vasopressin mediate the effects of early experience? *Proceedings of the National Academy of Sciences, 102*(51), 18247–18248.

Caspers, K. M., Cadoret, R. J., Langbehn, D., Yucuis, R., and Troutman, B. (2005). Contributions of attachment style and perceived social support to lifetime use of illicit substances. *Addictive Behaviors, 30,* 1007–1011.

Caspers, K. M., Yucuis, R., Troutman, B. and Spinks, R. (2006). Attachment as an organizer of behavior: Implications for substance abuse problems and willingness to seek treatment. *Substance Abuse Treatment, Prevention, and Policy, 1,* 32.

Cicchetti, D. and Rogosch, F. A. (1997). The role of self-organization in the promotion of resilience in maltreated children. *Development and Psychopathology, 9,* 797–816.

Coe, C. L., Lulbach, G. R., and Schneider, M. L. (2001). Prenatal disturbance alters the size of the corpus callosum in young monkeys. *Developmental Psychobiology, 41*(2), 178–185.

Davis, E. P. and Sandman, C. A. (2006). Prenatal exposure to stress and stress hormones influences child development. *Infants & Young Children, 19*(3), 246–259.

De Graaf-Peters, V. B. and Hadders-Algra, M. (2006). Ontogeny of the human central nervous system: What is happening when? *Early Human Development, 82*(4), 257–266.

De Wolff, M. S. and van Ijzendoorn, M. H. (1997). Sensitivity and attachment: A meta-analysis on parental antecedents of infant attachment. *Child Development, 68*(4), 571–591.

Fowden, A. L. and Forhead, A. J. (2004). Endocrine mechanisms of intrauterine programming. *Reproduction, 127,* 515–526.

Glover, V. and O'Connor, T. G. (2002). Effects of ante-natal stress and anxiety. *British Journal of Psychiatry, 180,* 389–391.

Gloviczki, P. J. (2004). Ceausescu's children: The process of democratization and the plight of Romania's orphans. *Critique: A Worldwide Journal of Politics, Fall,* 116–125.

Gordon, N. S., Burke, S., Akil, H., Watson, J., and Panksepp, J. (2003). Socially induced brain fertilization: Play promotes brain derived neurotrophic factor expression. *Neuroscience Letters, 341,* 17–20.

Hesse, E. and Main, M. (2000). Disorganized infant, child, and adult attachment: Collapse in behavioral and attentional strategies. *Journal of the American Psychoanalytic Association, 48*(4), 1097–1127.

Kapoor, A., Dunn, E., Kostaki, A., Andrews, M. H., and Matthews, S. G. (2006). Fetal programming of the hypothalamo-pituitary-adrenal function: prenatal stress and glucocorticoids. *Journal of Physiology, 572,* 31–44.

Lakatos, K., Toth, I., Nemoda, Z., Ney, K., Sasvari-Szekely, M., and Gervai, J. (2000). Dopamine D4 (DRD4) gene polymorphism is associated with attachment disorganization in infants. *Molecular Psychiatry, 5*(6), 633–637.

MacLean, K. (2003). The impact of institutionalization on child development. *Development and Psychopathology, 15,* 853–884.

McGeown, K. (July 8, 2005). *What happened to Romania's orphans?* Retrieved 5/23/07 from http://news.bbc.co.uk/1/hi/world/europe/4629589.stm

Mirescu, C. and Gould, E. (2006). Stress and adult neurogenesis. *Hippocampus, 16,* 233–238.

Mirescu, C., Peters, J. D., and Gould, E. (2004). Early life experience alters response of adult neurogenesis to stress. *Nature Neuroscience, 7*(8), 841–846.

Nelson, C. A. (2007). A neurobiological perspective on early human deprivation. *Child Development Perspectives, 1*(1), 13–18.

Nickerson, C. (November 11, 2006). Studies on orphans sees benefits in family care. *The Boston Globe* [Online], www.boston.com/news/world/articles/2006/11/11/study_on_orphans_sees_benefit_in_family_care/

O'Connor, T. G., Heron, J., Golding, J., Beveridge, M. and Glover, V. (2002). Maternal antenatal anxiety and children's behavioural/emotional problems at 4 years. *British Journal of Psychiatry, 180,* 502–508.

Ogawa, J. R, Sroufe, L. A., Weinfeld, N. S., Carlson, E. A., and Egeland, B. (1997). Development and the fragmented self: Longitudinal study of dissociative symptomatology in a nonclinical sample. *Development and Psychopathology, 9,* 855–880.

Perry, B. D. (1999). Memories of fear: How the brain stores and retrieves physiologic states, feelings, behaviors, and thoughts from traumatic events. In J. Goodwin and R. Attias (eds) *Splintered Reflections of Trauma.* Jackson, TN: Basic Books.

Perry, B. D. (2001). The neurodevelopmental impact of violence in childhood. In D. Schetky and E. Benedek (eds) *Textbook of Child and Adolescent Forensic Psychiatry* (pp.221–238). Washington, DC: American Psychiatric Press, Inc.

Rosenstein, D. S. and Horowitz, H. A. (1996). Adolescent attachment and psychopathology. *Journal of Consulting and Clinical Psychology, 64*(2), 244–253.

Salm, A. K., Pavelko, M., Krouse, E. M., Webster, W., Kraszpuski, M., and Birkle, D. L. (2004). Lateral amygdaloid nucleus expansion in adult rats is associated with exposure to prenatal stress. *Developmental Brain Research, 148*(2), 159–167.

Schore, A. N. (1997). Early organization of the nonlinear right brain and development of a predisposition to psychiatric disorders. *Development and Psychopathology, 9,* 595–631.

Schore, A. N. (2000). Attachment and the regulation of the right brain. *Attachment and Human Development, 2*(1), 23–47.

Schore, A. N. (2002). The neurobiology of attachment and early personality organization. *Journal of Prenatal and Perinatal Psychology and Health, 16*(3), 249–262.

Siegel, D. (2001). Toward an interpersonal neurobiology of the developing mind: Attachment relationships, "mindsight", and neural integration. *Infant Mental Health Journal, 22*(1–2), 67–94.

Siegel, D. J. (1999). *The Developing Mind.* New York: The Guilford Press.

Smyke, A. T., Koga, S. F., Johnson, D. E., Fox, N. A., Marshall, P. J., Nelson, C. A., *et al.* (2007). The caregiving context in institution-reared and family reared infants and toddlers in Romania. *Journal of Child Psychology and Psychiatry, 48*(2), 210–218.

Spangler, G. and Zimmermann, P. (1999). Attachment representation and emotion regulation in adolescents: a psycho biological perspective on internal working models. *Attachment & Human Development, 1*(3), 270–290.

Talge, N. M., Neal, C., Glover, V., and the Early Stress, Translational Research and Prevention Science Network: Fetal and Neonatal Experience on Child and Adolescent Mental Health (2007). Antenatal maternal stress and long-term effects on child neurodevelopment: how and why? *Journal of Child Psychology and Psychiatry, 48*(3/4), 245–261.

Trevarthen, C. (2001). Intrinsic motives for companionship in understanding: Their origin, development, and significance for infant mental health. *Infant Mental Health Journal, 22*(1–2), 95–131.

Tronick, E. Z., Cohn, J., and Shea, E. (1986). The transfer of affect between mothers and infants. In T. B. Brazelton and M. W. Yogman (eds) *Affective Development in Infancy* (pp.10–15). Norwood, NL: Ablex.

Waldinger, R. J., Seidman, E. L., Gerber, A. J., Liem, J. H., Allen, J. P., and Hauser, S. T. (2003). Attachment and core relationship themes: Wishes for autonomy and closeness in the narratives of securely and insecurely attached adults. *Psychotherapy Research, 13*(1), 77–98.

Weiss, B. and Bellinger, D. C. (2006). Social ecology of children's vulnerability to environmental pollutants. *Environmental Health Perspectives, 114,* 1479–1485.

Yamada, H., Sadato, N., Konishi, Y., Muramoto, S., Kimura, K., Tanaka, M., *et al.* (2000). A milestone for normal development of the infantile brain detected by functional MRI. *Neurology, 55,* 218–223.

8

The Influence of Attention Deficit Problems

Darryl Christian

Neuroscience provides insights into the ways attention is maintained and underscores attentional contributions to integrating perception, memory, emotions, decision-making, self-control, and relationships. Understanding the neurobiology of attention deficit disorders can assist clinicians in finding effective ways to help clients achieve integration and improved psychosocial functioning.

Attention determines how we experience the world. Internal feelings, thoughts, and emotions, as well as external sights, sounds, and sensations, compete for our unconscious and conscious attention. Without conscious attention or effort, perceptual, emotional, and behavioral responses to sensory stimuli embed in implicit memory. The responses happen pre-attentively as sensory stimulation begins an involuntary bottom-up process. Only when information reaches higher levels of processing can conscious voluntary top-down processes focus attention on forming explicit memories. Factual, semantic, or episodic memories contribute to a sense of self and autobiographical history (Fisher 1998; Grossberg 2001). Pre-attentive processes prepare and encode sensory information for selective use by higher cognitive processes that include attention and working memory (Schweizer 2001). Without attention, implicit memories, prompted by environmental or internal triggers—not by conscious effort–may be re-experienced. Implicit memories are not accompanied by a sense of something being remembered, but rather are free-floating. Attention largely helps to integrate these experiences into a coherent personal narrative over time (Siegel 2006).

Attentional capacity and control is limited; we can only process so much information in a given period of time (Wood, Cox, and Cheng 2006). Alertness, processing speed, inhibition of competing information, genetic strengths and limitations, and development all impact our attentional capacity (Fisher 1998).

Deficits in attentional functioning result in problems that also significantly limit a person's ability to process and integrate emotional and interpersonal experiences (Siegel 2006). Sensory processing deficits cause problems in selection of sensory information while frontal cortex deficits lead to problems with top-down regulation of emotions and behaviors. Limbic deficits affect memory, behavioral control, and assessment of the emotional or memorial importance of events. Subcortical deficits result in bottom-up changes in attention, alertness, and energy (Fisher 1998; Serences and Yantis 2006; Figure 8.1).

The psychosocial challenges that affect people with attention-deficit disorders are examples of attentional systems gone awry, and are key areas of treatment for clinicians (Barkley 1995; Goldstein and Mather 1998; Safran 2002, 2003). Attention-Deficit/Hyperactivity Disorder (AD/HD) is the most common childhood neurobehavioral disorder, affecting 4 to 12 percent of children (American Academy of Pediatrics 2000). ADHD continues into adulthood for 60 percent of cases (Brown 2002).

Attentional difficulties are observable in art therapy tasks. The art content and art-making process can reveal problems with focus, motor control, memory, managing emotions, organization, sequencing, and decision-making (Safran 2003). Art-making has the potential to shape and integrate sensory processing and top-down control. Art processes can improve emotional well-being, develop cognitive skills, and enhance social interactions and relationships.

Attentional systems

Top-down goal-oriented cognitive processes utilize knowledge and expectations as well as memories and emotions to supervise attentional subcortical networks. Conversely, bottom-up alerting to salient sensory stimulation has the power to interrupt top-down cognitive tasks in order to attend to potentially dangerous, unexpected, or novel events (Corbetta and Shulman 2002).

Attention directed in a bottom-up fashion is driven automatically by sensory stimuli. We witness this vividly in client artwork. The nineteenth-century philosopher William James described involuntary attention to things that differ from the background: "Very intense, voluminous, or sudden…strange things, moving things, wild animals, bright things, pretty things, metallic things, blows, blood" (as cited in Corbetta and Shulman 2002, p.207). The strength of these images is influenced by relevance. Wild animals, blood, and blows are salient to human survival.

Brain imaging research hypothesizes three attentional networks that lead to behavioral choices: (1) an alerting system associated with sensory stimuli, arousal, and vigilance; (2) a predominantly bottom-up posterior orienting system that reflexively orients to and selects information from sensory stimuli; and (3) a voluntary top-down anterior executive control system involved in self-regulation of cognition and emotion through the strategic orienting to stimuli, and monitoring and resolving of conflict between brain areas (Nigg, Hinshaw, and Huang-Pollack 2006; Posner and Fan, in press; Rueda, Posner, and Rothbart 2004).

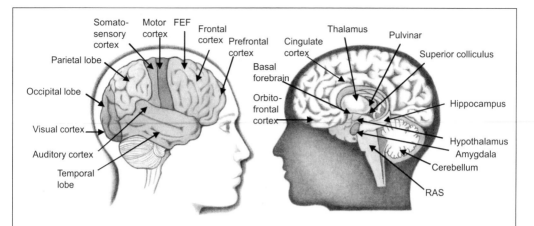

CORTICAL

FEF: Frontal Eye Field; *Frontal lobe*: reasoning, planning, movement, emotions, problem-solving; working memory; includes motor cortex; *Prefrontal cortex*: goal related thoughts and actions, e.g. inhibition of motor response (impulse control), working memory, voluntary attention; *Temporal lobe*: auditory processing, speech, memory, visual processing; *Occipital lobe*: processing of visual stimulus; includes visual cortex; *Somatosensory cortex*: orientation, processing of, and transfer of sensory information to the motor cortex; *Parietal lobe*: integration of sensory information; spatial "where" processing; manipulation of objects; automatic response associations; working memory.

SUBCORTICAL STRUCTURES

Basal ganglia (striatum): movement, behavioral response inhibition; *Basal forebrain*: memory and learning; produces and distributes acetylcholine to most of the cortex; alertness.

LIMBIC AND PARALIMBIC SYSTEMS

Cingulate cortex: receives input from the thalamus and cortex; links cortex, limbic, and motor areas; *Orbitofrontal cortex*: decision-making and reward; *Thalamus*: as a "gatekeeper" receives sensory information and sends it to cortex; receives information from the cortex; includes pulvinar; *Hypothalamus*: regulates autonomic nervous system; motivation; *Hippocampus*: memory and spatial movement; working memory; *Amygdala*: emotion, aggression and fear.

MIDBRAIN

Reticular activating system (RAS): a network in the brainstem that moderates consciousness, alertness, and arousal; *Superior colliculus*: automatically orients head movements toward auditory and visual stimuli.

BRAINSTEM

Locus coeruleus: produces norepinephrine, associated with alertness, body function, and the stress response, and enhances visual processing.

CEREBELLUM

Movement (excitatory), attention, habitual actions, balance; *Left hemisphere*: detail processing; *Right hemisphere*: global processing.

Figure 8.1 Brain structures involved in the attentional systems. Drawing by Jennifer Kirk.

The alerting system

The alerting system is characterized by sensitivity to sensory stimuli and by regulation of states of arousal/alertness and vigilance/sustained attention. Alertness refers to an ability to respond to potential stimuli while sustained attention refers to an ability to wait and maintain task focus over time. Alerting moderates the posterior orienting system as well as the anterior executive system, and contributes to the earliest self-regulation functions in infants (Nigg *et al.* 2006). Alerting is associated with the thalamus and with right frontal and right parietal cortices, which contribute to global processing (Posner, DiGirolamo, and Fernandez-Duque 1997; Posner, Rothbart, and Rueda 2003; Sohlberg and Mateer 2001). Alertness typically results in a faster but less accurate response. Sustained attention is hypothesized to be mediated by acetylcholine produced by the basal forebrain, which recruits the anterior executive attentional system and enhances sensory, perceptual, and spatial processing (Sarter, Givens, and Bruno 2001). Norepinephrine from the locus coeruleus also increases the rate of selection of visual information for processing (Posner and Petersen 1990). Alerting is enhanced by cues indicating *when* an event will take place (Posner and Fan, in press). As an example of its moderating functions, alerting may interrupt and recruit the orienting system or executive system processes when a stimulus is relevant to a task (Corbetta and Shulman 2002; Sarter *et al.* 2001).

The posterior orienting system

Attention is oriented through cues to *where* an event will take place (Posner and Fan, in press). The orienting system provides a spatial context for objects and facilitates unconscious aspects of visuo-motor skills (Baars 1999) through the dorsal visual *where* pathway. Orienting requires shifting attention, either covertly (without eye movements) or overtly (with eye movements). The superior colliculus and thalamic pulvinar inform posterior brain areas involved in orienting. The superior parietal, the frontal eye fields, and superior colliculus may be part of a bilateral system involved in both covert and overt orientation, where the right hemisphere is responsible for global orienting and the left is responsible for detailed orienting (Corbetta and Shulman 2002; Fisher 1998; Posner *et al.* 1997; Posner and Fan, in press). Neuronal activity in the right parietal is enhanced when attention is given to the spatial location of a stimulus. If more visual and tactile detail is needed, the lower ventral visual pathway is recruited (Posner and Petersen 1990). The lower ventral system, the *what* pathway, involves information flow from the occipital lobe to the temporal lobe. It associates information with emotional saliency (Shipp 2004). Automatic spatial orienting and perceptual selection of information are two functions of the posterior attentional system (Nigg *et al.* 2006).

The anterior executive system

Executive attention helps resolve conflict between brain areas; it involves planning, decision-making, error detection, and creating novel responses. The executive system is most active when the degrees of complex discrimination are greatest. The anterior frontal attentional network—the frontal cortex, basal ganglia, and anterior cingulate cortex—is vital when a non-habitual response is needed. Conflict resolution also engages working memory processes associated with hippocampal and prefrontal regions (Posner *et al.* 1997, 2003). The thalamus plays an important role in this dopamine-mediated wide network; it targets and selects information from the brainstem and from the cortex for processing by higher-level structures (Sohlberg and Mateer 2001).

Controlled attentional processes involving working memory are conscious, slow, and require effort. Processing is explicit and voluntary. Controlled attention modulates and enhances sensory processing. Top-down activation of sensory areas can be utilized in the therapeutic use of imagery (e.g. art therapy, sports psychology, visualization) to enhance task performance (Posner *et al.* 1997). Working memory training for children with AD/HD decreased symptoms of AD/HD and led to cognitive improvement that generalized to other non-trained tasks (Klingberg, Forssberg, and Westerberg 2002). Results were achieved by the use of computer image tasks, like video games, that enhance sensory discrimination and help develop cortical plasticity in sensory and motor areas. Improvements in working memory also correlated with reduced motor movements.

Top-down and bottom-up systems work in concert so that relevant information is favored. At the level of the retina and visual cortex, the selection process for attention appears to be based on sensory stimulus and recognition of features such as discontinuities, edge orientation, luminance, contrast, and movement. The frontal, temporal, and parietal cortices identify objects and assign meaning to stimuli, suppressing unrelated and unattended responses. Thus, coherent representation depends upon coordinated neural activity directed by attentional processes (Serences and Yantis 2006; Treue 2003).

Art therapy may activate attention through training, repetition, control, and coordination. The manipulation of media in order to draw or sculpt requires a similar progression. Attentional sequences involved in making and creating art may be generalized to daily life activities. Furthermore, executive attention mediates the conflicting responses brought on by art media, visual stimulation, and the resulting motor and emotional reactions. Art therapy can lead to enhanced integration and growth through active engagement during a creative and novel response context.

Development cues attentional maturation

Changes in the brain are also affected by genetic and environmental experiences that determine which neuronal connections will survive and be strengthened. These changes shape attentional abilities. Maturation at the cellular level includes changes in the number of neuronal connections in the brain through the elimination of unnecessary neuronal connections and synaptic pruning. Throughout critical periods of development, maturation strengthens neuronal connections by myelinating neural axons, which increases the speed, efficiency, and synchronicity of information transmission between cells and across structures. Myelinated neurons are known as white matter in the brain. Maturation also increases performance of grey matter, which refers to unmyelinated neurons responsible for processing information. The denser the grey matter, the easier information is processed, since more pathways form between neurons (Satz 1993). Maturation refines the functioning of specific brain regions. Attentional structures mature in a sequence from posterior (back) to anterior (front) brain areas. The progressive growth mirrors Piaget's cognitive developmental stages that culminate in the appearance of formal operational thinking, which is dependent upon the ability to sustain attention (Day, Chiu, and Hendren 2005). Attentional gains are associated with improved emotion and memory processing, executive functioning, empathy, working memory, and impulse control (Luna and Sweeney 2004; Munakata, Casey, and Diamond 2004; Sabbagh 2006). The prefrontal areas of the cortex responsible for executive attention myelinate after the somatosensory and visual cortices responsible for orienting have developed. Skill building, like learning to use language during development, reflects myelination of neurons. Basic sensory structures and functions involved with alerting are developed before those structures involved in orienting and integrating them are myelinated (Gogtay *et al.* 2004). Some subcortical areas that modulate behavioral responses are on-line at birth, or shortly after, and play a primary role in determining saliency (Posner and Fan, in press). Emotions (amygdala, at birth), memories (hippocampus, two to three years), and motivation (hypothalamus, at birth) contribute, with or without awareness, to the attentional importance of stimuli. At the subcortical level of processing, attention is internally and voluntarily driven by memory, fears, and motivation (Fisher 1998; Johnson and Weisz 1994).

Emotion and memory are capable of exerting powerful influences on the processing of sensory material. For example, abused children show signs of changes in perception and attention due to past trauma. Physically and emotionally abused children who are acutely aware of signs of anger or threat have difficulty taking their attention away from an angry face (Munakata *et al.* 2004). Emotions also bias attention to perception of mood-congruent stimuli (Phillips *et al.* 2003). When the words or faces people encounter are consistent with their current mood, decision-making is faster and requires less sensory evidence (Johnson and Weisz 1994).

Adolescents have a harder time performing certain executive tasks. Decision-making tasks utilize the prefrontal cortex (PFC) and require much more effort from adolescents than from adults. Maturation of the executive function continues through adolescence and into the twenties. If an unexpected event occurs during an already demanding problem-solving situation, adolescents may exhaust their developing prefrontal resources for planning and impulse control and return to habitual or impulsive behaviors (Sabbagh 2006). For example, when an adolescent, who is focused, concentrated, and intent and appears to be having a good day working on an art task, suddenly throws down his pencil, gives up, and tears up the piece, it may be that prefrontal resources are exhausted. From a developmental perspective, spatial working memory becomes more integrated and efficient as it becomes distributed across brain regions by the end of adolescence (Sabbagh 2006).

Attention contributes to learning flexible responses. When we learn a new task, we engage in controlled, conscious, top-down attentional processes which require a great amount of energy. Over time, learning a specific task skill incorporates an automatic bottom-up attentional process, which consumes less effort and attentional energy (Fisher 1998). It is advantageous to respond to both external environmental demands and to internal demands in a flexible manner. Controlled attention enables us to develop the self-regulation that allows new ways of responding to create new patterns of neural activity and contribute to neural plasticity (Siegel 2006).

Controlled attention is associated with the function of the cingulate cortex, which is modulating attention, emotion, and motor responses (Rueda *et al.* 2004). The cingulate cortex development in later childhood is linked to executive control. The cingulate, connected to the medial frontal lobe, links emotional (limbic) and motor (cortex) areas. There is evidence that the developing neural executive attention network relates to development of self-regulation. Effortful top-down control modulates bottom-up reactions such as fear or stress responses.

The prefrontal regions are involved in focusing on tasks while decreasing interference from competing information. For instance, children seem to have more prefrontal cortex activation when attempting to inhibit motor responses. The result is a reduced ability for cortical inhibition of emotional responses from the amygdala. There appears to be a relatively long developmental period for the fronto-striatal network (frontal cortex to basal ganglia) that results in increased ability for response inhibition. The efficiency of these inhibitory functions affects other cognitive functions including motor and emotional control (Booth *et al.* 2003). While the ventral fronto-striatal network has a role in inhibiting habitual behaviors, the hippocampus is involved in learning new responses (Casey *et al.* 2002).

Effortful control plays a role in the development of conscience, pairing a reactive fear response, generated by the amygdala with prefrontal-driven behavioral and emotional self-regulation (Posner *et al.* 2003). An expression of sadness in another activates the amygdala and the anterior cingulate as part of the attentional network for the expression of emotion by others. The amygdala and cingulate cortex offer opportunities for socialization: one through a behavioral response to expressed emotion and the other through integrating internal attention with the emotional signals from the amygdala.

Attention deficits and dis-integration

Several general factors may account for the attentional deficits in AD/HD: dysregulation of the frontal cortex, dysregulation of subcortical structures, and dysregulation of the networks connecting the cortex and subcortical structures (Farone and Biederman 2002). Specific dysfunctions in the frontal-subcortical cortex affect regulation and inhibition of inappropriate actions by delaying immediate rewards, forming plans and concepts, keeping choices in mind, and selecting responses. Subcortical deficits affect automatic thinking and movement, focus, and procedural memory. Dopamine/norepinephrine regulation dysfunctions affect reward/pleasure regulation, arousal, and motivation. Cingulate cortex dysfunctions affect transfer of information between the cortex, motor, and limbic areas. Cerebellum dysfunctions affect procedural memory.

Arousal and alertness problems in AD/HD are related to dopamine (DA) and norepinephrine (NE) imbalance, disrupting communication across brain areas (Overmeyer *et al.* 2001). DA and NE imbalance are also associated with emotional disorders and complicate the accurate diagnosis of AD/HD, due to conditions such as anxiety, mood disorders, and substance use (Fisher 1998).

While the causes of AD/HD, specific diagnostic criteria, and associated neuroimaging findings are still researched (Castellanos and Tannock 2002; Halperin and Schulz 2006), the American Psychiatric Association (2000) has identified a hypothetical profile for the two main AD/HD subtypes. Based on the neurological differences and the critical maturation phases described earlier, there is a movement to separate the two subtypes into separate diagnoses (Nigg *et al.* 2006).

AD/HD, Predominantly Hyperactive-Impulsive Type, is a left-hemisphere disorder with dis-inhibition and inactivity of the frontal processes and subcortical connections. Disorganization, frustration, and impulsivity are typical. Stimulation is sought through risky and dangerous behaviors and substance use tends to be for stimulation. Social interactions and attachments are frequently superficial and difficult (Diamond 2005; Fisher 1998).

AD/HD, Predominantly Inattentive Type (or Attention-Deficit Disorder [ADD]) is a right-hemisphere disorder with parietal-sensory information processing and related spatial processing deficits in learning (including language). Deficits in working memory and arousal are predominant. Anxiety frequently co-occurs, encouraging self-medicating substance use for calming and self-soothing purposes. Anxious behaviors may be mistaken for hyperactivity. Behaviors may be attempts to self-arouse through stimulating activities. Social interactions can be difficult due to a need to please others. Both subtypes may be at work in AD/HD, Combined-Type (Diamond 2005; Fisher 1998).

Treatment considerations

Treatment that is informed by neuroscience insights on attention can impact the development of integrated mental functioning and positively contribute to more flexible, adaptive, coherent, energized, and stable mental processes (FACES) (Siegel 2006). Art therapists have used art therapy to increase attentional abilities and decrease impulsive behaviors (Smitheman-Brown and Church 1996), to provide psycho-educational support, to identify feelings and behaviors through non-verbal expression, to build socialization skills and self-esteem, and to provide for systemic and family support (Henley 1998; Safran 2002, 2003). Art therapists have recently begun to incorporate neuroscience insights into practice.

Safran (2002) has noted that artwork with clients with AD/HD has clinical value as a visual record that can be looked at again, allowing for further learning. The record of the artwork supports strengthening of memory, both working and long-term memory. Revisiting artwork can provide ongoing opportunities to process, rework, and integrate information about memory, emotions, and behaviors represented in its images.

Mandala drawing at the beginning of each session was shown to reduce impulsive behaviors (Smitheman-Brown and Church 1996). Malchiodi (1998) describes the positive effects of creating an image in a circle with homeless adolescents as improving focus and control of unfocused energies. The format provides a circular structure within the rectangular structure on the page that binds attention. A form within a page can sequence attention: it allows for the visual expression of whatever is in immediate attention; it allows for attention to visual-motor exploration and action without verbal cognitive demands, and it limits conflict and anxiety through presenting a semi-completed picture. Changing this directive by offering a choice of collage images to be used to fill in the circle could also engage the executive system through the introduction of choice and conflict. Offering a choice of tactile media would provide opportunities for continued controlled attention despite the emotional reaction that the tactile material could bring up. Progressing through a sequence of directive changes may help build controlled attention.

Children with AD/HD and ADD benefit in school settings from a reduction of classroom environmental distractions and stressors and from the structuring of lesson plans and schedules to fit attentional cycles and processing time constraints. Other beneficial accommodations utilize multi-sensory modalities and non-verbal learning strengths to engage children on a personal and emotional level (Jensen 1998) in a way similar to art therapy. Jensen also notes that movement and changes in location, either in the classroom or outdoors, engages the posterior attention system. Art therapists may be able to move around a room and incorporate movement into directives. Rotating the art piece or having a client pick up a picture and place it on a wall engages spatial orienting attention.

Educational therapy approaches help children with attention deficits benefit from scaffolding of tasks: a task broken into steps and stages. Art therapists can learn from cognitive rehabilitation treatment strategies that include a progression of tasks that build attentional skills and working memory (Sohlberg and Mateer 2001). For art therapists, making attentional and memory tasks explicit can assist a client to complete an art therapy intervention successfully (selecting a subject, selecting materials, drawing, adding words, etc.). Making implicit art therapy processes explicit may help decrease bottom-up responses and increase focus and top-down attentional capacity.

Assessment and treatment address performance in focused attention (responding to stimuli), sustained attention (vigilance and working memory), selective attention (ignoring distractions), and alternating and divided attention (mental flexibility). For art therapists, application of these principles begins with assessment, which may require referrals for psychiatric, psycho-educational, or cognitive assessment.

Neuroscience highlights the utility of sequencing art therapy interventions. For example, an adolescent boy has trouble at school. He is distracted (selective attention), has difficulty completing assignments (sustained attention and working memory), and impulsively leaves class (reactive responses). He is angry that he gets poor grades, so the therapist asks him to select three collage pictures that show how he feels about the situation. To get started, he is asked to write a title for the picture (a reminder that orients working memory to the task). The therapist provides an alerting cue, "Let's take about five minutes to find those pictures," and then provides time cues as work proceeds. Cues are provided if the client gets distracted with collage images or unrelated conversation: "Does that relate to this?" pointing at the picture title. Images are assembled and glued down (orienting and executive attention). Orienting questions such as "What do you...?" or "Is something missing?" help focus alerting attention to relevant visual information. The therapist is attentive to emotional reactions and memories that emerge. Pictures are added to show salient responses. The therapist supports self-regulation by the executive system by attending to the client's competing attentional responses. The therapist is especially alert to habitual responses or actions that might usurp executive attention. Another directive, "Let's add some pictures to show what's going on around you in the class," or "Add something that shows what you do when you feel like this," orients attention onto finding new but relevant information that may help in executive conflict resolution. The next task, "Write some words for each picture," is a step toward explicit integration of material that has emerged. Finally, a review of the artwork and process supports integration. Art therapy interventions build on the client's strengths and target attentional skills in a developmental progression that also incorporates real-life demands.

Summary

Neurobiology research assists in understanding the complex development and interaction of neural systems involved in attention and AD/HD. Consequently art therapists can provide an environment that supports the development of executive attentional skills that in turn lead to flexible, adaptive, coherent, energized, and stable functioning. Art products serve as an external integrating work space for internal processes, conflicts, and problem-solving. As research helps clarify our knowledge of brain systems and attention deficits, art therapists are called upon to integrate these new insights thoughtfully and creatively into art therapy practice.

References

American Academy of Pediatrics. (2000). Clinical practice guidelines: Diagnosis and evaluation of the child with attention-deficit/hyperactivity disorder. *Pediatrics, 105*(5), 1158–1170.

American Psychiatric Association. (2000). *Diagnostic and Statistical Manual of Mental Disorders, 4th Edition Text Revision.* Washington, DC: American Psychiatric Association.

Baars, B. J. (1999). Attention versus consciousness in the visual brain: Differences in conception, phenomenology, behavior, neuroanatomy, and physiology. *The Journal of General Psychiatry, 126*(3), 224–233.

Barkley, R. A. (1995). *Taking Charge of ADHD.* New York: Guilford Press.

Booth, J. R., Burman, D. D., Meyer, J. R., Lei, Z., Trommer, B. L., Davenport, N. D., *et al.* (2003). Neural development of selective attention and response inhibition. *NeuroImage, 20,* 737–751.

Brown, T. E. (2002). DSM-IV: ADHD and executive function impairments. *Advanced Studies in Medicine, 2*(25), 910–914.

Casey, B. J., Thomas, K. M., Davidson, M. C., Kunz, K., and Franzen, P. L. (2002). Dissociating striatal and hippocampal function developmentally with a stimulus-response compatibility task. *Journal of Neuroscience, 22*(19), 8647–8652.

Castellanos, F. X. and Tannock, R. (2002). Neuroscience of attention-deficit/hyperactivity disorder: The search for endophenotypes. *Neuroscience, 3,* 617–628.

Corbetta, M. and Shulman, G. L. (2002). Control of goal-directed and stimulus-driven attention in the brain. *Nature Reviews Neuroscience, 3,* 201–215.

Day, J., Chiu, S., and Hendren, R. L. (2005). Structure and function of the adolescent brain: Findings from neuroimaging studies. *Adolescent Psychiatry, 29,* 175–215.

Diamond, A. (2005). Attention-deficit disorder (attention-deficit/hyperactivity disorder without hyperactivity): A neurologically and behaviorally distinct disorder from attention-deficit/hyperactivity disorder (with hyperactivity). [Electronic version] *Development and Psychopathology, 17*(3), 807–825.

Farone, S. V. and Biederman, J. (2002). Pathophysiology of attention-deficit/hyperactivity disorder. In K. L. Davis, D. Charney, J. T. Coyle, and C. Nemeroff (eds) *Neuropsychopharmacology: The Fifth Generation of Progress* (pp.577–596). Philadelphia, PA: Lippincott Williams & Wilkins.

Fisher, B. C. (1998). *Attention Deficit Disorder Misdiagnosis.* Boca Raton, FL: CRC Press Publisher.

Gogtay, N., Giedd, J. N., Lusk, L., Hayashi, K. M., Greenstein, D., Vaituzis, A. C., *et al.* (2004). Dynamic mapping of human cortical development during childhood through early childhood. *Proceedings of the National Academy of Sciences, 101*(21), 8174–8179.

Goldstein, S. and Mather, N. (1998). *Overcoming Underachieving.* New York: John Wiley & Sons, Inc.

Grossberg, S. (2001). Linking the laminar circuits of visual cortex to visual perception: Development, grouping, and attention. *Neuroscience and Biobehavioral Reviews, 25,* 513–526.

Halperin, J. M. and Schulz, K. P. (2006). Revisiting the role of the prefrontal cortex in the pathophysiology of attention-deficit/hyperactivity disorder. *Psychological Bulletin, 132*(4), 560–581.

Henley, D. (1998). Art therapy as an aid to socialization in children with ADD. *American Journal of Art Therapy, 37,* 2–12.

Jensen, E. (1998). *Teaching with the Brain in Mind.* Alexandria, VA: Association for Supervision and Curriculum Development.

Johnson, M. K. and Weisz, C. (1994). Comments on unconscious processing: Finding emotional in the cognitive stream. In P. M. Niedenthal and S. Kitayama (eds) *The Heart's Eye: Emotional Influences in Perception and Attention* (pp.145–164). San Diego, CA: Academic Press.

Klingberg, T., Forssberg, H., and Westerberg, H. (2002). Training of working memory in children with ADHD. *Journal of Clinical and Experimental Neuropsychology, 24*(6), 781–791.

Luna, B. and Sweeney, J. A. (2004). The emergence of collaborative brain function. *Annals of the New York Academy of Sciences, 1021,* 249–309.

Malchiodi, C. A. (1998). *The Art Therapy Sourcebook*. New York: McGraw-Hill.

Munakata, Y., Casey, B. J., and Diamond, A. (2004). Developmental cognitive neuroscience: Progress and potential. *Trends in Cognitive Sciences, 8*(3), 122–128.

Nigg, J. T., Hinshaw, S. P., and Huang-Pollack, C. (2006). Disorders of attention and impulse regulation. In D. Cicchetti and D. Cohen (eds) *Developmental Psychopathology* (2nd edition, pp.358–403). New York: Wiley.

Olesen, P., Westerberg, H., and Klingberg, T. (2004). Increased prefrontal and parietal activity after training of working memory. *Nature Neuroscience, 7*, 75–79.

Overmeyer, S., Bullmore, E. T., Suckling, J., Simmons, A., Williams, S. C. R., Santosh, P. J., *et al.* (2001). Distributed grey and white matter deficits in hyperkinetic disorder: MRI evidence for anatomical abnormality in an attentional network. *Psychological Medicine, 31*, 1425–1435.

Phillips, M. L. Drevets, W. C., Rauch, S. L., and Lane, R. (2003). Neurobiology of emotion perception I: The neural basis of normal emotion perception. *Biological Psychiatry, 54*, 504–514.

Posner, M. I., DiGirolamo, G. J., and Fernandez-Duque, D. (1997). Brain mechanisms of cognitive skills. *Consciousness and Cognition, 6*, 267–290.

Posner, M. I. and Fan, J. (in press). Attention as an organ system. In J. Pomerantz (ed.) *Neurobiology of Perception and Communication: From Synapse to Society. The IVth DeLange Conference.* Cambridge: Cambridge University Press.

Posner, M. I. and Petersen, S. E. (1990). The attention system of the human brain. *Annual Review Neuroscience, 13*, 25–42.

Posner, M. I., Rothbart, M. K., and Rueda, M. R. (2003). *Brain Mechanisms and Learning of High Level Skills*. A paper presented at a meeting on Brain and Education, Vatican City, November 2003.

Rueda, M. R., Posner, M. I., and Rothbart, M. K. (2004). Attentional control and self-regulation. In R. F. Baumerister and K. D. Vohs (eds) *Handbook of Self-regulation: Research, Theory, and Applications* (pp.283–300). New York: Guilford Press.

Sabbagh, L. (2006). The teen brain, hard at work. *Scientific American Mind, 17*(4), 20–25.

Safran, D. S. (2002). *Art Therapy and AD/HD: Diagnostic and Therapeutic Approaches*. Philadelphia, PA: Jessica Kingsley Publishers.

Safran, D. S. (2003). An art therapy approach to attention-deficit/hyperactivity disorder. In C. A. Malchiodi (ed.) *Handbook of Art Therapy* (pp.181–192). New York: Guilford Press.

Sarter, M., Givens, B., and Bruno. J. P. (2001). The cognitive neuroscience of sustained attention: Where top-down meets bottom-up. *Brain Research Reviews, 35*, 146–160.

Satz, P. (1993). Brain reserve capacity on symptom onset after brain injury: A formulation and review of evidence for threshold theory. *Neuropsychology, 7*, 273–295.

Schweizer, K. (2001). Preattentive processing and cognitive ability. Intelligence [Electronic Version]. Retrieved 12/23/06 from www.accessmylibrary.com/coms2/summary_0286-10738382_ITM.

Serences, J. T. and Yantis, S. (2006). Selective visual attention and perceptual coherence. *Trends in Cognitive Sciences, 10*(1), 38–45.

Shipp. S. (2004). The brain circuitry of attention. *Trends in Cognitive Sciences, 8*(5), 223–230.

Siegel, D. J. (2006). An interpersonal neurobiology approach to psychotherapy: Awareness, mirror neurons, and neural plasticity in the development of well-being. *Psychiatric Annals, 36*(4), 248–256.

Smitheman-Brown, V. and Church, R. P. (1996). Mandala drawing: Facilitating growth in children with ADD or ADHD. *Art Therapy Journal of the American Art Therapy Association, 13*(4), 252–259.

Sohlberg, M. M. and Mateer, C. A. (2001). *Cognitive Rehabilitation: An Integrative Neuropsychological Approach*. New York: Guilford Press.

Treue, S. (2003). Visual attention: the where, what, how and why of saliency. *Current Opinion in Neurobiology, 13*, 428–432.

Wood, S., Cox, R., and Cheng, P. (2006). Attention design: Eight issues to consider. *Computers in Human Behavior, 22*, 588–602.

9

Memory and Art

Robin Vance and Kara Wahlin

Memory involves recalling and recombining patterns of internally or externally cued information. We don't store all the detailed features of a friend's face, but rather the basic shapes of that face (Biederman and Kalocsai 1997). Memories are groups of interlinked neurons that fire together to reveal information. When neural cells fire together, the interlinking strengthens the networks of neurons and enables them to convey informa- tion more efficiently (Carlson 2001). Memory exists throughout the brain, although types and the quality of memories depend on the complementary and/or competitive functioning of different brain regions (Baddeley *et al.* 2000).

The brain's left hemisphere has an assertive influence on memories whereas the brain's right hemisphere demonstrates an accepting influence (Carter 1998). The left hemisphere is the center for language comprehension and expression as well as being prone to positive and pro-social emotions. It holds our explicit conscious memories. It coordinates the conscious, social side of our experience—problem-solving, coping with conventions, and detecting probabilities in our environment and in our emotional-social presentation. Verbal working memory has been shown by neuroimaging experiments to take place in the left hemisphere of the prefrontal cortex, whereas visuo-spatial memory takes place in the right hemisphere of the prefrontal cortex, as well as in the parietal lobe (Walter *et al.* 2003; Figure 9.1).

Producing emotions, reading facial expressions, and utilizing visual-spatial and musical abilities are largely right brain processes. Visuo-spatial memory activates the right hemisphere of the prefrontal cortex, as well as the parietal lobe (Walter *et al.* 2003). The parietal coordinates experiences of the body in real and in imagined space. Robin Vance, an artist and art therapist, reports that she moves as she makes the art. Music at times facilitates her movement. She describes movement as opening a necessary door. Robin suspects that moving towards implicit unknown somatic memories enlists her right hemisphere, leaving the left's sequential planning and problem-solving behind. Shifting into a time-free zone, she can update, remember and forget the content and process of feeling states and narratives. Letting go of outdated, unused, emotionally charged memories, she moves into unrecognized territories of self-awareness. Her sym- pathetic nervous system becomes benignly aroused, increasing norepinephrine and

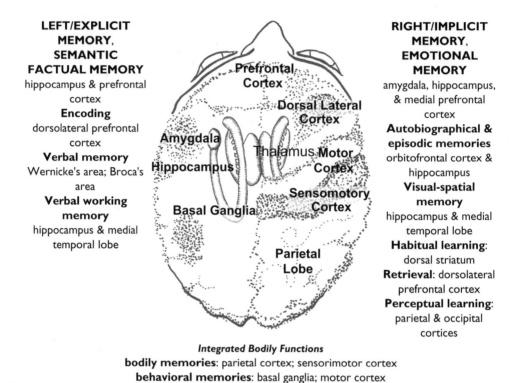

Figure 9.1 Hemispheric lateralization of memory.

memory functions. Moving away from anxiety and/or loss states, which negatively impact memory, towards positive excitation, arouses memory (Figure 9.2).

Dance interlinks art-making and memory. Movement invites making new memories and forgetting background memories. The picture's velvety dark background represents unconscious and maybe implicit memories, but more specifically, right hemispheric emotionally charged memories. There is something inviting and comforting in the velvety darkness, like a deep sleep, as well as frightening. The dark is unknown, attractive and repulsive at the same time. Tendrils of neurons, organ-pods, and paint dripped on the black velvet background signify forgetting, the falling away of non-repeated excitations and blocking of neural networks. They represent events that are no longer marked as significant or emotionally meaningful. After all, what would happen to us if we could not forget? Surely, our minds would implode. According to decay theory, information decays because it has not been retrieved or accessed over a long period of time, as it was probably not useful (Altmann and Gray 2002; Byrnes 2001).

The experience of making *Dance* was talismanic and reduced Robin's reoccurring back pain. She moved to forget pain, gratified with making new memories and focusing on the pleasure and joy of discovery. Forgetting may also involve the proactive processes

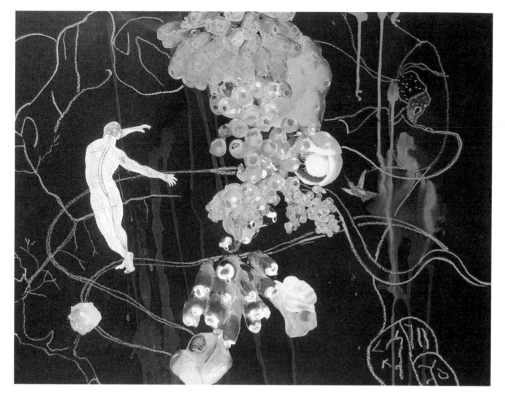

Figure 9.2 Dance. *A yellow-greenish figure is shown with his back to the viewer. He is dancing in an ambiguous space: to his right is a cascade of fuchsia, orange and blue sea squirts, and flower parts. Close by, a brown hummingbird swoops to drink. An image of a doubled pair of hands is part of the cascade, fingers tightly interlaced in a prayerful gesture. The background is a velvety black, out of which neuron-like tendrils weave amongst teal paint drips and pale outlines of bladder-shaped pods and organs. Robin Vance, 25″ × 19.5″. Media: Xeroxed collage on paper, gouache, and oil pastel.*

of intrusion, or interference, as new information conflicts with or overshadows older information (Byrnes 2001). In this instance, forgetting can be construed in terms of strengthening existing coping pathways while doing the art helps distract from the pain (procedural memory). Discovery engages hippocampal and amygdala functioning. Movement stimulates endorphins and dopamine. Joy activates a sense of pleasure and involves the rewarding access of dopamine along with serotonin. Creating new and strengthening existing neural pathways is central to clinicians.

The formation of memories

The formation of memory is experience-dependent. Learning and memory involve the long-term potentiation (LTP) of neurons. First noted in the hippocampus and cortex, the process occurs throughout the nervous system (Sapolsky 2005). Potentiation strengthens a synaptic connection so that a neural pathway is more easily and quickly stimulated, requiring less effort for the brain to recall a memory or react to a stimulus. Action potentiation of the neuron involves the release of calcium and the shift of potassium from within the cell (Kalat 2004).

Repeated release of the excitatory neurotransmitter glutamate into synapses containing N-methyl D-aspartic acid (NMDA) receptors cause a second glutamate receptor to become excited by calcium released at the site, decreasing neural thresholds for excitation. Then, four main mechanisms happen to make the potentiation long lasting for 50 years and more: First, the calcium influx allows stored receptors to come online; second, these receptors remain activated for a longer time; third, the actual shape of the neuronal dendrite changes, which makes the excitation spread more widely; and, last, neurotransmitters, known as retrograde neurotransmitters, release and travel backwards across the synapse, causing more glutamate to be released. Potentiating neural networks forms the basis for the profound complexities in the interconnecting billions of cells in the nervous system (Carlson 2001; Figure 9.3).

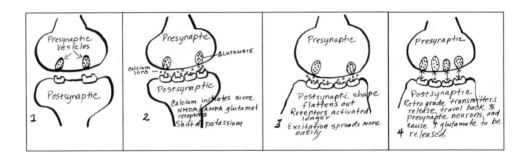

Figure 9.3 Mechanisms of long-term potentiation.

Implicit memory

Implicit memory does not require conscious awareness. It directs actions, reactions, and body responses with little or no conscious effort, involving multiple brain structures (Figure 9.1). The amygdala, hippocampus, and medial prefrontal cortex support fear conditioning and emotional memory, the basal ganglia and motor cortex support behavioral memory, the parietal and occipital cortices facilitate perceptual memory, and the parietal cortex stores bodily memories (Carlson 2001). Implicit memories refer to somatic/bodily, perceptual experiences, which include memories of how things looked or smelled as well as our emotions and moods at the time. Behavioral types of experiences also contribute to our implicit sense of who we are. *Changeling*, depicted on the cover page, arouses an implicit sense of body parts, utilizing collage and juxtaposition of the pieces (cover). *Changeling* is about putting many parts into wholeness. Some of the parts suggest implicit memory. Robin reports feeling that they arise from her body as somatic eddies, waves of sensation, and even the absence of feelings. Other parts are semantic memories; facts, concepts, and beliefs from a social life lived within a community, with shared histories, and traditions. Procedural memory, a form of implicit memory, is also utilized in collage making. Whereas cutting and pasting of the collage elements are automatic and non-declarative, titling the collage requires conscious efforts.

The emotional vividness elicited by the attractive and repulsive combinations of form and function invites viewers to explore the boundaries of their belief systems. Verbal interpretation may further move the observer and artist to new understanding and new memories. Research shows that memories triggered by emotionally-laden liter-ature arouse affect-prompted readers to resonate cognitively and emotionally with the mind of the author (Oatley 2003). Kara and Robin engaged in creating newer narratives of the art. Both found how artworks can shift between several interpretations as they evoke many forms of emotional memory. When resonating with memories of being connected (non-alone) or like others, Robin noticed that autobiographical memory, the distinctly personal memory that makes me into myself, strengthened her sense of self.

Implicit memory doesn't require conscious processing for either encoding or retrieval. When an infant is exposed to a loud noise, that sound is unconsciously, auto-matically linked to a sense of fear and perhaps a startle reaction. When the infant hears a loud noise in the future, she is automatically startled and afraid. Due to evolutionary demands, the brain works to anticipate, constantly shaping information about the future or present based upon past perceptions and models. Implicit memory primes us for survival from threats of all kinds (Cozolino 2002; LeDoux 2002; Siegel 1999). By one year of age, many patterns of implicit memory are firmly built into the brain. Repeated attachment experiences, positive or negative, are juggled in the neural networks of the brain, so much so, that they become personality traits of the person. This juggling happens automatically—outside of recall—and informs who we are and who we will become (Siegel 2001; Figure 9.4).

Implicit memory builds up unconscious generalized summaries of experiences, which help us learn from the past, anticipate future experiences, and quickly react to survival threats (Siegel 1999). Implicit memory forms mental models responsible for themes underlying the stories we tell, the in-between-the-lines qualities in our narra-tives. Unconscious processing influences behaviors, feelings, and thoughts (Siegel 1999). We may believe that our decisions are based on our objective review of available data and possible choices, but mostly our decisions about who we are and what we do are based upon the bubbling up of quick implicit memories, sensations, and projections.

Hidden, unconscious, implicit memory structures tend to be conservative and ego-centric—they hold onto memories that have worked thus far to ensure survival, so we persevere in attending to what supports our beliefs and ignore what contradicts them; this is belief perseverance. This is why negative self-beliefs persist and even why racial prejudice tends to endure despite evidence to the contrary (Cozolino 2002).

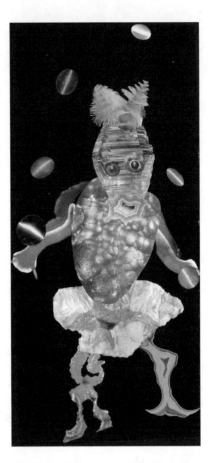

Figure 9.4 Juggler. *The figure sways, absorbed in maintaining her balance to accommodate the juggling of many spinning balls. Her head and torso are shimmery rainbow hues. Her nudibranch arms are fuschia, one leg green and the other blue. Robin Vance, 19.5" × 44". Media: Xeroxed collage on paper.*

Explicit memory

Explicit memory is the conscious access to remembering, which evolves with the development of language expression and comprehension at 18 months. Explicit memory brain structures include the medial temporal lobe, parts of the hippocampus, and the orbitofrontal cortex (Kalat 2004; Figure 9.1).

There are different types of explicit memory. The semantic-factual memory involves the memory of the meaning that we assign to an image of a colorful butterfly wing that we insert into a collage image of the self (Figure 9.5).

Semantic memory is encoded in the left hippocampus and the left prefrontal cortex (Figure 9.1). Semantic memories feel experientially different from other types of explicit memory because they are mostly anchored in language and come from left hemispheric activation centers.

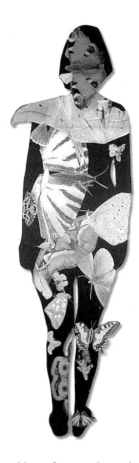

Figure 9.5 Butterfly. *Spotted and striped butterflies crowd in and around the black silhouette of the artist's body. They vibrate with flight, delicately probing the body with proboscises, transitory beauty: blues, oranges, and pinks. Robin Vance, 18" × 59.5". Media: Xeroxed collage on gatorboard.*

Episodic memory, another type of explicit memory, maps and binds together pieces of semantic memory. Semantic memory tells you what a spring butterfly looks like, while episodic memory tells you about the first spring butterfly you saw last spring. All new experiences of butterflies will modify that semantic representation of a butterfly. Robin's memories are further modified by the memory of how the butterflies surrounding her body felt. Did her memory of her body as heavy or light change? Autonoetic self-aware or self-perceiving autobiographical memory also updates through experience (Figure 9.5).

Autonoetic awareness of episodic memory coordinates with information from other multi-layered, cerebral lobes. Spatial information stored in the posterior parietal lobe becomes sequenced and organized while executive functions arise from prefrontal regulation of diffuse brain processes, negotiating self-awareness, social insight, and limbic feelings (Siegel 1999). Autonoetic memories are the implicit, non-declarative memories that involve sensory information and perception of episodic events.

Episodic memory sequencing probably stems from the hippocampal role of cognitive mapping. This enormously enhancing survival skill provides us with the ability to make four-dimensional models of ourselves in the world across time. In the second year, children begin expressing a more sophisticated view of themselves. They start showing a sense of time dependent upon knowing the order in which things happen (Siegel 1999, 2001). By two years of age, narratives between parents and children become co-constructed at a rate of 2.2 per hour during regular conversations. The stories connect, give meaning, and translate reality. Parents, being self-aware at this point, teach their children self-awareness by encouraging their kids to share their own narratives (Cozolino 2002).

Autobiographical memory, a subtype of episodic memory, presents the unique sense of one's self in the past, present, and future. Autobiographical memory encodes in the right hippocampus and the right orbitofrontal cortex. Autobiographical memory is a mental time travel (Siegel 2001). Autobiography includes memories of specific personal events, such as when one first used paint in school; memories of general art-making events; a gestalt of making art over the years; or personal facts such as the United States President when you were born. Emotions intensify memories. Emotional situations yield especially enduring and vivid memories known as flashbulb memories. These can happen in response to an outstanding public event that powerfully impacts millions, like Princess Diana's tragic death in 1997, or in response to a personal event (Kandel 2006; LeDoux 2002; Pillemer 1998; Van der Kolk 1996). The common features of flashbulb memories are a high degree of surprise, high consequentiality, and repeated verbal and mental rehearsal, with strong persistence. They return you to somewhere else like *Jumping Through*. The visceral intensity of *Jumping Through* bypasses normal constraints, and puts experiencing directly into emotional appraisal (Figure 9.6).

The amygdala is highly involved in the emotional intensification of explicit memory and its appraisal. The probing anemone tentacles of *Changeling* stir the appraisal of the psychological interactions of emotion and memory (cover image). The evaluation is largely unconscious because the engaged limbic areas activate unconsciously. Emotional arousal causes the amygdala to stimulate adrenaline and noradrenaline release from the adrenal medulla activating the brain, and further stimulating the amygdala (LeDoux 2002). Through connections with the hippocampus, the amygdala increases consolidation of explicit memories created during emotional arousal. Later, these vivid memories of the original event are easily retrieved. The amygdala stores memories about threatening situations in its own network and contributes to the formation of new explicit hippocampal memory formations (LeDoux 2002). *Changeling* is expected to arouse an emotional reaction in viewers that will contribute to seeing the amalgamation of the collage cutouts as a new whole (cover page).

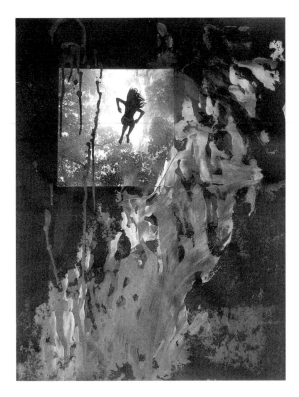

Figure 9.6 Jumping Through *is about amassing one's personal agency to risk crossing into unknown cognitive or emotional territories. The figure jumps into a light source that bathes the piece in blues and greys. Robin Vance, 19.5" × 25.5". Media: Xeroxed collage, gouache, and tempera on paper.*

Autobiographical memory is less about truth than one's expectations of what various memories should be like (Tulving 2002). Older schemas and positive or negative expectations enslave and subordinate autobiographical memory mechanisms. All spatial/temporal/perceptual information is first interpreted by semantic memory where our beliefs about such details and the unique qualities of specific experiences are kept, awaiting encoding. General beliefs and expectations determine what is retrieved. They include sensory inputs and implicit theories about how people, including oneself, are; the nature of memory, wishes, and desires that become automatically activated during our experiences. Both true and false memories form in the same way. Folk wisdom suggests that we remember what we remember because we believe what we believe (Windhorst 2005). We tend to assume that choices, which are the outcomes of memory, are more beneficial or attractive than non-choice options. We tend to distort reality so that I believe what I choose is the best and what is mine is good (Mather, Shafir, and Johnson 2003). In making art products, clients activate many procedural and autobiographical choices while forming a visual narrative. Therapeutic encouragement reinforces their sense of agency, and art-making allows clients to adjust past views/beliefs about their abilities to express themselves. Successful art-making enhances the memory of self as capable.

The process of recollection itself modifies memories. In *Dance*, internal and external cues, as well as explicit and implicit memories of color and form, find abstract and concrete expression (Figure 9.2). In the artist's mind, the art qualities mingle and interface with the declarative intentions of the artists and with other unpredictable cues, like somatic representations of pain. Vivid original memories and highly relived memories almost always have strong visual images associated with them (Rubin, Schrauf, and Greenberg 2003). Salient visual imagery triggers working memory adding to older, stored information. Therefore, the memory of events, especially emotionally charged events, often differs significantly from what actually happened. We continually rework modified memories (LeDoux 2002; Siegel 1999). *Dance* reminds us that a memory is a pattern of networks that interact amongst themselves and with neurons from other networks (Figure 9.2). Art pieces are continuous reconstructed memories. The involvement of divergent networks provides for unique connections (Sapolsky 2005) that can be accessed by creativity.

Working memory/rehearsal/priming

Working memory is our capacity to hold temporarily onto information that is useful in completing a task as we are performing that task and updating our memories. *Dance's* central cascade displays the temporary machinations of working memory during which a variety of representations from implicit memory are recalled, recognized, and thus updated (Figure 9.2).

Initially, neural activation of our perceptual system lasts about a quarter to a half second. From numerous, varied sensory items, only selected items occupy working memory for about half a minute, providing there's no further rehearsal (D'Esposito and Postle 2002). Images or words processed by working memory may be encoded in and then stored to long-term memory. Functional magnetic resonance imaging (fMRI) shows hippocampal involvement in long-term memory formation a few years after memories are stored in the frontal lobes. However, it seems that the entorhinal cortex, a subcortical area just below the orbital frontal cortex and adjacent to the midbrain structures, sustains memory consolidation processes for up to 20 years (Haist, Gore, and Mao 2001; Figure 9.1). Working memory, short-term memory and long-term memory are regulated by separate brain subsystems. Sometimes these memory, systems utilize the same brain structures, and at others, different brain structures. Supported by a vast variety of molecular mechanisms, some appear to be linked (McDonald, Devan, and Hong 2004).

The strength of one's working memory correlates with one's capacity to learn and to manipulate new information (Gathercole and Alloway 2006). Thinking about something, we reflect upon the present and recall items from the past, as illustrated in

Juggler (Figure 9.4). Our cognitive process allows us to link various representations and juggle them, within the prefrontal cortex. Linkage is essential for short-term memory. Short-term memory does not require the protein production that long-term memory needs. Instead, it relies on the functional connections amongst neural networks (Siegel 2001).

Scientific studies suggested that working memory is a function of three different functional components: the phonological loop juggling and retaining auditory linguistic material; the visuo-spatial sketchpad holding onto visual and spatial representations that are like moving balls; and the episodic buffer using information stored in long-term memory about how to juggle and integrate information into the logic and decision-making process of working memory. The central executive system in the brain supports the processing of working memory (Gathercole and Alloway 2006).

Rehearsal, part of the phonological loop of working memory, involves silent practicing of phonological/auditory representations in order to refresh an individual's understanding of an utterance or auditory stimulation. Rehearsal increases the potential for a working memory to become long-term memory. In a therapeutic or academic context, rehearsal can be invoked by encouraging an individual to practice using a word at first vocally (i.e. repeating a word after reading it) and then shifting to a sub-vocal rehearsal of the word (Gathercole and Alloway 2006).

Stress has a strong effect on working memory. When stress hormones are released, working memory may be inhibited. High levels of stress significantly inhibit working memory and are associated with continuous cortisol release that can diminish hippocampal volume (Elzinga and Roelofs 2005; Sapolsky 2004). A small amount of stress promotes short-term memory function. Experiments show that elevated levels of cortisol without high levels of stress do not result in impaired working memory (Elzinga and Roelofs 2005).

Constant amygdala arousal can also change processing in the sensory cortex due to its part in all its stages of processing stressors. Amygdala overload obstructs our normal ability to focus on one thing at a time, and ignore irrelevant stimuli. A damaged amygdala allows implicitly processed, unconscious emotional stimuli to slip into working memory and into consciousness in overwhelming ways (LeDoux 2002; Sapolsky 2004).

Long-term memory

Consolidation is the development of long-term memories resulting from the repetitive stimulation of neural connections in the brain over months or even years. Every time a memory is activated, neural connections constructing the memory are stimulated and the neural network is strengthened. During consolidation, memory location shifts in the brain from the hippocampus to the entorhinal cortex and then the neocortex. Long-term memory seems to take place in the hippocampus, entorhinal cortex, perirhinal cortex, parahippocampal cortex, and amygdala of the medial temporal lobe. Early in consolidation, networks in the medial temporal lobe are stimulated, strengthening connections between and within neocortical areas. Some researchers believe consolidation requires a non-conscious activation or rehearsal process that allows representations to be stored in the cerebral cortex. Consolidation of memory, the repetition of neural networks, situates long-term memory permanently in the prefrontal cortex. The constellation of *Figure Group* exemplifies rehearsal amplifications (Figure 9.7).

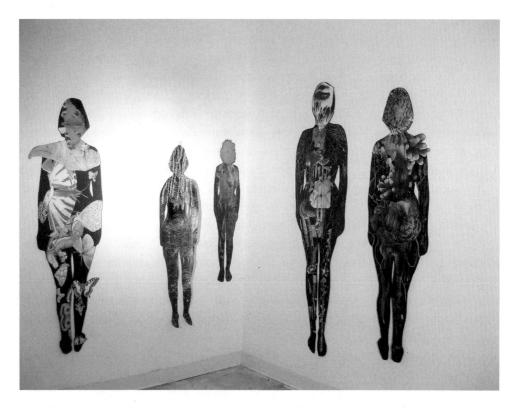

Figure 9.7 Detail of Figure Group. *The figures represent different aspects and phases of Robin's life and personality. The changing scale contributes to a view of how the long-term sense of self changes over time with rehearsal. Robin Vance, Media: Gouache, tempera, oil pastel, xeroxed collages on gatorboard.*

Consolidation requires that various records integrate during memory storage processes (Eichenbaum 2001; Haist *et al.* 2001), thereby freeing the hippocampus from the need for retrieval. Without focal attention, items are encoded implicitly (Siegel 2001). The process of making sense of the day's activities is believed to be dependent upon the rapid-eye-movement of the REM sleep stage. Older people often remember the events of their youths in detail but have difficulty with new information. That's because long-term memories distributed throughout the cortex are less sensitive to the aging effects than short- and medium-term memories. Records are the products of consolidation. Neural records are stored in both visual and verbal formats, making it possible for someone to remember the ocean in a variety of ways (Figure 9.8).

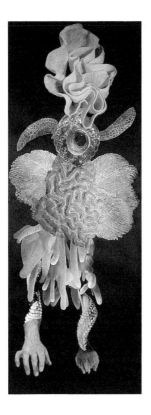 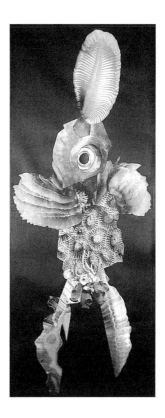

Figure 9.8(a)–(b) Ocean Selves 1 and 2. *Robin refers to these images as self-portraits before evolution into human form, enjoying the ocean as a coral/fish/sea squirt being. Every underwater hue is in evidence: livid oranges, blues, pinks, and green. Robin Vance, Ocean Self 1: 19.25"×53", Ocean Self 2: 19.5"×58". Media xeroxed collages on paper.*

Ocean Selves 1 and 2 displays Robin's memory of swimming in the Pacific Ocean, drawn from the ocean's darkness and memories of sea creatures from vacations, movies, and books. They recall her overall somatic feeling of being in the ocean. The strength of a neural record refers to how often someone uses a particular record. If it is strong, it is easily accessible to recall with conscious thought. A high-strength record is something well consolidated into long-term memory and often primed, such as an individual's first name. Priming a recent and frequent exposure to a stimulus connects it to a record or neural network. When an individual is primed to a stimulus, the records or neural networks that inform the individual's understanding of that stimulus are more easily accessible (Byrnes 2001).

Recognition is the non-verbal or implicit understanding an individual holds of a record, such as in *Ocean Selves* where clues to swimming experiences with sea creatures are juxtaposed (Figure 9.8). In recognition, the individual has prior somatic experience. Sensory inputs, visual, taste, smell, and touch, inform recognition. Recognition can be understood as an external experience that we match seamlessly with an internal representation like when someone sees a familiar person (Byrnes 2001).

Summary

In this chapter we recognized how memory systems were expressed in art-making. The artwork can be an expression of several types of memories as it engages multiple cognitive and perceptual neural pathways processes. The serious play of the art process updates memories, and supports a broader and more flexible personal agency. Our work afforded us the opportunity to re-remember the self.

References

Altmann, E. M. and Gray, W. D. (2002). Forgetting to remember: The functional relationship of decay and interference. *Psychological Science, 13*(1), 27–33.

Baddeley, A., Bueno, O., Cahill, L., Fuster, J., Ixquierdo, I., McGaugh, J., *et al.* (2000). *The Brain Decade in Debate: I. Neurobiology of Learning and Memory. Brazilian Journal of Medical and Biological Research, 33*: 993-1002.

Biederman, I. and Kalocsai, P. (1997). Neurocomputational bases of object and face recognition. *Philosophical Transactions of the Royal Society: B series, 352*(1358), 1203–1219.

Byrnes, J. P. (2001). *Minds, Brains, and Learning: Understanding the Psychological and Educational Relevance of Neuroscientific Research.* New York: Guilford Press.

Carlson, N. R. (2001). *Physiology of Behavior.* Boston, MA: Allyn and Bacon.

Carter, R. (1998). *Mapping the Mind.* Los Angeles, CA: University of California Press.

Cozolino, L. (2002). *The Neuroscience of Psychotherapy: Building and Rebuilding the Human Brain.* New York: W. W. Norton & Co.

D'Esposito, M. and Postle, B. R. (2002). The neural basis of working memory storage, rehearsal, and control processes: Evidence from patient and functional magnetic resonance imaging studies. In L. R. Squire and D. L. Schacter (eds), *Neuropsychology of Memory* (pp.215–224). New York: Guilford Press.

Eichenbaum, H. (2001). The long and winding road to memory consolidation. *Nature Neuroscience, 4*(11), 1057–1058.

Elzinga, B. M. and Roelofs, K. (2005). Cortisol-induced impairments of working memory require acute sympathetic activation. *Behavioral Neuroscience, 119*(1), 98–103.

Gathercole, S. E. and Alloway, T. P. (2006). Practitioner Review: Short-term and working memory impairments in neurodevelopmental disorders: Diagnosis and remedial support. *Journal of Child Psychology and Psychiatry, 47*(1), 4–15.

Haist, F., Gore, J. B., and Mao, H. (2001). Consolidation of human memory over decades revealed by functional magnetic resonance imaging. *Nature Neuroscience, 4*(11), 1139–1145.

Kalat, J. W. (2004). *Biological Psychology* (8th edition). Belmont, CA: Thomson/Wadsworth.

Kandel, E. R. (2006). *In Search of Memory: The Emergence of a New Science of Mind.* New York: W.W. Norton & Co.

LeDoux, J. (2002). *Synaptic Self: How Our Brains Become Who We Are.* New York: Penguin Group.

McDonald, R. J., Devan, B. D., and Hong, N. S. (2004). Multiple memory systems: The power of interactions. *Neurobiology of Learning and Memory, 82*(3), 333–346.

Mather, M., Shafir, E., and Johnson, M. (2003). Remembering chosen and assigned options. *Memory and Cognition, 31*(3), 422–433.

Oatley, K. (2003). Creative expression and communication of emotions in the visual and narrative arts, In R. J. Davidson, K. R. Scherer, and H. H. Goldsmith (eds) *Handbook of Affective Sciences* (pp.481–502). New York: Oxford University Press.

Pillemer, D. B. (1998). *Momentous Events, Vivid Memories.* Cambridge, MA: Harvard University Press.

Rubin, D. C., Schrauf, R. W., and Greenberg, D. L. (2003). Belief and recollection of autobiographical memories. *Memory and Cognition, 31*(6), 887–901.

Sapolsky, R. M. (2004). Stressed-out memories: A little stress sharpens memory. But after prolonged stress, the mental picture isn't pretty. *Scientific American Mind, 14*(5), 28–34.

Sapolsky, R. (2005). *Biology and Human Behaviors: The Neurological Origins of Individuality,* Part I (2nd edition). Chantilly, VA: The Teaching Company.

Siegel, D. (1999). *The Developing Mind: Toward a Neurobiology of Interpersonal Experience.* New York: Guilford Press.

Siegel, D. (2001). Memory: An overview, with emphasis on developmental, interpersonal, and neurobiological aspects. *Journal of the American Academy of Child and Adolescent Psychiatry, 40*(9), 997–1011.

Tulving, E. (2002). Episodic memory: From mind to brain. *Annual Review of Psychology, 53*, 1–25.

Van der Kolk, B. (1996). *Traumatic Stress: The Effects of Overwhelming Experience on Mind, Body, and Society.* New York: Guilford Press.

Walter, H., Bretschneider, V., Gron, G., Zurowski, B., Wunderlich, A. P., Tomczak, R., *et al.* (2003). Evidence for quantitative domain dominance for verbal and spatial working memory in frontal and parietal cortex. *Cortex, 39*(4–5), 897–911.

Windhorst, C. (2005). The slave model of autobiographical memory. *Cognitive Processing, 6*(4), 253–265.

10

Couples Art Therapy:
Gender Differences in Neuroscience

Jessica Tress Masterson

Why won't he listen to me? Why does she discuss a problem endlessly and then become angry when I quickly try to solve it? I'm frustrated with his simplicity; why does he insist on doing things one at a time, so methodically? Why does she become emotionally bonded by sex and I feel unaffected? Why does he make decisions quickly instead of talking things over with me? How neurobiological gender differences contribute to these miscommunications assists in modifying couples art therapy directives (Kwiatkowska 1967; Landgarten 1981; Riley 1991; Wadeson 1973) and helps provide more effective art therapy couples counseling.

Gender-based differences in brain functioning produce psychological changes in behavior that last a lifetime (Bear, Connors, and Paradiso 2002; Hiller 2004). From infancy, there is evidence of a verbal preference in the female brain and an action preference in the male brain (Cahill 2005). Infant boys track moving objects better, while infant girls recognize family faces more easily. High levels of testosterone predispose infant boys toward more aggressive and energetic activities (LeVay 1994). Infant girls respond differently than boys to frustration. Throughout the lifespan, girls are more likely to enlist the support of others while boys tend to approach problem-solving more independently (Zakriski, Wright, and Underwood 2005). Overall, evolutionary processes led male and female brains to develop characteristics associated with common gender roles: females as mothers/nurturers and males as hunters/gatherers (Blum 1998; Cahill 2006; Wood and Eagly 2002).

Female biases: brain structures, functions, and behaviors

An adult woman's corpus callosum is 25 percent larger than a man's, with 15 percent more blood flow to the brain (Gurian 2003; Figure 10.1).

Because the corpus callosum supports communication between right and left hemispheres, this difference allows female brains to more easily connect feelings to words, make language out of emotional experiences, and use less activity than males in process-

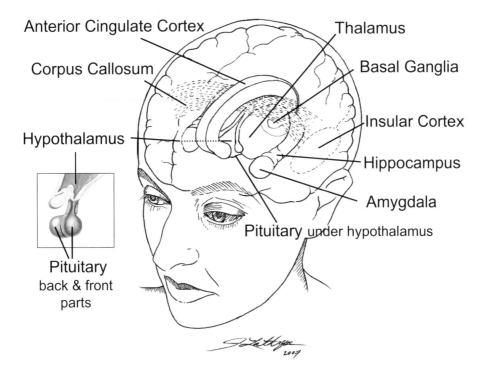

Figure 10.1 Midbrain and limbic diagram. Illustration by Jennifer Lathrope.

ing sensory information. It may take less effort for women to feel emotions and put them into words than for a man (Baron-Cohen 2003; Cahill 2005). Female brains have a strong capacity for communication and multi-tasking, and use high levels of brain activity to navigate three-dimensional problem-solving tasks (Kimura 2004). The female prefrontal cortex is larger and matures earlier than the male's. The size difference helps modify the amygdala's urges and allows women to practice impulse control, patience, the ability to sit still, relate to others, and concentrate for longer time periods (Brizendine 2006). Women have livelier and bulkier insulas, a brain area which processes intuitive feelings. They tend to rely more on insight and are better able to infer and translate non-verbal clues, as well as access instinctual thoughts (Brizendine 2006). A woman's anterior cingulate cortex, located above the corpus callosum and involved with cognitive skills of balancing judgments and concerns, is larger than a man's. Therefore, women may experience higher levels of worrying, moodiness, and stress than men (Brizendine 2006). Women have strong neural connections in their temporal lobes that lead to detailed memory, acute listening skills, and highly sensitive hearing (Gurian and Stevens 2004).

The amygdala, the emotional brain, is smaller in women, with more neural linkage to the frontal cortex, which may lead to decreased aggression, ease at regulating emotions, enhanced impulse control, and intense awareness of fear responses. These differences may contribute to women taking fewer chances on average. Women also typically remain emotionally centered and able to decipher emotional cues at an instinctual level. They, on average, are more inclined to self-imposed worry when depressed (Hall *et al.* 2004). Differences in amygdala size may also contribute to differences in how men and women experience empathic experiences (Gurian 2003).

The learning and emotional memory center of the brain, the hippocampus, is larger in women, heightening their ability to recall emotional memories and landmark physical environments. Women navigate a course by observing familiar objects; men approximate space (Cahill 2005; Kimura 2004). Women may remember emotional details, colors, textures, and designs, as well as visualize and verbalize their memories more easily (Brizendine 2006). Due to hippocampal differences, a woman's learning ability may be impaired under stress while a man's may be enhanced (Wood and Shors 1998); however, chronic stress causes less damage to a woman's hippocampus (Cahill 2006).

The pituitary gland and the hypothalamus regulate hormones throughout one's life. Many affect gender and pregnancy. The secretion of different amounts of serotonin and oxytocin by the hypothalamus shifts one's ability to bond emotionally (Gurian 2003; Janov 2000). The female hypothalamus responds to high hormone levels by triggering additional secretions. Higher hormone levels dramatically affect behavior and may stimulate gender-related communication differences not explained by context or circumstance. The male hypothalamus may contribute different effects as well (Moir and Jessel 1991). Psycho-educational information on female-male brain neurochemistry and brain structures is helpful for therapists and clients as it contributes to mutual understanding.

Male biases: brain structures, functions, and behaviors

Testosterone exerts strong influences upon the male system, furthering development of compartmentalized and lateralized brain hemispheres (Baron-Cohen *et al.* 2005). With a smaller corpus callosum, higher testosterone levels, and less hemispheric integration, a man's ability to complete one task and then systematically move on to the next is enhanced. Testosterone surges sway right hemisphere functioning toward spatial ability preferences, influencing the development of technical skills and mechanical exploration (Baron-Cohen *et al.* 2005; Geiger and Litwiller 2005; Kimura 2004; LeVay 1994). Hemispheric specialization helps men excel at tasks involving navigational aptitude and the ability to retrace a route taken only once (Baron-Cohen, Lutchmaya, and Knickmeyer 2004; Geiger and Litwiller 2005; Kimura 2004). Testosterone encourages risk tolerance in men, as well as the tendency to seek excitement and high-risk activities

(Discovery Channel 2003). Testosterone levels contribute to goal-focused and quick decision-making behaviors as well as to a tendency for problem-solving. Men may also more readily enjoy mechanical activities, and may more easily compartmentalize emotions than women (Gurian and Stevens 2004).

The male hippocampus, a structure related to memory functions, is especially facile during spatial tasks (Baron-Cohen 2003; Cahill 2005; Kimura 2004). This inherent bias leads men toward action, instead of verbal explanation (Gurian 2003). Due to higher secretion of testosterone, the hypothalamus is typically larger in the male brain, which is related to spatial skills development (Baron-Cohen 2003). The male sex drive is also stimulated by visual-spatial information; hence, the male propensity towards pornographic material (Fisher *et al.* 2002).

Emotion starts with limbic responses that are more directly connected to the right hemisphere. The production of speech, as well as differences between meanings of words or symbols, are more directly processed in the left hemisphere. Speech is also processed by tone, pausing, and metaphorical meanings, which are right hemisphere functions. With fewer hemispheric connections, men use more of the brain's energy to process emotional content and verbalize emotions. Men have fewer neural connections in their temporal lobes, resulting in less detailed emotional memory, and may feel less comfortable processing facial emotions. Men tend first to recognize a face before figuring out the emotion; women process both simultaneously (Proverbio *et al.* 2006). The amygdala is usually larger in men, with fewer links to the frontal lobes. This distinction leads to increased aggression; higher heart rate; quick, aggressive action in arousing situations; and decreased ability to regulate emotions and impulses (Cahill 2005). During emotional stress, men may also use more analytical thinking to make systematic connections, whereas women may tend to rely on emotional memories (Hall *et al.* 2004).

The different approaches to dealing with events, some of which are delineated above, often lead to mis-attuned couples communication and may further complicate personal circumstances and environmental stressors.

Couples directives

Wadeson (1973) described the following advantages for couples art therapy: (1) working on a task together can immediately provide a renewed, shared sense of fun and pleasure; (2) drawing provides a concrete object to encounter, study, react to, and use for clarification/review; and (3) revealing the genuineness of unexpected material in the artwork challenges the couple's beliefs and assists the therapist's work.

Four directives were examined for gender influences: the Non-Verbal Joint Drawing (Wadeson 1973), the Abstract of the Marital Relationship (Wadeson 1973), the Two-Dimensional Bridge Drawing (modified from Gladding 1997) and the Three-Dimensional Bridge Sculpture (modified from Landgarten 1981). The editors, Noah and Richard, participated as consultants for the inquiry.

Gender responses to unknown situations

The Non-Verbal Joint Drawing directive (Wadeson 1973) asks a couple to draw a picture together without verbal communication. Drawing together without words may be an unfamiliar request for the couple. The request can stimulate a sense of loss of control in either participant and stress the joint decision-making methods used by the couple. Amygdala reactions may also shift problem-solving styles used by each gender (Tranel *et al.* 2005). Lack of familiarity with art therapy directives may stir unsafe and threatening emotions. Such feelings reflect right hemisphere activations, found subsequent to the stress responses in both genders.

Richard, a neuroscience expert and an art therapy novice, asked many role-play questions to figure out how to relate to the context before trying out the Non-Verbal Joint Drawing. He thought his responses reflected an attempt to gain control over unfamiliarity, reduce stress, and use systematic thinking, typical of how men problem-solve. Noah concurred. She had experienced similar goal-centered approaches to art therapy by other males in couples art therapy. Male brains generally lateralize, using left hemisphere dominance more than females. The dominance is expressed through linear cause-and-effect reasoning (Cahill 2005). As the directive is designed to facilitate emotional expression and interaction in couples, the possibility that its non-verbal nature may stimulate more angst in males than females needs to be considered. One hypothesis is that males who encounter unfamiliar contexts with sparse organizing cues choose to create specific and tangible goals to reduce stress. However, men typically become more open to learning while under stress (Shors *et al.* 2001; Wood and Shors 1998); therefore, the Non-Verbal Joint Drawing may provide a growth-oriented experience more than an expression of a man's conscious view of his relationship.

The female stress response differs. Reduced amygdala size and reactivity, along with a more active and enlarged corpus callosum, which facilitates better hemispheric communication, helps women verbally and emotionally fill in an unfamiliar directive. Consequently, females may find it easier and less stressful to participate in art therapy. Stress and a need for precise cues may be reduced and may lead a female to produce a more creative expression of the relationship. However, if a heightened stress response occurs, the flight or fight response may bring forth anger or withdrawal (Shors *et al.* 2001; Wood and Shors 1998). These differences suggest challenges in evaluating whether a couple's responses are more about their gender differences or a reaction to the unexpected request to participate non-verbally.

Drawing images of contents known to both partners such as faces, hands, and flowers reflect activated shared memory processes associated with hippocampal learning (Tulving 2002). Shared, known imagery invites couples to build common ground as a part of their interactive process. Abstract unknown content may activate amygdala-based emotions such as fear or anxiety (LeDoux 2003). Unknown imagery in couples' non-verbal joint drawing may stimulate distancing or challenge their ability to work together abstractly. Each type of drawing reveals the nature of the couple's ability to process new events together. The consultants reported that their attempt at creating a Non-Verbal Joint Drawing brought up significant emotional material, exposing gender differences in creative approaches, relationship interactions, stress responses, and individual processing.

Since gender-based stress reactions are triggered differently, the couples' emotional interaction may be significantly heightened by the Non-Verbal Joint Drawing directive. Consequently, for high conflict couples, it may be more appropriate first to offer the opportunity to engage in a joint verbal drawing. Sequencing the art directives appropriately may reduce some stress and help explore gendered contributions to joint decision-making and communication.

Relationship isolation and marital expectations

In the Abstract of the Marital Relationship Drawing directive (Wadeson 1973), each partner is asked individually to draw an abstract picture of their marital relationship and to title the drawing when finished (Figures 10.2 and 10.3).

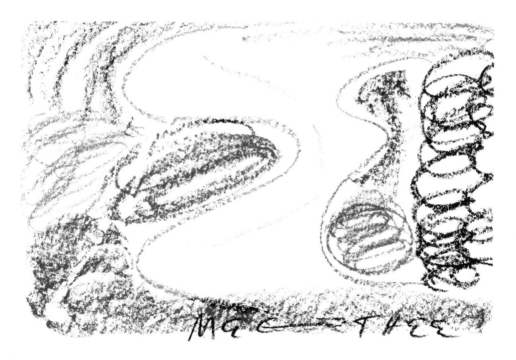

Figure 10.2 Me ⟵⟶ Thee: *male's drawing (Marital Relationship Drawing—Wadeson 1973). On the Me side are circular shapes of bright green, hot pink, and orange. In the center of the drawing, there is a blue and orange boundary with white space in the middle. On the Thee right side of the drawing are tight spirals of hot pink, red, and dark blue with a sky blue shape at the top. Across the bottom of the drawing is a heavy orange bar wherein the title, written in dark blue, is placed (Richard, role-play).*

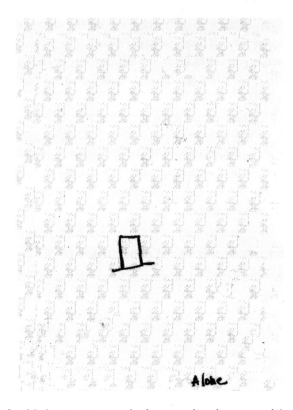

Figure 10.3 Alone: *female's drawing. Image and title in a medium brown pastel (Noah, role-play).*

Exploring the couples' drawings in relationship to each other rather than focusing on the individuals' point of view helps illustrate couples' relationships (Figures 10.2 and 10.3). Interpersonal practices can reveal relational aspects, stress, and coping mechanisms, as well as help couples define gender differences and pull together to change struggles. The role-play-consultation comparison between the highly expressive, drawing *Me* ←—→ *Thee*, and the smaller, solitary image in *Alone*, exemplifies these principles.

Me ←—→ *Thee*, characterized by strong colors and intermingling shapes, contrasts with *Alone*'s small, outlined hat-looking object. Comparing *Me* ←—→ *Thee* and *Alone* suggests that a common ground or bond is not evident to help address relational difficulties. *Me* ←—→ *Thee* may represent pleasure in the art process, reduced stress, and a creative interaction between non-verbal and representative processes—perhaps a bilateral brain response. *Alone* suggests withdrawal or a flight reaction, high stress, and therefore a fear-based amygdala reaction. The bleak landscape drawn in *Alone* seems to reflect diminished bonding (oxytocin) and reward-based (dopamine) functions necessary for females to diminish stress. Discussion revealed that this image represented unexpressed emotional overload, potentially right hemispheric overwhelm. Hypothetically, this reflected an impact of deficit oxytocin levels normally needed to diminish stress. Stimulating oxytocin by heightening one's sense of connectedness is a typical female right brain response to stress (Brizendine 2006; Taylor *et al.* 2000). At a time of relational stress, this kind of drawing may reflect either heightened awareness of internal stress and/or attunement to relational difficulties. *Alone* may be more representative of the here-and-now relationship becoming unmanageable and of an ensuing stress response. In contrast, *Me* ←—→ *Thee* suggests an attempt to self-organize in the moment, paying attention to abstraction and utilizing color, texture, and shape. The art reflects a playful intrapersonal frame of mind that strives for control over any stress response. *Me* ←—→ *Thee* reflects hope, with a goal of inclusion, yet includes a defense against the stressors revealed in felt, but unexpressed, differences. The role-play may have activated reward-based, problem-solving circuitry seeking excitation and relief through an imagined connectedness. The verbal titling of the art helped in exploring these two very different drawings, underscoring the need for verbalization in building coherence.

The way each partner copes with disagreement and isolation may reflect gender-based differences. Discord can increase stressful interactions and additional friction reflecting gender-based, stress response differences (Shors *et al.* 2001; Wood and Shors 1998).

During the creation of the artwork and the discussions, each partner's stress reactions may have been activated, surfacing different coping skills. During stress, women often turn to other women for relief (Taylor *et al.* 2000). If the therapist is a female, the female partner may turn to her for support, attempting to reduce her stress, rather than work within the relationship. Or, as in *Alone*, she may retreat in reaction to fear-based response. As stress increases in women, the ability to communicate may diminish and flight or fight responses activate, whereas early stressors may motivate men to become emotionally active and utilize risk-taking behaviors, such as forthright verbal communication (Shors *et al.* 2001; Wood and Shors 1998). Gender-based differences in coping with stress may play a part in a couple's withdrawal from each other and their eventual isolation. Each may defend him/herself from the source of the stressful experience, which may be perceived as the other person. The identification of these tensions is one of the first crucial steps in couples art therapy.

Building bridges two- and three-dimensionally

The two-dimensional (2-D) bridge directive asks couples to draw together using verbal communication to create a bridge between their differences (Gladding 1997), whereas the three-dimensional (3-D) bridge sculpture involves the use of clay and verbal communication (Landgarten 1981). The consultants discussed how the 2-D directive may

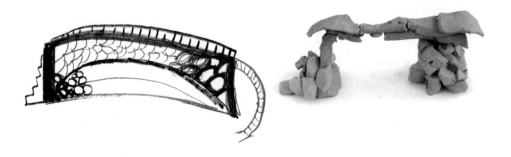

Figure 10.4 (left) and Figure 10.5 (right) Two- and three-dimensional bridge images (role-play).

produce more conflict than the 3-D directive, which reveals how verbal and emotional interactions can be altered depending upon the media used (Figures 10.4 and 10.5). The 2-D directive may seem vague and contradictory to male clients since the term "bridge" has multiple meanings which may be hard to conceptualize as a two-dimensional drawing. Ambiguity and abstraction may lead to a defensive mindset from the start, prompting questions like, "Don't give me any kind of abstraction, how am I going to solve this thing?" and "What are the differences we are trying to bridge?" A male might think in practical, structural terms and look for precise directions to solve the question logically. However, different individual and male responses may occur that express variation in mental functioning and problem-solving found along a continuum from male to female.

Communicating verbally while working creatively may increase frustration experienced by men. There are three tasks going on simultaneously: working creatively, communicating verbally, and combining words with emotions. Male brains tend to lateralize to one hemisphere (Baron-Cohen 2003; Kimura 2004), making this kind of multi-tasking potentially difficult. For females, communicating verbally while working creatively may be easier, as multi-tasking reflects an inter-hemispheric communication capacity found in female brains (Brizendine 2006).

A woman may experience her male partner's concentration on the task as a refusal to interact, possibly perceiving it as abandonment (although he may not realize that she interprets his lack of verbal interaction as a personal rejection). She also may not recognize his task-oriented focus as his way of joining. Her perception of the interaction removes one of the simpler female-based means for reducing stress: the tend-or-befriend response (Taylor *et al.* 2000). The satisfaction the woman derives from the bridge building directive may be more related to the experience of working together, whereas the man's satisfaction may arise from the drive to complete the bridge successfully (Gurian 2003). Similar differences for husbands and wives in attaining marital satisfaction have been noted by several researchers (Gottman and Krokoff 1989; Kriegelewicz 2006; Robin, Caspi, and Moffit 2000).

The 3-D directive (Figure 10.5) provides concrete objectives, which could alleviate some of the difficulties posed by the 2-D directive. Working three-dimensionally may offer a more tangible sense of completion along with a product to own. The accessibility of 3-D media creates a fluid, easily altered situation, where even without words, communication can occur. The purpose in this 3-D directive is to erect a bridge. The opportunity to work flexibly occurs from media that allows creative changes to be made. Potentially, this promotes balanced left and right hemispheric involvement in both genders. Male partners may prefer the end product of this work and understand that goal as part of the initial directive. Thus, the directive may appeal to the male brain, which tends towards working within the mechanical, spatial-kinesthetic centers, as well as valuing concrete 3-D objects (Gurian 2003). Women are more likely than men to hold emotional or internalized representations of their relationship. Increased cross-hemispheric interactions and social networking facilitated by their larger corpus callosum may be responsible for the difference (Brizendine 2006). Visualizing relational differences may stimulate emotional involvement for a woman, allowing her to work fluidly with either media.

Following a 2-D directive with a 3-D directive can contribute to increased familiarity with the art requests and may reduce potential stressors, thereby facilitating more communication and/or satisfaction. Repeating a couples' directive while utilizing another media may help undo tension and communication issues. Sequencing similar yet different directives can build familiarity of context, reduce stress, and increase anticipation of mutual success.

Differences vibrate through interpersonal relationships over time and may create long-term stress. The challenge for art therapists is to disentangle couples from these recursive layers of interpersonal stress. The 3-D directive offers help by engaging more physical senses and motor skills than drawing. The task's requirements facilitate resolution of a sympathetic nervous system (SNS) flight or fight response more easily for males than females. Manipulating 3-D media and striving to complete a tangible product can provide a felt sense of mastery and control, which reduces stress. Working in a 3-D format activates the right hemisphere, which is also more directly connected into the autonomic nervous system (Schore 1994). Hypothetically, the 2-D directive verbal exchanges could impact the SNS more than the 3-D manipulation of the clay. The bridge directive may reveal different gender-based solutions to stressors utilized by couples, thus providing the art therapist with a window into the role of stress and its tolerance during the relating process. When partners have the opportunity to reduce stress responses that are related to gender differences, they can be more available to each other.

Seating arrangement

Structuring the therapeutic environment, primarily the seating arrangement of the couple with the art therapist, may also activate gender-based brain responses (Figure 10.6).

If the couple is seated in the side by side seating arrangement (Figure 10.6), the partners' access to each other's emotional, facial expressions is more limited. Visual and auditory fields are functionally lateralized. Therefore, the hemisphere that processes stimulation in any of these fields interprets the stimulation differently. A left hemisphere interpreting what is seen in the right visual field of both eyes will be biased to supply missing cues intellectually, increasing a likelihood of interpretive associations (Cozolino 2002). In the seating chart, this biases the partner on the right of the other. The right hemisphere in the other will sense unfolding emotions perceived by left visual fields in both eyes, and establish emotional resonance with the expressions seen creating an affective bias. The left ear shows a bias towards information processing, while the right ear displays an advantage in processing emotional cues (Kalat 2004; Sininger and Cone-Wesson 2004). To overcome this, each partner must face the other fully to

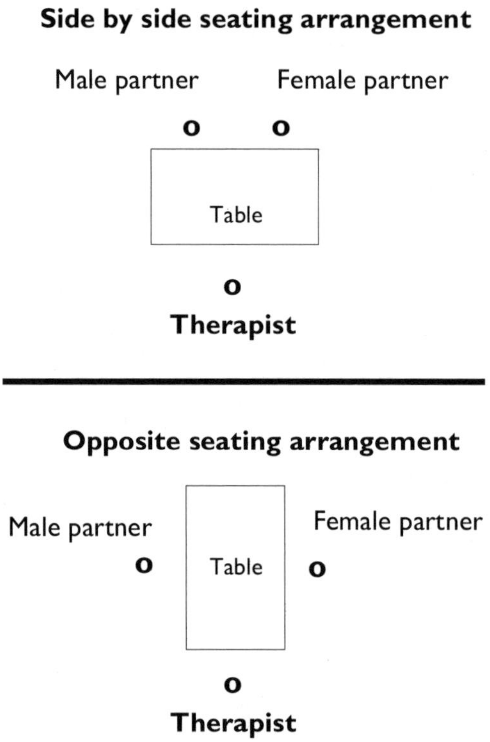

Side by side seating arrangement

Male partner   Female partner

o   o

Table

o
Therapist

Opposite seating arrangement

Male partner   Female partner

o   Table   o

o
Therapist

Figure 10.6 Seating arrangements. Side by side seating arrangement: Couple next to each other with therapist across from couple (top). Opposite seating arrangement: Couple across from each other with therapist at end of table (bottom).

neutralize these biases (Figure 10.6). For example, a right-handed woman seated to a right-handed man's left will have to turn to her right to address him fully. Otherwise, her right visual hemi-field biases the processing of his actions, thus facilitating more non-emotional left hemispheric sensing; vice versa if she sits to his right. Possibly, a woman's increased inter-hemispheric communication facilitated by her larger corpus callosum may moderate this. If so, she may experience less bias in sensing his presence. A man seated to the woman's right would turn toward his left to address her fully, predisposing a right hemisphere bias (Gazzaniga 1995). Increased right hemispheric activation in a man, along with the non-verbal aspects of the directive, may increase his anxiety due to the gender-based left hemisphere bias in male functioning.

An opposite seating arrangement (Figure 10.6) may facilitate fuller processing of emotions. In the opposite seating arrangement, each partner can see and respond to the other's whole face and the art. The amygdala, the gateway to emotional processing (Appleton and Mishkin 1986), and SNS-based stress responses are more easily stimulated in this arrangement. The amygdala is very reactive to faces (Phelps and LeDoux 2005). Full processing of facial expressions allows each partner and the therapist to access and respond to the other's emotions more easily. However, men and women may lateralize and interpret facial expressions differently (Proverbio *et al.* 2006). Therefore, depending upon the degree of conflict between the couple, sitting opposite each other may become overwhelming, in which case a side by side seating arrangement may be a good alternative.

The consequences of both seating arrangements should be considered during therapy. However, the therapist also needs to attune to how each person in couples therapy is seated relative to the therapist. Hemispheric communication and interpretive biases exist in reading the therapist's face as well as in listening to the therapist's voice.

Gender-based therapeutic inquiry

Acknowledging gender differences allows therapists to understand conflict more confidently in the light of gender specifics without exciting blame or defensiveness. Specific gender-based questions may further help reveal how couples regulate their differences circumstantially and during stress responses. The inquiry may help couples accept their differences and acknowledge relationship conflicts while more readily alleviating blame and guilt (Table 10.1).

Discussing these questions as well as exploring the art's titles offers significant insights for understanding the way creative work affects gender-biased brains. Dialogue is integral to gender-based inquiries. Emotional responses and non-verbal body language have been found to be more directly processed in the right hemisphere (Schore 2001), while verbal language processing dominates left hemisphere functioning (Gurian and Stevens 2004). Verbalization allows creative material to move from non-verbal to verbal, and therefore also allows the emotion to travel from the limbic

Table 10.1 Questions for therapeutic inquiry.

Examples of gender-based therapeutic inquiry questions

- Did you feel the need to organize the picture or sculpture? Did it seem abstract, confusing, or okay?
- Was letting the picture unfold in front of you acceptable or did you prefer a pre-planned outcome approach?
- Did you prefer working with specific familiar images and/or with unknown and abstract novel images?
- Was the 3-D exercise more or less satisfying than the 2-D exercise?
- Was the art interaction with your partner an opening of intimate communication? Why or why not?
- Did the art interaction contribute to your stress? If so, which feelings did you experience?
- How did talking before, during, and after the art directives work for either of you?

system to the right prefrontal orbital lobe across the corpus callosum to the left hemisphere (Cozolino 2002). Without making the switch back to the verbal area, done by titling the artwork, emotions may remain cycling in continuous, unconscious, action circuits resulting in relational conflict.

Couples' relational stages

Additional areas of inquiry may arise from understanding which biologically driven relational stages—lust, romantic passion, or attachment—the couple may be experiencing. The lust stage can provoke romantic obsession, developed primarily to ensure reproduction of the species (Aron *et al.* 2005). Lust is driven primarily by the sex hormones: testosterone, vasopressin, estrogen, and oxytocin, all of which cause men and women to bond differently (Fisher *et al.* 2002). Differing hormonal levels and responses explain why men and women often misinterpret the emotional significance in intimate sexual contact.

The romantic passion stage evolved to facilitate the need for bonding and caring of children. Serotonin, dopamine, norepinephrine, and oxytocin play important roles at this time (Diamond 2003). During this stage, couples spend many hours together building an emotional union and focusing upon mates' positive qualities. Oxytocin is released by both sexes during sexual activity promoting a romantic love bond. Increased levels of dopamine in the central nervous system cause couples to believe their love object, the other person, is unique, and thoughts of being with another partner often disappear (Fisher *et al.* 2002). Due to the intense bonding, it is less likely that couples will present for therapy during this stage of relating.

The attachment stage is signified by a longer lasting commitment and bond, which helps keep couples together when they have children. Attachment phases are associated with close body contact, separation anxiety, and a sense of calm, security, and peace with a partner of choice. In most couples, passionate love and sexual attraction tend to fade as attachment grows (Fisher *et al.* 2002). Unless couples transition to an attachment phase, it is quite likely they will break off the relationship and start searching for a new mate as this stage begins. Once attachment is formed and infatuation has diminished, hormone levels return to a balance (Bartels and Zeki 2003).

Summary

There are multiple advantages to incorporating clinical neuroscience information with art therapy practices. Sensitivity to gender-based media preferences and fine tuning directives contribute to enhanced communication. Gender-based relational stress may emerge through gender sensitive inquiry and reveal itself in the couple's seating arrangement and in the art. Exploring the couple's relational stages helps determine which biochemistry changes contribute to vulnerabilities in the couple's relationship. Finally, taking into account the therapist's gender and providing psycho-education about gender-related differences may serve to make art therapy with couples more balanced and successful.

References

Appleton, J. P. and Mishkin, M. (1986). The amygdala: Sensory gateway to the emotions. In R. Plutchik and H. Kellerman (eds) *Emotion: Theory, Research and Experience (3)* (pp. 281–299). Orlando, FL: Academic Press.

Aron, A., Fisher, H., Mashek, D. J., Strong, G., Haifang, L., and Brown, L. L. (2005). Reward, motivation, and emotion systems associated with early-stage intense romantic love. *Journal of Neurophysiology, 94*, 327–337.

Baron-Cohen, S. (2003). *The Essential Difference, the Truth About the Male and Female Brain.* New York: Basic Books.

Baron-Cohen, S., Hackett, G., Knickmeyer, R. C., Raggatt, P., Taylor, K., and Wheelwright, S. (2005). Gender-typed play and amniotic testing. *Developmental Psychology, 41*(3), 517–528.

Baron-Cohen, S., Lutchmaya, S., and Knickmeyer, R. (2004). *Prenatal Testosterone in Mind.* Cambridge, MA: Massachusetts Institute of Technology.

Bartels, A. and Zeki, S. (2003). The neural correlates of maternal and romantic love. *NeuroImage, 21*, 1155–1166.

Bear, M. F., Connors, B. W., and Paradiso, M. A. (2002). *Neuroscience: Exploring the Brain* (2nd edition). Baltimore, MD: Lippincott Williams & Wilkins.

Blum, D. (1998). *Sex on the Brain, the Biological Differences between Men and Women.* New York: Penguin Books.

Brizendine, L. (2006). *The Female Brain.* New York: Morgan Road Books.

Cahill, L. (2006). Why sex matters for neuroscience. *Nature Reviews Neuroscience.* AOP, published online May 10, 2006.

Cahill, L. (2005). His brain, her brain. *Scientific American*, 40–47.

Cozolino, L. (2002). *The Neuroscience of Psychotherapy.* New York, London: Norton.

Diamond, L. M. (2003). What does sexual orientation orient? A biobehavioral model distinguishing romantic love and sexual desire. *Psych Review, 110*, 173–192.

Discovery Channel (2003). *Science of the Sexes: Different by Design;* DVD. Silver Spring, MD: Discovery Communications.

Fisher, H. E., Aron, A., Mashek, D., Li, H., and Brown, L. L. (2002). Defining the brain systems of lust, romantic attraction, and attachment. *Archives of Sexual Behavior, 31*, 413–419.

Gazzaniga, M. S. (1995). Principles of human brain organization derived from split-brain studies. *Neuron, 14*, 217–228.

Geiger, J. F. and Litwiller, R. M. (2005). Spatial working memory and gender differences in science. *Journal of Instructional Psychology, 32*(1), 49–57.

Gladding, S. T. (1997). The creative arts in groups. In H. Forester-Miller and J. A. Kottler (eds) *Issues and Challenges for Group Practitioners.* Denver, CO: Love.

Gottman, J. M. and Krokoff, L. J. (1989). Marital interaction and satisfaction: A longitudinal view. *Journal of Consulting and Clinical Psychology, 57,* 47–52.

Gurian, M. (2003). *What Could He Be Thinking? How a Man's Mind Really Works.* New York: St. Martin's Press.

Gurian, M. and Stevens, K. (2004). With boys and girls in mind. *Educational Leadership, 62*(3), 21–26.

Hall, G. B., Witelson, S. F., Szechtman, H., and Nahmias, C. (2004). Sex differences in functional activation patterns revealed by increased emotion processing demands. *Neuroreport, 15,* 219–223.

Hiller, J. (2004). Speculations on the links between feelings, emotions and sexual behavior: Are vasopressin and oxytocin involved? *Sexual and Relationship Therapy, 19*(4), 393–412.

Janov, A. (2000). *The Biology of Love.* New York: Prometheus Books.

Kalat, J. W. (2004). *Biological Psychology* (8th edition). Belmont, CA: Thomson/Wadsworth.

Kimura, D. (2004). Human sex differences in cognition: Fact not predicament. *Sexualities, Evolution and Gender, 6*(1), 45–53.

Kriegelewicz, O. (2006). Problem-solving strategies and marital satisfaction. *Polish Psychiatry, 2*(40), 245–259.

Kwiatkowska, H. Y. (1967). Family art therapy. *Family Process, 6*(1), 37–55.

Landgarten, H. B. (1981). *Clinical Art Therapy, a Comprehensive Guide.* New York: Brunner/Mazel Publishers.

LeDoux, J. (2003). *Synaptic Self: How Our Brains Become Who We Are.* New York: Penguin Group.

LeVay, S. (1994). *The Sexual Brain.* Cambridge, MA: Massachusetts Institute of Technology.

Moir, A. and Jessel, D. (1991). *Brain Sex: The Real Difference between Men and Women.* New York: Dell Publishing.

Phelps, E. A. and LeDoux, J. E. (2005). Contributions of the amygdala to emotion processing: From animal models to human behavior. *Neuron, 48,* 175–187.

Proverbio, A. M., Brignone, V., Matarazzo, S., del Zotto, M., and Zani, A. (2006). Gender differences in hemispheric asymmetry for face processing. *BMC Neuroscience, 7,* 44.

Riley, S. (1991). Couples therapy/art therapy: Strategic interventions for family of origin work. *Art Therapy, 8*(2), 4–9.

Robin, R. W., Caspi, A., and Moffit, T. E. (2000). Two personalities, one relationship: Both partner's personality traits shape the quality of their relationship. *Journal of Personality and Social Psychology, 79,* 251–259.

Schore, A. N. (1994). The experience dependent maturation of a regulatory system in the orbital prefrontal cortex and the origin of developmental psychopathology. *Development and Psychopathology, 8,* 59–87.

Schore, A. N. (2001). The effects of early relational trauma on right brain development, affect regulation, and infant mental health. *Infant Mental Health Journal, 22,* 201–269.

Shors, T. J. and Levner, B. (2003). Estogen-medicated effects on depression and memory formation in females. *Journal of Affective Disorders, 74,* 85–96.

Sininger, Y. S. and Cone-Wesson, B. (2004). Asymmetric cochlear processing mimics hemispheric specialization. *Science, 10*(305), 1581.

Taylor, S. E., Klein, L. C., Lewis, B. P., Gruenewald, T. L., Gurung, R. A., and Updegraff, J. A. (2000). Behavioral response to stress in females tend-and-befriend, not fight or flight. *Psychological Review, 107*(3), 411–429.

Tranel, D., Damasio, H., Denburg, N., and Bechara, A. (2005). Does gender play a role in functional asymmetry of ventromedial prefrontal cortex? *Brain, 128,* 2872–2881.

Tulving, E. (2002). Episodic memory: From mind to brain. *Annual Review of Psychology, 53,* 1–25.

Wadeson, H. (1973). Art techniques used in conjoint marital therapy. *American Journal of Art Therapy, 12*(3), 147–164.

Wood, W. and Eagly, A. H. (2002). A cross-cultural analysis of the behavior of women and men: Implications for the origins of sex differences. *Psychological Bulletin, 128*(5), 699–727.

Wood, G. E. and Shors, T. J. (1998). Stress facilitates classical conditioning in males, but impairs classical conditioning in females through activational effects of ovarian hormones. *Proceedings of the National Academy of Sciences USA, 95*(3), 4066–4071.

Zakriski, A. L., Wright, J. C., and Underwood, M. K. (2005). Gender similarities and differences in children's social behavior: Finding personality in contextualized patterns of adaptation. *Journal of Personality and Psychology, 88*(5), 844–855.

Part III

In Praxis

11

Circles of Attachment:
Art Therapy Albums

*Joanna Clyde Findlay, Margarette Erasme Lathan,
and Noah Hass-Cohen*

In my Haitian culture, Creole words most often used to describe an infant are terms of endearment: ti pitite, little one, the baby; ti moun, the little person. I recall the same words being used to describe older children as, in my case, eight-year-old twin girls. My twin sister, Joelle, and I would often be yelled after by passersbys: "gade ti pitit yo" (Hey little ones, look at the little ones). This was de rigueur in our native country. Children remain little ones from birth to ten.

A baby's brain delights in expressed feelings of love, excitement, and pleasurable experiences with mom, dad, and the community. She learns to self-calm if there is someone there to help guide and take that journey with them. Once self-calming behaviors are mastered, the baby masters sleeping through the night, the toddler explores her environment with ease, the three-year-old shares toys with peers at the park, the four-year-old tolerates frustrations with more patience, the ten-year-old engages in pro-social behaviors, the adolescent develops meaningful friendships, and the securely attached adult engages in trust-based relationships. When such a woman gets married and has babies of her own, she parents with an emphasis on attuned moments of love, holding, and positive emotion. (Margarette Lathan)

Introduction

Margarette Lathan showcases what infant, toddler, and adult attachment relatedness may look like. Noah Hass-Cohen and Joanna Clyde Findlay describe and show three-dimensional cloth-based attachment journals created by adult art therapists in training. Joanna, a trained MARI® Mandala practitioner (Kellogg 2002), found that spontaneous circles seemed to coalesce visuals with attachment states of mind as represented in Kellogg's 13 stages. We three authors, daughters and mothers, felt that writing about the theory had helped us earn a more secure attachment. This sensitive developmental framework allows therapists to connect emotionally with clients with any attachment style. Writing about formative child attachment years, and making art about attachment states, provide rich training opportunities for art therapists.

Attachment theory

Attachment theory has emerged as a main paradigm for understanding the infant's, the child's, and the adult's personal and interpersonal psychosocial world (Bowlby 1988; Main 2000; Siegel 1999; Sroufe 2000). Attachment represents systems of proximity-seeking behaviors generated by parent/child interactions that develop and maintain across the lifespan. They comprise an innate system that organizes motivation, emotion, memory, and ways of making sense of interpersonal relationships. Thus, attachment theory provides an overarching foundation for human relatedness; it bridges therapeutic approaches organized around early developmental experiences and here-and-now, non-pathological systems viewpoints. Bowlby's (1969, 1973, 1980) attachment theory represents a clear departure from classical and other contemporary psychological approaches, since it evolved from an ethological approach, which is the study of animal behaviors in their natural setting. Simulated laboratory settings furthered its application to understanding human behavior (Ainsworth *et al.* 1978).

Approximately ten years after Bowlby originated his theory, Margaret Ainsworth worked with mother-child dyads using a "strange situation" research paradigm. Dyads were observed through a one-way mirror or on videotape as mother and child separated and reunited in a room full of toys. Ainsworth observed and assessed the dyad based upon the mother's communication process with the child and the child's response to the mother, both verbally and non-verbally, during the moments of separation and reunion. How each member of the dyad managed a stranger entering and confounding the mother/child environment was included in the assessment. Ainsworth coined the terms *secure* (B) and *insecure* as two main organized categories of attachment theory. The insecure type divided into the avoidant style (A), and ambivalent-resistant style (C). Later Mary Main and Judith Solomon added a disorganized/disoriented attachment style (D; 1990).

The nature of the infant attachment to the primary caregiver evolves into the principal internal working model of attachment used throughout childhood and adulthood (Fraley 2002; George, Kaplan, and Main 1996; Main and Solomon 1990). Caregiver gestures, tone of voice, eye contact, touch, facial expressions, and the intensity, timing, and physical proximity of his or her non-verbal affect all contribute significantly to building the sense of feelings of a secure base (Siegel and Hartzell 2003). As conflicts and mis-attunements arise during the dyad's early life, the caregiver can effectively repair the breech by co-regulating and reintroducing an attuned communication. The resulting resonance reflects the child's feelings, and provides the predictable exchanges that the child craves (Schore 1994, 2001). Accordingly, a child may have a different attachment style with each caregiver.

Adult attachment styles internalize the repetitive and meaningful expectations built during formative caregiver and intimate partnerships into complex, feeling-based working models. Life-enduring attachment patterns may alter during very negative experiences or very positive ones. The adult attachment styles are categorized as secure, dismissive, preoccupied, and disorganized (Main and Goldwyn 1998). As a result, if an adult expressing an insecure internal working model forms an ongoing intimate relationship with a person utilizing a secure internal working model, the insecurely attached person may become more resilient over time. Unconscious internal models of attachment successfully change with successful long-term relationships in marriages and are vulnerable to trauma and chronic psychosocial stressors (Hesse 1999). Therefore, child and adult attachment styles describe states of mind aroused in the face of attachment-related stress rather than absolute brain structures and/or unremitting personalities (Main 2000).

A therapist, a mate, a friend, an adult sibling, or other therapeutic relationships may also positively influence an insecure individual's interpersonal functioning and help attain a more flexible and resilient, *earned*-secure level of relating (Siegel 1999). *Earned* attachment categories represent integrated interactional processes that allow adults to interrupt familial patterns leading to insecure attachment (Main 2000). Art therapy training can assist art therapists in working towards an earned attachment status.

Art therapy pathways to earned secure attachment

The precise process whereby internalized positive change in attachment security is achieved and how the process of change can be measured continues to be investigated (Roisman, Fortuna, and Holland 2006; Roisman *et al.* 2002). An individual's ability to talk about the distressing events and relationships of childhood coherently defines the essence of earned secure attachment. People expressing an earned secure status can talk about early distressing events because of either consistent or ameliorative support from caring adults (Roisman *et al.* 2002; Weinfield, Sroufe, and Egeland 2000). *Earned* attachment represents a functional internal change that empowers coherent talking about a distressing past as well as a deeper capacity for trust in relational contexts.

In an effort to help facilitate an earned secure attachment style, master's-level art therapy trainees were given a class assignment: create a cloth attachment album and visually showcase the four principal attachment categories. The use of fabrics called upon an experiential, kinesthetic understanding of the styles. The choices of textures, beyond color or design, called forth reactions to the tactile experiences in the sensory images.

Visual and verbal conversations emerged regarding warmth and closeness, coldness and fulfillment, and/or dissatisfaction with attachment experiences. The albums were shared in small, supportive group settings, which helped process feelings aroused by visiting each attachment visual (Figure 11.1).

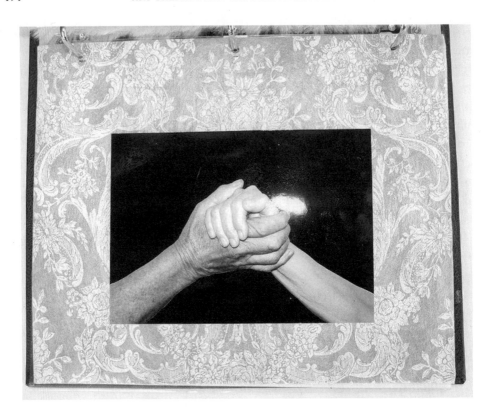

Figure 11. 1 Final image from attachment album. "I had very negative reactions to the avoidant and ambivalent images, and felt a sense of pain and despair when working on the disorganized image. Each piece brought about a strong emotional response so it was very helpful to end with a personal visual and written reflection. The final image is the photograph of my parents' hands. It is about a couple's ability to survive many years of life together with compassion." Jessica Tress Masterson.

In a supportive environment, the truthful quality and succinct quantity of verbal and visual expressions can positively contribute to discourse coherence (Grice 1975, 1989). In the process of art-making, art therapists in training sometimes recognize that they feel more secure, and notice that they have transited from an earlier insecure attachment style into an earned secure attachment. Our experiences as educators have shown us that helping art therapy trainees clarify, order, and enhance the relevance of their narratives through art can contribute to a contingent *earned* discourse.

Dyadic secure organized patterns of relatedness

Classifications of child and adult attachment styles may at times distract from understanding that attachment style expresses the outcome of a previous dyadic process that may be attempted in future dyadic processes. The corresponding child-adult attachment style classifications are: secure child to secure adult; avoidant child to dismissive adult;

ambivalent-resistant child to preoccupied adult; and disorganized/disoriented child to disorganized adult (George *et al.* 1996).

The secure dyad is seen in their commitment and valuing of their attachment-related experience (Main 2000). The relationship between caregiver and baby provides repeated experiences of feeling connected, protected, and understood (Siegel and Hartzell 2003). A securely attached child experiences the caregiver as empathic, reflective, and sensitive to his or her state of being (Fonagy 2002; Siegel and Hartzell 2003). The caregiver intuits his/her child's inner life, senses the child's feelings and conveys a secure state of mind to the child. On average, 55–67 percent of the non-clinical population achieves this state of secure attachment (Siegel 1999). A securely attached infant learns lifelong self-calming, self-regulating patterns, enhancing its ability to integrate its sensed world.

Margarette, an art therapist, felt herself feeling increasingly safe and relaxed as she watched Dihanna and her mother. Dihanna is a 26-month-old Latina girl. Dihanna's mother, Daniella, is emotionally available, perceptive, and responsive. One can feel her absorption and delight as she beams while Dihanna smiles, showing her mother a newly acquired skill. Daniella is tuned to her child's body, emotions, and state of mind. Dihanna recognizes her mother as her soother, her co-regulator. When Dihanna falls asleep in the session, Danielle covers her with a much-used blanket. Dihanna's way of being expresses, *I count on my mom to be there, to smile and cuddle me, to feed and soothe me when I need her.* Mother and child, when attuned to one another, enter a state that others who are outside of their interactive realm may feel awkward about interrupting.

The album art therapy directive asks for art therapist trainees to be open, to learn and to experience every attachment style through the art. When asked to describe the cloth album's secure attachment style page, art therapy trainees often reached for textures of comfort and warmth. The baby's cuddly blanket is frequently evoked and the trainee is drawn to touch and caress the piece with gentleness.

Even before turning album pages, the cover of the album may spontaneously capture the art therapist's relationship with attachment. Several thought to show their understanding of attachment as a private container of security and safety. For example, Andrea used the image of a house as a cover for her album. Both Andrea and Jennifer applied universal symbols often evoked directly or indirectly by art therapists (Figures 11.2 and 11.3).

A secure experience is also suggested by Andrea's and Jessica's choice of an attractive soft material that beckons to be touched (Figures 11.4 and 11.5). Inside the house album, the universal symbol of a circle is used as the holding space (Figure 11.4). MARI® Mandala methods focus on images within the circles as relating to an intrapersonal psychic snapshot in time, space, and in relationship to others (Kellogg 2002). The album's cloth images suggest the usefulness of mandalas to describe attachment as an interpersonal dynamic experience. The structural aspects of their cloth images used to describe secure attachment (Figures 11.4 and 11.5) successfully

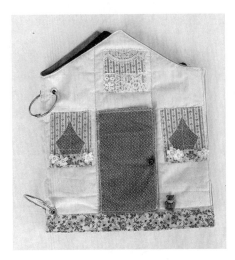

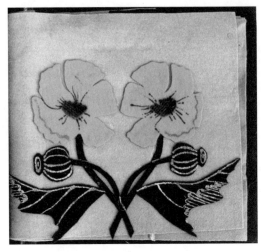

Figure 11.2 House attachment album by Andrea Lewis. The house is cozy and welcoming with a door that opens and shuts.

Figure 11.3 Flowers attachment album by Jennifer Lathrope. Secure attachment is represented by two intertwined flowers.

communicate the orderly quality of the organized secure-insecure attachment styles (A, B, C; Ainsworth *et al.* 1978). MARI® Mandala training underscores how a checker board's fine mesh symbolizes organized early bonding qualities (Figures 11.3 and 11.4; Stage 1; Kellogg 2002). MARI® Mandala Stage 1 speaks to security versus insecurity in early maternal bonding. Andrea's circle with its tiny checkerboard combines the focus on maternal bonding with a color known as "Mother Mary Blue" which, according to Kellogg, is a color of trust. The sewn hem adds a radiating quality to the image, further enforcing a transcendent sense.

Jessica wrote that the mother's and child's open palms facing up in the photograph signify trust and protective holding, allowing the child to explore her world (Figure 11.5). The mother's hands and the child's hands echo each other, illustrating a fine attunement. The hands and arms that cut across the page forming a symmetrical split (illustrating Stage 6 as presented in Kellogg 2002) suggest a struggle in the movement towards autonomy, while the dyad's hands form a circle within the boundaries of the square photograph representing a high level of function and integration (illustrating Stage 7; Kellogg 2002). Such a combination of archetypal structures implies that the movement to secure attachment may require effort and involve internal conflict resulting in re-attunement. This image conveys increased earned-secure status, as it implies a struggle leading towards a new level of consciousness.

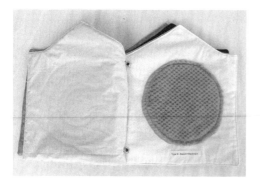

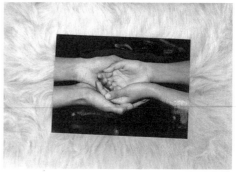

Figure 11.4 Secure attachment style by Andrea Lewis. A mother noted how her school-aged children delighted in the sky-blue fleecy fabric, wanting to keep the image for themselves.

Figure 11.5 Secure attachment style by Jessica Tress Masterson.

Dyadic organized-insecure: adult preoccupied and child resistant/ambivalent patterns of relatedness

The adult with an insecure-preoccupied attachment style does not have a consistently stable internal model of trust (George *et al.* 1996). As a baby, this adult could not gauge the parent's emotional state. One minute, the parent was emotionally attuned, and the next, the parent was preoccupied with his or her own inner turmoil, or intruding into the baby's internal state. The baby was constantly attempting to lure the caregiver back to their previous attuned state. She builds a pattern of being preoccupied with the caregiver. As an adult, she may compulsively try to please his/her partners or friends. During that process, she is prone to feeling under-appreciated because she has overextended. Insecure-preoccupied adults are worried with the nature of their relationships and anxiously wonder about undesirability and love. Insecure attachment patterns reflect an unreliable base from which the person explores the world, that is, parent/child interactions have eroded the basis for confident, assured exploration. Child ambivalent-resistant attachment patterns account for 5–15 percent of the non-clinical population (Siegel 1999).

Three-year-old Tyrone stood silently clinging to his mother Shari's leg, as she told him to greet Margarette with a hug. She effusively described the situation at home, her relationships and Tyrone's impossible behavior, in intimate detail. Tyrone listened, staying close by, noticing the toys as Shari began to talk more about herself and her own parents. Just as Tyrone tentatively explored the toys at her feet, Shari turned and picked him up onto her lap. Tyrone began to cry, pushed her, and then would not get down. The dyad presented with mutual anxiety and uncertainty. Communication was awkward, mis-attuned and created relational distress. Margarette felt the anxiety. She was unable to track Shari's reactions and she observed that Tyrone could not be soothed. An inner representation of his dilemma might sound like this:

> I don't know what to expect from you; sometimes you can remember to feed me and cuddle me, but at other times you are in another world, forgetting that I am hungry and cold, forgetting that I need you to talk gently to me and to love me. Repeated experiences like this will turn me into an anxious child. I will cling to you and not leave your side in order to be sure that you will come back for me. This morning you did not come back when you said you would, and you did not come back the day before after saying, "I will be right back."

The three-dimensional fabric representations of the child's resistant ambivalent category poignantly describe the misattunement of such an experience. In her teddy bear album, Marissa created an internal pocket or a grab-bag for whatever unpredictable textures will be present: a scrap of soft wool; a crinkled ribbon, or a fabric with sandpaper roughness. She empathically grasped and communicated that the anxious child reaches into the pockets and makes do with whatever scraps are available.

Within the safety of the mandala circle, symbol and color can express the vulnerable dependency and neediness of the insecure ambivalent attachment category (Figure 11.6). Andrea's bright pink fetal shape upon a dark brown circle communicates the demanding needs of a young child in relationship to the low self-esteem of its nurturer, where the child's needs are unmet and perverted (characteristics of Stage 4, Kellogg 2002). This archetype warns of future dependency vulnerabilities in relationships or with substances. In Jennifer's image, the dynamic is similarly strong (Figure 11.7). The child poppy is large in its neediness, turning towards the fragment of a mother with an anxious screaming light fuchsia halo (Kellogg 2002; Figure 11.7).

Dyadic organized-insecure: adult dismissive and child avoidant patterns of relatedness

As a baby, this individual could not rely on her mother to be there because her caregiver's actions were unpredictable. Insecure attachment patterns reflect an unreliable base from which the child explores the world. On average, in low risk populations, avoidant attachment styles have been found in 20–30 percent of the population (Siegel 1999). Living in fear of being rejected, the dismissive adult rejects others first and finds that trusting others is difficult. Adults with a dismissive style judge others as undependable and relationships as not safe. Others are felt as threatening to stability and control. An adaptive defensive response can be seen. Intimacy and closeness are avoided. However, this is still an organized response to a pattern of unreliability that is predictable and consistent.

Rosa, nearly two-and-a-half years old, entered the room and charged towards the toys, going from one toy to another. Clemencia, her mother, was a petite woman who did not

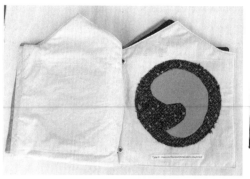

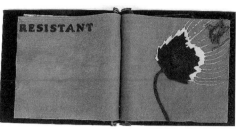

Figure 11.6 Insecure resistant-ambivalent attachment by Andrea Lewis. The needy fuschia pink fetal shape finds itself in a dark, mis-attuned home.

Figure 11.7 Insecure resistant-ambivalent attachment by Jennifer Lathrope. The child poppy turns for attunement to the frazzled maternal fragments. Its needs remain unmet.

engage with her daughter's activities. Margarette observed that when Rosa attempted to approach her mother, she stopped mid-way and returned to a toy. When Clemencia looked at Rosa, Rosa turned away and seemed to enter her own world, engrossed with the toys. Clemencia described a difficult personal history, idealizing her parents and feeling rejected by them. Despite her best intentions, Clemencia was emotionally unavailable to her daughter. Rosa adapted by avoiding closeness and emotional connection to her mom.

> When you are not aware of what is going on with me, I begin to fend for myself. I feign independence even though I crave your touch and your gaze. Experiencing this type of parental style during my first three years of being out of the womb will decrease my capacity to self-regulate. I will have difficulty sleeping. I will be anxious and unforgiving. If you leave me in a room full of strangers, I will not cry for you because I could never count on you to respond to me anyway. I have not experienced reciprocal attunement—I cannot trust adults to give me what I need (emotional feedback and attunement).

The art depictions of the avoidant category from the training exercises potently captured the block to resolving the child's emotional needs. The exploration of this category evoked deeper, darker colors. The art helped deepen the future therapists' intuition about how it may feel for Rosa and Clemencia.

Jennifer's visual dynamic portrays rigidity (Figure 11.8). The adult scarlet poppy is the center of the story with the vulnerable young flower, unopened, drooping and turning away, needing to fend for itself—the young bud unable to open and flower. Within the mandala, the target shape denotes a striving for control (Stage 5, Kellogg

2002). Dark rings of ochre, red brown, dark brown, and purple in Andrea's circle evoke the powerful target defenses that Kellogg (1992) describes as being fed by low self-esteem and wounding (Figure 11.9). Describing this style as an attachment relationship, it connects the parental use of force to consequences experienced by the child. The color of the young poppy bud is a sickly green (Kellogg 1992), reinforcing its vulnerability. Both album pages communicate the inherent dynamic of this attachment style; the parental control dominates the child (Figures 11.8 and 11.9).

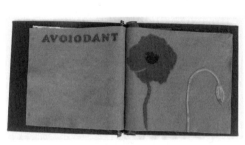

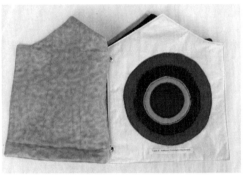

Figure 11.8 Avoidant attachment by Jennifer Lathrope. The full-grown poppy blazes as the young flower turns away.

Figure 11.9 Avoidant attachment by Andrea Lewis. The circle holds the tension of a rigid target that strives for control and defense.

Dyadic child and adult disorganized patterns of relatedness

The disorganized/disoriented attachment category reflects terror responses that impact the relating process, whether provoked by the primary caretaker in the infant or the infant in his or her parents. Brief bouts of chaotic and contradictory behaviors in the mother/child dyad become manifested by the child in response to psychosocial stressors in general. Disorganized/disoriented attachment patterns may occur under very stressful conditions within dyads classified as avoidant, secure, and ambivalent-resistant in non-stressful moments. Thus, disorganized/disoriented attachments may manifest as two different attachment categories: one during stressful psychosocial situations and another in non-stressful situations. High risk abused children studies show 55–80 percent of children with disorganized attachment have terror responses to their attachment figures (Siegel 1999).

As a baby, this adult was terrified by his or her attachment figure, or able to create terror in the caregiver. Unable to be soothed, fright, dread, and/or menacing were part of this dyad's daily experience. This bind creates an inexorable paradox: the safe haven has also become the threat. Sometimes this baby will freeze in shock, not knowing how to respond to his or her caregiver's alarming behaviors. In an observation protocol to assess infant attachment style, the baby, unable to flee, would be stuck between reaching out to and avoiding the terrorizing or terrified attachment figure. As an adult, his or her sense of safety will have been shattered. The disorganized person controls, punishes others, and may express dissociative behaviors derivative of trauma. Disturbing patterns of behaviors and significantly impaired social functioning may develop, leading to diagnoses such as conduct disorder, antisocial personality disorder, borderline personality disorder, post-traumatic stress disorder (PTSD), and Dissociative Identity Disorder (DID) (Lyons-Ruth and Jacobvitz 1999).

The baby repeatedly experiences communication in which the mother's behavior is overwhelming, frightening, and chaotic (Main and Hesse 1990). The child is disoriented, frightened:

> My mom can never read my cues. She becomes upset when I become upset. She never comforts me. I will never be able to tolerate and regulate my intense emotions, because she cannot regulate her own. I startle easily; if you look at me the "wrong way," you will petrify me and I will fall apart. Sometimes I am in a daze and refuse to look in to people's eyes. I avoid your gaze because you may scare me with your eyes. My mom scares me with her rageful affect and eyes every day of my life. So why should I look at you and communicate with you.

Four-year-old Porcha's relationship with her mother is very conflicted. Her mother Louise says she has up to 20 severe outbursts a day. She does not want to hold her mother's hand on the bus or in the street, and runs away from her in the mall, putting her at risk for injuries and falls. Louise suffers from bi-polar disorder with a history of psychiatric illness, homelessness, and her own early foster placement because her mother could no longer care for her and her siblings. Louise repeatedly shared with Margarette that she had contemplated giving Porcha up for adoption or foster care. She feels insulted when she picks Porcha up from her sitter as Porcha will always ignore her and/or bypass her and run into the street. On the bus, Porcha tantrums often and Louise has to physically restrain her.

In therapy, Porcha was very quiet, her eyes quickly scanning the room. However, Louise automatically prompted her to behave. Margarette immediately felt unease and an awareness of a heightened non-verbal tension between mother and child. Louise looked at her child with disdain and Porcha's body crumpled and sagged.

> When you gaze into my eyes, I am petrified by your face and the unpredictability of your actions. I only know that I never get my needs met by you. You horrify me and I retreat into aggressive and defiant behavior because you leave me alone for a few minutes when I tantrum. Then and only then can I feel a tiny respite from the chaos that envelops our lives.

For art therapist trainees, the visual depiction of the disorganized style evoked strong images of fragmentation and violence. Palette color choices moved to dark and/or were polarized with dominant blacks and dark grays. It was fear-arousing even to think of manifesting this category. The textures of the cloth were rough, torn, or harmful. One album's page was penetrated by three-inch carpenter nails, unseen from above, but ferocious from the side. Another hid the threat of tiny, almost invisible sewing pins. The images are no longer structured and organized; there is an absence of a center characterized by the fragmentation of Stage 11 (Kellogg 2002).

In Jennifer's album, disorganized attachment was depicted as either the frightening, withered skeletal roots of the poppy plant or the blown out shell of its seed pod—both disoriented and unable to be nurtured (Figure 11.10). To Joanna, the structure suggested a tangled web or shattered circle (characteristic of Stages 1, 11; Kellogg 2002). According to Kellogg, the web speaks to the crisis in early bonding and the shattered pod to the sense of disintegration and chaos. Andrea chose to shatter the psychic mandala space into black textured shards. The fragments are mirrored, describing the dynamic associated with this stage that can be dangerously attractive and that, like a mirror, deflects deep examination (going into Stage 11, Kellogg 2002; Figures 11.10 and 11.11). The disorganized attachment category is an attachment state that can periodically exist within an overall organized category. Lee and Georgina were able to help glimpse the disorganized dynamic in an organized insecure ambivalent-resistant category (Figures 11.12 and 11.13). Both effectively used fabric to show this mobility.

Figure 11.12 shows a green sweater. Lee took scissors to the garment; its sleeve is missing; the neck is vast; and could smother the self. The symbol is profound. Clothing constitutes our outer interface with the world. It should protect us and meet our needs for comfort. Similarly, the dependent child can be left precariously dangling from a thread above a shiny, almost reflective silk surface (Figure 11.13). Georgina used a coppery, shiny silk to represent the attractive and compelling maternal figure. She offers no warmth or comfort and evokes a strong defensive shield to deflect feelings (Kellogg 2002).

The full story: emergent coherence through attachment album making

> The process of creating the albums included a final reflective art visual page. This gave us the opportunity to reflect upon our own childhoods and, for some, our parenting experiences. Our final reflection pages expressed a range from integration to ambivalence. The solution to painful memories could be found on an unfinished page, symbolic of the chance to achieve earned, secure, attachment. The emergence of insight was woven and collaged into the albums and coherence to the visual story was often apparent throughout. Perhaps we all have experienced at least moments of each attachment style. (Lathrope 2007)

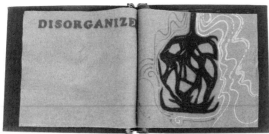

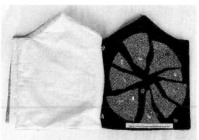

Figure 11.10 Disorganized attachment by Jennifer Lathrope. The caretaker cannot nurture, full of anxiety, dead ends and ruptures.

Figure 11.11 Disorganized attachment by Andrea Lewis. The mandala represents deep unconscious fragmentation in dark and seductive colors.

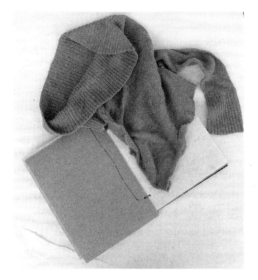

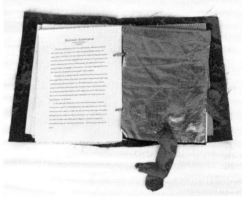

Figure 11.12 Disorganized attachment by Lee Ignacio. The sweater does not hold its shape. It is cut off; it does not meet the need to clothe the body, it is lacking in some places.

Figure 11.13 Disorganized attachment by Georgina Marshall. The child dangles from a thread, outside the album, desiring the shiny silky surface; however, is unable to connect.

The therapist-artists were invited to share their experience, lay the cloth album out in a small group with their peers, turn the pages, talk and discuss. The multiple ways of engaging with attachment theory and their own personal reactions allowed the therapists-in-training a process of supportive, integrated learning to promote truthful and collaborative expression. It can pave the way to earned secure attachment measured by contingent and coherent autobiographical narrative (Hesse 1999; Main 2000). Grice (1975, 1989) generated an over-riding Cooperative Principle and four maxims for the kind of consistent and collaborative discourse associated with the development of *earned* secure attachment (Table 11.1). Jennifer's statement is an example of a truthful statement as she recognizes how she has experienced at least moments of each attachment style. It is succinct, complete and relevant.

Table 11.1 Grice maxims.

Maxim	How it is expressed
Quality	Be truthful and have evidence for what you say
Quantity	Be succinct, yet complete
Relation	Be relevant or perspicacious
Manner	Be clear and orderly

The album cloth journals can also offer a therapeutic experience. In a deeply personal manner, Britta used the creation of the album as a reparative journey. She made a tiny felt baby for each attachment style. The baby was tucked in a fabric bed, with its own small blanket texturally reflective of the attachment style whilst facing collage images of inter-action of babies and mothers (art not shown). Under each flap where a baby was, she placed a collage of relevant images offering a reparative attachment experience for the baby. The album was a clear narrative with an intentionally organized sequence of the stages reflecting a truthful personal story.

In summary, engaging with the four attachment categories through reading, writing, cloth albums, personal reflections and discussions offers the art therapist trainees a unique opportunity to learn, experience and integrate an important model facilitating understanding human relatedness. Either sewing or gluing cloth echoes the concept of earned secure attachment, as the action mirrors how, in therapy, one examines elements of one's life and experience and then puts the pieces back together. The requirement to experience different attachment dynamics vicariously offers a profound path for clinicians not only to prepare themselves professionally, but to deepen their individual work and move towards greater coherence.

The Attachment Cloth Album Directive was created by Noah Hass-Cohen in memory of her father, Josef Hass 1924–2005.

1. Make an album with at least five pages. One page for each of the four attachment categories. The last page will be a reflection.

2. Make an image/s for each attachment style. The primary media is cloth.

3. A book format is needed. One must be able to turn pages in space. There are no size limitations. The last reflection page is also an image.

4. Underneath each image or across from it give a title for the attachment style of the image.

5.   Include a three to five page written paper explaining how each image goes with each attachment style. Reflect on your text and imagery using Grice's maxims.

6.   Include a two page written reflection discussing your personal interaction with the material and how you may directly, or in a modified fashion, use attachment albums with clients.

References

Ainsworth, M. D. S., Blehar, M. C., Waters, E., and Wall, S. (1978). *Patterns of Attachment: A Psychological Study of the Strange Situation*. Hillsdale, NJ: Lawrence Erlbaum Associates, Inc.

Bowlby, J. (1988). *A Secure Base: Parent-Child Attachment and Healthy Human Development*. New York: Basic Books.

Bowlby, J. (1969/1982). *Attachment and Loss: Vol. 1. Attachment*. New York: Basic Books.

Bowlby, J. (1973). *Attachment and Loss: Vol. 2. Separation*. New York: Basic Books.

Bowlby, J. (1980). *Attachment and Loss: Vol. 3. Loss*. New York: Basic Books.

Fonagy, P. (2002). Understanding mental states, mother-infant interaction, and the development of the self. In J. M. Maldonado-Duran (ed.), *Infant and Toddler Mental Health: Models of Clinical Intervention with Infants and Their Families* (pp.57–74) Washington, DC: American Psychiatric Publishing.

Fraley, R. C. (2002). Attachment stability from infancy to adulthood: Meta-analysis and dynamic modeling of developmental mechanisms. *Personality and Social Psychology Review, 6*(2), 123–151.

George, C., Kaplan, N., and Main, M. (1996). *Adult Attachment Interview* (3rd edition). Unpublished manuscript, Department of Psychology, University of California, Berkeley.

Grice, H. P. (1975). Logic and conversation. In P. Cole and J. L. Moran (eds) *Syntax and Semantics: Speech Acts* (pp.41–58). New York: Academic Press.

Grice, H. P. (1989). *Studies in the Way of Words*. Cambridge, MA: Harvard University Press.

Hesse, E. (1999). The adult attachment interview: Historical and current perspectives. In J. Cassidy and P. R. Shaver (eds) *Handbook of Attachment: Theory, Research, and Clinical Applications* (pp.395–433). New York: Guilford Press.

Kellogg, J. (1992). Color therapy from the perspective of the great round of mandala. *The Journal of Religion and Psychical Research, 15*(3), 138–146.

Kellogg, J. (2002). *Mandala: Path of Beauty* (3rd edition). Bellair, FL: ATMA, Inc.

Lathrope, J. (2007). Personal Communication.

Lyons-Ruth, K. and Jacobvitz, D. (1999). Attachment disorganization: Unresolved loss, relational violence, and lapses in behavioral and attentional strategies. In J. Cassidy and P. R. Shaver (eds) *Handbook of Attachment: Theory, Research, and Clinical Applications* (pp.520–554). New York: Guilford Press.

Main, M. (2000). The organized categories of infant, child, and adult attachment: Flexible vs. inflexible attention under attachment-related stress. *Journal of the American Psychoanalytic Association, 48*(4), 1055–1096.

Main, M. and Goldwyn, R. (1998). *Adult Attachment Scoring and Classification System* (version 6.3). Unpublished scoring manual, University of California at Berkeley.

Main, M. and Hesse, E. (1990). Parents' unresolved traumatic experiences are related to infant disorganized attachment status: Is frightened and/or frightening parental behavior the linking mechanism? In M. T. Greenberg, D. Chicchetti, and E. M. Cummings (eds) *Attachment in the Preschool Years: Theory, Research, and Intervention* (pp.161–182). Chicago, IL: University of Chicago Press.

Main, M. and Solomon, J. (1990). Procedures for identifying infants as disorganized/disoriented during the Ainsworth Strange Situation. In M. T. Greenberg, D. Cicchetti, and E. M. Cummings (eds), *Attachment in the Preschool Years: Theory, Research, and Intervention* (pp.121–160). Chicago, IL: University of Chicago Press.

Roisman, G. I., Fortuna, K., and Holland, A. (2006). An experimental manipulation of retrospectively defined earned and continuous attachment security. *Child Development, 77*(1), 59–71.

Roisman, G. I., Padron, E., Sroufe, L. A., and Egeland, B. (2002). Earned secure attachment status in retrospect and prospect. *Child Development, 73*(4), 1204–1219.

Schore, A. N. (1994). *Affect Regulation and the Origin of the Self: The Neurobiology of Emotional Development*. Hillsdale, NJ: Lawrence Erlbaum Associates, Inc.

Schore, A. N. (2001). The effects of a secure attachment relationship on right brain development, affect regulation, and infant mental health. *Infant Mental Health Journal, 22*, 7–66.

Siegel, D. J. (1999). *The Developing Mind: How Relationships and the Brain Interact to Shape Who We Are*. New York: Guilford Press.

Siegel, D. J. and Hartzell, M. (2003). *Parenting From the Inside Out: How a Deeper Self-understanding Can Help You Raise Children Who Thrive*. New York: Tarcher/Putnam Books.

Sroufe, L. A. (2000). Early relationships and the development of children. *Infant Mental Health Journal, 21*(1–2), 67–74.

Weinfield, N. S., Sroufe, L. A., and Egeland, B. (2000). Attachment from infancy to early adulthood in a high-risk sample: Continuity, discontinuity, and their correlates. *Child Development, 71*(3), 695–702.

12

Immunity at Risk and Art Therapy

Joanna Clyde Findlay

Immunity at risk can be understood as the multi-directional interplay of the neural, immune, and endocrine systems in response to stress (Daruna 2004). There are mutual receptor mechanisms for hormones, neurotransmitters and white blood cells/lymphocytes (Lekander 2002). Synapses between immune and neural cells are found in lymphoid tissue. The interface of sympathetic nerves with immune cells in the gastrointestinal tract (Pert 1999) further contributes to integrated bodily responses to physical, psychosocial, environmental, and infectious stimuli. For example, the body interprets the activity of cytokines, a type of lymphocyte messenger, as an internal signal of sickness (Lekander 2002), while regulatory centers of the brain respond by inducing rest, sleep and even depression (Lekander 2002; Figure 12.1).

The price of stress: physical, endocrine and immune function

Long-term stress increases the release of glucocorticoids from the adrenal glands. Glucocorticoids, cortisol, can indiscriminately kill lymphocytes (white blood cells) via a process that causes the cells to synthesize a suicide protein. Glucocorticoids compromise the immune response or cause it to spiral into autoimmunity when the immune system mistakes a normal part of the body for an invader and attacks it (Sapolsky 1998; Figure 12.1).

The effect of chronic hypothalamus-pituitary-adrenal (HPA) driven stress on the functioning of the immune system is significant. Glucocorticoid immune suppression causes shrinkage of the thymus gland via reduction in the formation of new lymphocytes that constitute thymic tissue (Sapolsky 1998).

Bodily damage can result from an enduring HPA response. Related pancreas dysfunction can cause insulin dependent-diabetes with vascular damage, increased epinephrine release contributes to atherosclerosis, and cardiac arrest may result from the breakdown of the body's hardware. Older adults whose immune systems are already compromised due to age-related diseases (Kiecolt-Glaser *et al.* 2002a) suffer the greatest repercussions.

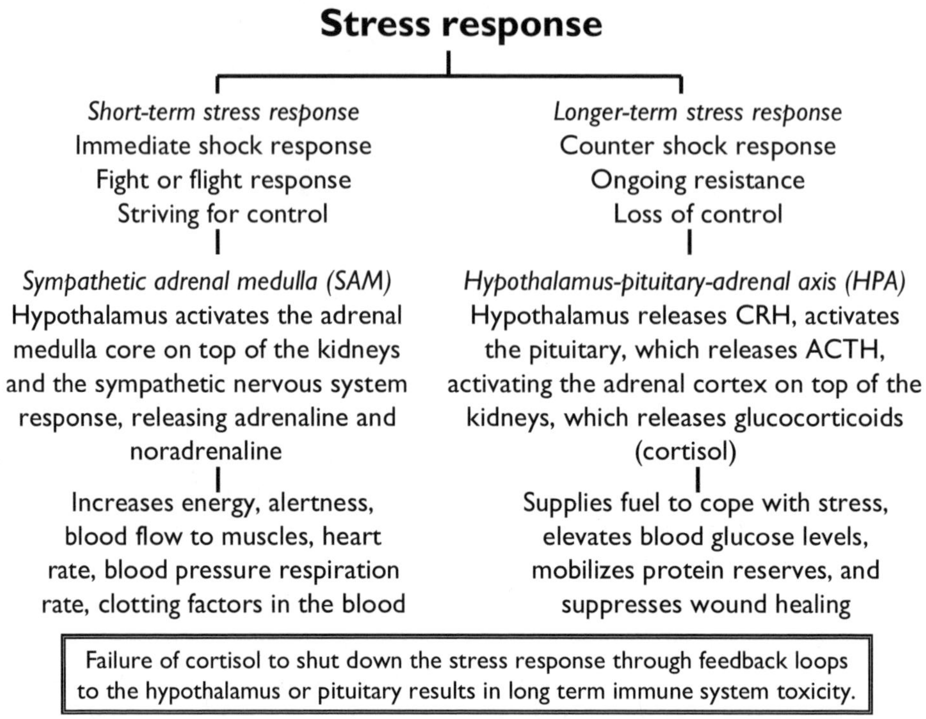

Stress response

Short-term stress response	Longer-term stress response
Immediate shock response	Counter shock response
Fight or flight response	Ongoing resistance
Striving for control	Loss of control
Sympathetic adrenal medulla (SAM) Hypothalamus activates the adrenal medulla core on top of the kidneys and the sympathetic nervous system response, releasing adrenaline and noradrenaline	Hypothalamus-pituitary-adrenal axis (HPA) Hypothalamus releases CRH, activates the pituitary, which releases ACTH, activating the adrenal cortex on top of the kidneys, which releases glucocorticoids (cortisol)
Increases energy, alertness, blood flow to muscles, heart rate, blood pressure respiration rate, clotting factors in the blood	Supplies fuel to cope with stress, elevates blood glucose levels, mobilizes protein reserves, and suppresses wound healing

Failure of cortisol to shut down the stress response through feedback loops to the hypothalamus or pituitary results in long term immune system toxicity.

Figure 12.1 Effects of the stress response. Mild elevations in glucocorticoids enhance memory during short-term stress, dendritic spine stimulation makes synapses hyperresponsive and delivers more energy via glucose to brain. Unremitting glucocorticoid release causes the death of hippocampal dendrites and neurons contributing to memory loss. CRH: corticotropin releasing hormone; ACTH: adrenocorticotropin hormone.

Distress-related immune function may be one core mechanism behind a diverse set of health risks associated with negative emotions (Ryff and Singer 1998). Depression can also provoke the release of pituitary and adrenal hormones that can dysregulate the immune system. Negative emotions contribute indirectly to immune dysregulation by increasing proinflammatory cytokine production (Kiecolt-Glaser *et al.* 2002b). The interplay is multi-directional as stress, diseases, anxiety or anxious imagery may exacerbate chronic stress. Distress may provoke substantial delays in wound healing and enhance the risk for infection (Kiecolt-Glaser *et al.* 2002b). For example, three days before an important exam, students' wounds healed 40 percent slower than during summer vacation (Lekander 2002).

Individuals who experience non-remitting stress often have multiple behaviors that put them at greater risk: poorer sleep, propensity to substance abuse, poorer nutrition and less exercise (Lekander 2002). These behaviors, together with endocrinological and immunological consequences, can become cyclically patterned behaviors that cause still greater distress.

Psychoneuroimmunology and cancer

The internal drama of our valiant immune response is seen in magnified *before, during* and *after* images of our cellular defense against a cancer cell (Lennart 1973; Nilsson 1985; Figure 12.2).

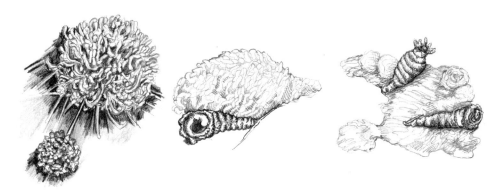

(a) The tiny prickly killer cell moving close to a huge cancer cell

(b) The killer cell morphs to extend itself, releasing its potent toxin kiss to kill the cancer cell

(c) The cancer cell is destroyed leaving its entrails extruding, awaiting the macrophages' clean

Figure 12.2 (a)–(c) The Death of a Cancer Cell. *Art by Joanna Clyde Findlay* .

Cancer is most likely a result of alterations in the genetic machinery of a cell, where the normal growth-regulating genes change into oncogenes, giving the message to proliferate wildly (Yaha 2001). Depending on the type of cancer, a suppression of immune activity allows cancer cells to multiply and divide undetected (Kiecolt-Glaser *et al.* 2002c). Cancers caused by chemical carcinogens (e.g. lung cancer) may be less influenced by psychological, behavioral and immunological factors than cancers associated with a virus such as the Epstein Barr virus, which are immunogenic. Specifically, decreased lymphocyte proliferation and reduced natural killer (NK) cell cytotoxicity, or cell damaging capacity, are associated with stress. Interferon is a crucial regulator of NK cells, stimulating their growth and differentiation, as well as enhancing their ability to destroy target cells. There is evidence that even momentary stress such as taking an exam has modulated the synthesis of the immune messengers interleukin-2, leaving students with weakened immunity (Kiecolt-Glaser *et al.* 2002c; Figure 12.3).

NK cells, killer T cells, macrophages and B cells facilitated by interferons and interleukins are natural healing, cancer fighters. Compelling evidence exists for the role of immune cells, such as NK cells, in resisting the progression of metastatic tumors, the migration and growth of malignant cells at sites far from their origin (Kiecolt-Glaser *et al.* 2002c). Evidence among rodent models showed that social stressors not only increased NK cytotoxicity, they also enhanced metastasis of transplantable tumors (Sapolsky 1998). Bereaved spouses had elevated cortisol and decreased natural killer activity (Irwin, Daniels and Weiner 1987). Psychological distress was also linked to effects on cellular repair and apoptosis, or disintegration of cells into the membrane (Kiecolt-Glaser *et al.* 2002c).

Empirical evidence linked the development of breast cancer with the effects of a prolonged HPA axis response (Spiegel 1999). High serum levels of dehydro-epiandrosterone, a correlate of HPA axis activity, predicted the subsequent development of breast cancer nine years later in normal postmenopausal women. In patients operated on for breast and stomach carcinoma, the failure of morning cortisol levels to decrease within two weeks after admission was associated with shorter survival times (Spiegel 1999). However, the link between stress and cancer does not necessarily imply causality. Increased levels of cortisol and sensitivity to stress may be attributed to prior premorbid conditions and/or genetic vulnerability.

Enhancement of immune function

Social support and psychotherapy factors appear protective and were linked to improved self-care behavior, sleep, relaxation, exercise, nutrition, medical compliance, and changes in biological pathways of disease and resistance (Achterberg, Dossey, and Kolkeimer 1994; Spiegel 2002). Positive feelings, thoughts and attitudes associated with neocortical function and the availability of spiritual resources were associated with better health and altered autonomic activity and immune function (Daruna 2004).

There has been a shortage of evidence about the neocortical-immune axis (Tuohy 2005). However, recent research indicated a direct neocortical influence on migration of mature T cells from the thymus regulating production of mature CD4+ and CD8+ cells (Moshel, Durkin, and Amassian 2005). Rat research showed that electrical stimulation of a rat's left temporo-parieto-occipital cortex during its behaviorally active night time period caused increased levels of circulating T cells, but not NK or B cells (Moshel *et al.* 2005). The implication that individual cortical processing (Tuohy 2005) may regulate immunity substantially is exciting. The implication is that therapeutic interventions that contribute to regulation of affect and cognitions can regulate immunity. One of the most robust findings is the positive impact of personal relationships on immune and endocrine regulation (Kiecolt-Glaser *et al.* 2002b). Medical students who reported better social support mounted stronger responses to the hepatitis B vaccine than those with less support (Kiecolt-Glaser *et al.* 2002a). Individuals with fewer social ties were

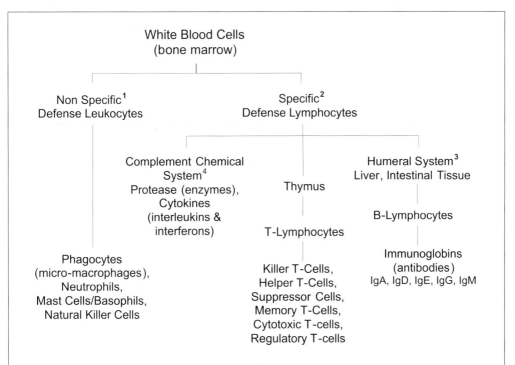

White Blood Cells
(bone marrow)

Non Specific[1]
Defense Leukocytes

Specific[2]
Defense Lymphocytes

Complement Chemical
System[4]
Protease (enzymes),
Cytokines
(interleukins &
interferons)

Thymus

T-Lymphocytes

Humeral System[3]
Liver, Intestinal Tissue

B-Lymphocytes

Phagocytes
(micro-macrophages),
Neutrophils,
Mast Cells/Basophils,
Natural Killer Cells

Killer T-Cells,
Helper T-Cells,
Suppressor Cells,
Memory T-Cells,
Cytotoxic T-cells,
Regulatory T-cells

Immunoglobins
(antibodies)
IgA, IgD, IgE, IgG, IgM

[1]*Non Specific Defense:* Foreign pathogens, (viruses/bacteria) are detected by white blood cells, (WBC-leukoocytes) produced in the bone marrow. Leukocytes (phagocytes-micro/macrophages-, neutrophils, mast cells basophils-, natural killer cells), engulf and destroy pathogens. During the process (phagocytosis) the pathogens are labeled for future identification. Natural killer cells play a role in cancer & viral defense; they stun, insert cellular material into the cancer cell and paralyze it.

[2]*Specific Defense:* T lymphocytes mature in the thymus (killer cells, helper cells, suppressor, memory T, cytotoxic T and regulatory T cells). Killer T cells & cytotoxic cells exterminate specific viruses, bacteria or cancer cells. During inflammatory responses helper T cells excrete chemicals (cytokines-interleukins/interferons) causing killer T cells to replicate and eradicate the viral memory. Suppressor & regulatory cells signal to stop immune response thus limiting destruction of the self.

[3]*Humeral System:* Immune responses generate antibodies and immunological memory. Antibodies (immunoglobins IgA, IgD, IgE, IgG, IgM) mature in the bone marrow. They fit the invader, immobilize it, and signal to the neutrophils which devour it. Memory cells retain response memories for antigens.

[4]*Complement System:* A chemical cascade (proteases, enzymes & proteins) activates antibodies to clear pathogens, marks them for destruction and triggers the specific defense system. Chemicals coat the surface of the invader and trigger recruitment of inflammatory cells to clear neutralized antigens.

Figure 12.3 Immune system summary chart.

more susceptible to more respiratory viruses (Cohen *et al.* 1997). In a sample of HIV (human immunodeficiency virus) positive men, low perceived emotional support related to a more rapid decline in CD4+ T cells, an important marker in progression of HIV infection (Kiecolt-Glaser *et al.* 2002b).

Evaluation of the efficacy of cancer group psychotherapy suggested that affective and interpersonal factors play a pivotal role in the mind-body connection (Spiegel and Cordova 2001). Metastatic breast cancer patients who received one year of support-ive-expressive group therapy reported lower mood disturbance, anxiety, maladaptive coping responses and pain, as compared to the control group who received educational materials only. A ten-year follow-up evaluated the effect of this group intervention on survival (Spiegel *et al.* 1989). The patients in the intervention group lived an average of 18 months longer than the control group, even when differences in prognostic clinical indicators or medical treatment received were controlled.

A crucial component of social support is the direct confrontation of fears of dying and death, and the expression of emotions such as fear, sadness, and anger in a support-ive group setting (Spiegel and Cordova 2001). Women with advanced breast cancer who used affect regulation strategies became expressive without being more hostile. Even at a time when they were coping with debilitating treatment, pain, and loss of function, they benefited by experiencing enhanced coping (Giese-Davis *et al.* 2002).

The use of art therapy in symptom and pain control for cancer patients has been recently explored (Nainis *et al.* 2006). Significant reductions in eight out of nine symptoms measured by the Edmonton Symptom Assessment Scale, including the global distress score and the Spielberger-State Trait Anxiety Index, were found after one hour art therapy sessions. Subjects reported comfort with the process and reduced subjective experience of stress.

Imagery research

Based on brain imaging studies, expectancies of sensory stimulation or internal imagery seem to share the same brain circuits as sensory stimulation or external images (Ganis, Thompson, and Kosslyn 2004; Martindale 1990). Similarly, immune system function may shape internal images (Hass-Cohen 2006). Research on the precise connections between imagery, the nervous system, and the immune system is hard to find. Mental imagery literature hypothesizes that imagery can be an expression of the immune system response to stress (Bach 1990; Hass-Cohen 2003; Malchiodi 1999; Naparstek 1994; Rossman 2002). Images are a non-verbal way to find out about automatic thoughts, and to utilize active imagery in order to move from frozen fragmented representations to coherent narratives (Beck 1995).

Active imagery is *personal, vital* and *action-oriented* (Hass-Cohen 2006); it can be deliberately, consciously manipulated and expressed for purposes of change (Beck 1995). Vivid and salient memories are recorded as visual, sensory mental data (Pillemer

1998). The hippocampus, in the limbic brain, is pivotal for accessing images of personal explicit memories (Sapolsky 1998). When working with such memories in cognitive behavioral therapy, a significant part of the work is to translate the imagery into words. In art therapy, vividly recorded images are directly expressed onto paper and can be manipulated with and without words, thus changing the internal landscape. The work contributes to increasing control and decreasing the experience of stress, facilitating cognitive restructuring and possibly contributing to more balanced immune function.

Personal imagery was found to impact change positively (Conklin and Tiffany 2001). Detailed person-specific imagery increased positive mood and suppressed craving; personal details of smokers' images added coherency and underscored the available resources for help, while becoming deepened with specific symbolism.

There are different ideas as to how affect and visual imagery link. Some views suggest that the special relationship of imagery and emotion relates to evolutionary needs. Visual imagery is an older representation system than language, and might be available to express basic emotions, such as fear and disgust derived from direct sensory experience (Kosslyn, Ganis, and Thompson 2001). Affective-laden personal events, unlike generic classes of events, may be stored in the form of images in autobiographical memory (Conway 2001). It could be that imagery has emotional effects because it mimics real-life perceptual events and has privileged access to episodic memories (Conway 2001). These views suggest that imagery is associated with greater affective responses regardless of the type of emotion involved. While there is a paucity of empirical evidence to support the widespread clinical assumption connecting mental imagery and emotion, Holmes and Matthews (2005) showed that imagery of aversive events is indeed associated with greater anxiety reactions than encoding the same information verbally. Consequentially, using imagery to regulate emotions and to affect the activated HPA axis stress response may reduce damaging glucocorticoid levels and speaks to the advantages of art therapy.

Visualization training for participants with diseases that depress the immune system showed increases in neutrophils (WBCs) over a 90-day period in 20 patients with cancer, AIDS (acquired immune deficiency syndrome) and viral infections (Donaldson 2000). The participants received 30 minutes of audio training which included verbal suggestions, relaxation and visualization instructions. Individuals also received training in generating self-healing mental images that matched their disease. A positive, statistically significant improvement for dermatomyositis, an immune microvasculopathy disorder, was attributed to treatment with meditation and visualization (Collins and Dunn 2005).

Visualization may enhance the ability of patients with medical problems to become mindful about their physical activity, emotional responses, cognitive ideation, and consciousness (Donaldson 2000). Visualization is probably also effective because the human body cannot fully distinguish between a physical experience and a vivid mental experience (Siegel 1986).

Targeted visualization can produce specific physiological responses (Donaldson 2000). In 1929, Jacobsen showed that visualization can induce firing of appropriate neurons related to bodily activity. In a study of mental weight lifting exercises, muscle tension levels increased relative to suggested increases in the weight that was mentally lifted (Shaw 1940). Athletes' use of imagery to regulate their motivation and arousal levels were studied extensively (Gregg and Hall 2006). Imagery ability measures indicated that motivational arousal and mastery could be psychometrically correlated with competitive athletes' successful use of imagery skills. Purposeful self-created images are rated for clarity, ease with which they are seen, emotional valance, feel of the movement, and sense of control (Gregg and Hall 2006). Autogenic training, using relaxation (Jacobsen 1929; Kabat-Zinn 1990) and visualization of body part or organ functioning in a normal way (Achterberg *et al.* 1994) are adjunctive treatments for medical disorders.

Art therapy principles of imagery

Achterberg (1985) summarized six general research findings on imagery and physiology:

> Images relate to physiological states; images may either precede or follow physiological changes, indicating both a causative or reactive role; images may be induced by conscious, deliberate behaviors, as well as by subconscious acts (electrical stimulation of the brain, reverie, dreaming etc.); images can be considered as the hypothetical bridge between conscious processing of information and physiological change; images can exhibit influence over the voluntary (peripheral) nervous system, as well as the involuntary (autonomic) nervous system. (p.115)

Personal symbolic art expression most likely allows sensory routes to speak directly to the limbic brain. Individuals' belief systems are reflected in the level of imagery absorption and manipulation, which infuses the imagery with sensory potency (Malchiodi 1999). The value of using affect-laden, personalized imagery is also underscored in guided imagery practices (Achterberg 1999; Achterberg *et al.* 1994; Battino 2000; Naparstek 1994).

The exploration of the interconnections between the immune, neural, and endocrine systems through imagery is a personal account of the disease. The art expressions show how the individual makes sense of the disease and how it affects their sense of self. The art expression of the disease story is further revealed by the clients' responsiveness to the art, the therapist, and the art directive. Six art therapy dynamic principles assist in exploring the interconnectivity (Hass-Cohen 2005).

First, considering the *Vividness* of the client-created image is central. Its vitality and clarity for the creator indicate affect expression and regulation. Second, the image is placed on a continuum of *Coherency Versus Fragmentation*: does it have visual and narrative cohesiveness? This reflects the individual's personal autobiographical perception of the illness. Third, how does the client relate to the image as an expression of self-agency, or convey *Mastery and Control* concerning the problem? Fourth, where is the image on a spectrum from *Dynamic Versus Static*: is it showing a fixed state with regards to the problem, or is it change- or action-inherent? Dynamic imagery reveals the sense of freedom or ability to take action in relation to the related stress response. Fifth, how developed is the imagery's *Degree of Symbolism*: has it become part of an integrated individualized language for the creator? What is the function of an integrated right and left brain capacity to form language about the problem? Lastly, what *Resources—Psychological Support, Personal and Interpersonal Assistance* are depicted and are able to be called forth, and how does the full information from the six principles coalesce with diagnostic impressions and prognostic expectation (Table 12.1)?

Table 12.1 Imagery principles can assist the art therapist in forming diagnostic impressions and in furthering mental health outcomes.

Principle	*What to look for*
Vividness	Image's vitality and clarity indicate affect expression and regulation
Coherency Versus Fragmentation	Image's visual/content/narrative cohesiveness reflects the individual's personal autobiographical perception of his or her illness
Mastery and Control	How does the client relate to the image as an expression of self-agency with regards to the problem?
Dynamic Versus Static	Is the image showing a fixed state with regards to the problem or is it change- or action-inherent? This relates to the ability or sense of freedom to take action in relation to the related stress response
Degree of Symbolism	Is the imagery part of an integrated individualized language for the creator? What is the function of an integrated right and left brain capacity to language about the problem?
Resources—Psychological Support, Personal and Interpersonal Assistance	What internal and external resources are both depicted and called forth?

Case study

Jim, a 38-year-old Caucasian man, wanted to work with imagery as part of a holistic treatment for his recent diagnosis of thyroid cancer. He had a malignant tumor measuring 12mm by 5mm by 5mm. Although removal of his thyroid and a lifetime of chemically regulated endocrine treatments had been recommended, he decided to coordinate alternative approaches to healing, while keeping in touch with his conventional doctor. From the start, we established our goal of working with imagery for healing, rather than the curing of his disease (Achterberg *et al.* 1994). During the eight-month period that he came to weekly art therapy sessions, he was also in traditional psychotherapy, consulted a Chinese herbal doctor, pursued a raw food diet and exercised.

In response to Jim's initial anxiety and description of the multiple stressors in his life, I taught him a progressive muscle relaxation protocol, using deep breathing, visual identification and amplification techniques. In support of his stress management strengths, I asked him to draw his *Safe Place* (Figures 12.4 and 12.5).

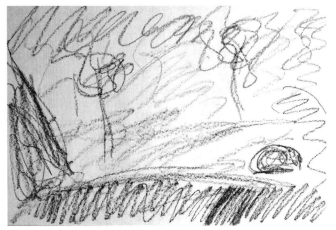

Figure 12.4 Safe Place, *with red-tumor-dot. Pastel.*

Figure 12.5 Self-Portrait, *terrified self-portrait. Pastel.*

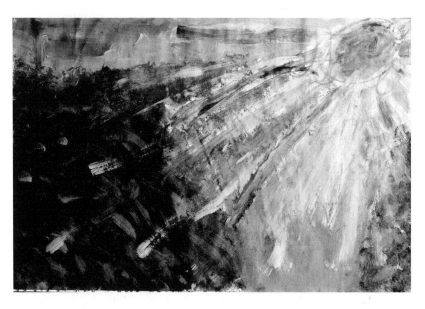

Figure 12.6 Enhanced Safe Place. *Paint.*

Jim described *Safe Place* as a secluded, fertile, green garden he knew and loved. I noticed that in the bottom right corner, there was a small mark. A round, red dot visually evoked the image of the tumor. The symbol of an alien dot being nurtured in Jim's safe haven expressed his urgent need to address the tumor. Jim's anxiously rendered self-portrait also suggested that the act of making art was stressful to him. Making art can be initially stressful, which opens the door to psychoneuroimmunological therapeutic work. In this context, the aroused sympathetic nervous system response can be easily controlled by finding a safe media, putting the image away, or altering it. Oftentimes this short burst of adrenaline promotes a good feeling. In this manner, over time, the HPA axis can be convinced that the stress is indeed only short term and the person increases their stress management skills.

By teaching relaxation and breathing techniques as well as facilitating the individual's *mastery and control* over the art media and his or her experience of stress and emotions, levels of oxytocin can be increased. Oxytocin is a hormone in the brain and blood, related to breast feeding, social contact and physical touch. The therapist's empathic resonance, mindfulness and holding environment stimulate an oxytocin response, calming the stress response.

During the application of relaxation strategies and identification of self-healing images, sunlight and light became Jim's core safety images. *Enhanced Safe Place* (Figure 12.6) shows how switching to paint from pastels augmented the vividness of Jim's image of healing. Outside of therapy Jim was able to generalize and use the image of light to bring about a sense of calm and safety.

The change of media from pastel to paint permitted a more visible *dynamic action* (Table 12.1) to permeate the safe garden, where the red dot was no longer represented. Inherent to the application of the six imagery principles was a continuous assessment of Jim's level of absorption with image-making. It seemed that Jim was not particularly comfortable working with pastels and paint, and these materials were acting as stressors. Indeed once he began to doodle with colored clay, it became clear that his engagement with his own personal symbolism grew deeper. There was more depth and detail to the work and he became engrossed in manipulating the clay (Figures 12.7 to 12.10).

Sunlight was an early symbol for Jim for healing and light. *Sunlight* is two-dimensional and contains a darkened twisting center. The same symbol later manifested in clay and paper, *Healing Light*, was even more satisfying for him. It shows the light flowering, radiating and emanating in three-dimensional space with increased *coherency* and integration (Table 12.1). The kinesthetic action of rolling out dots and twisting tendrils of light in colored clay became an almost ritualized practice in each session. Subsequently, clay was conditioned as safe and reassuring. Jim would pick up the clay and start to doodle with it automatically, almost before we had identified our goal for the session. Safe art therapy practices with concrete manipulation of materials offers actual kinesthetic and symbolic belief of control which, according to Pennebaker (1997), correlates positively with resiliency and life expectancy. Principles regarding optimism versus

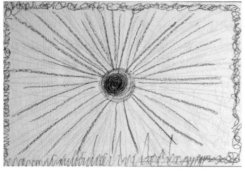

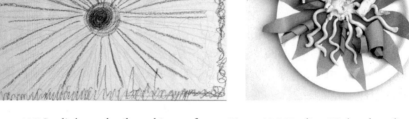

Figure 12.7 Sunlight, *early oil pastel image of healing light, with anxious dark lines in the center.*

Figure 12.8 Healing Light, *three-dimensional sun with yellow clay and green construction paper.*

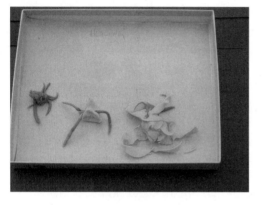

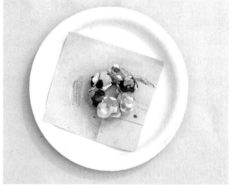

Figure 12.9 Three Stages of Healing, *the visual story of the penetration and consumption of Jim's tumor in colored clay.*

Figure 12.10 All Is One, *a circle of small colored clay balls assembled from multiple tiny colored balls.*

learned helplessness offer robust findings in terms of mental health (Kemeny 1994). Such an experience of security allows the client to develop new thoughts and experience new emotions within a safe relationship.

The improved fit with the media naturally facilitated Jim's *deepening symbolism* (Table 12.1). Our sessions exclusively devoted to working with healing imagery became the ritual that allowed not only powerful, detailed acts of mind and body focus, but overall reduction of anxiety, depression, and feelings of helplessness. Sometimes the clay expressions were abstract journeys with color; at other times he sculpted disintegrating clay tumors.

One session began with Jim making the small, life-size, tight red and bright pink ball of his tumor. It looked large and frightening. I encouraged him to show the process of its obliteration. Jim then made a dramatic progressive depiction of the body of the tumor being penetrated and eaten up by the twisting reach of the life-force of green and then yellow light. The emotional impact for Jim was great. He had visualized, created, externally seen and experienced the annihilation of his tumor (Figure 12.9).

When I subsequently showed Jim biological images of the working of his killer cells and macrophages, he was stunned to realize the remarkable biological accuracy of his spontaneous images. This connection may be contributed to by the thalamus connected to the hypothalamus in the brain, which receives biologically correct imagery from the somatosensory cortex (Hass-Cohen 2003).

Jim's visual language became less tentative, emboldened in size and certainty of form, expressing his increased affect expression regulation, dynamism and coherency. Our conversations reached places where we could explore the merits and demerits of conventional treatment and tentatively make meaning of Jim's current life story challenges. Jim's mastery of the clay intensified his personal symbolism. To make *All Is One* (Figure 12.10), Jim spent the heart of the session rolling tiny ball after tiny ball of colored clay. He then delicately rolled out each ball into a wispy tendril. When he had a mass of worm-like colors, he lightly assembled five separate balls from gently collected strands, finally pressing them more firmly into balls, and finishing by uniting the balls into a ring. At the time, he could not articulate this process. His hands and the material led him. Yet his title, *All Is One*, spoke impressively of the restoration of harmony, of the gathering of the pieces, of the making wholes of the fragments. As Achterberg *et al.* (1994) remind us, we can understand disease as a rupture in life's harmony and healing as a coming together. Jim and I parted company after eight months, and I believe he had begun to put his life back together again.

Four years later, we met to review and touch base. Jim chose *All Is One* (Figure 12.10) and *Three Stages of Healing* (Figure 12.9) as his favorite art pieces. Jim also told me there was no tumor left. Three months after diagnosis and his holistic treatments, it reduced by 28 percent, and after six months, it was 60 percent smaller. At his last check up, his regular doctor, who had originally found the tumor, told him that no remnant of the cancer remained.

Jim recalled our work together by describing how before our work he had experienced disconnects between his physical body and his self. He said that he was now as conscious, analytical, and physical as before, but had made a long lasting direct connection between his mind and body. He felt that with imagery and visualization he could and did manifest change and light in his body. I asked Jim if he would like to make something visual about this reflection. He once more worked with clay and made an image of the sun/light (Figure 12.11).

Jim reviewed his previous work, which he had not looked at for four years. He was amazed to see that in *Illumination* (Figure 12.11) he had incorporated the same light-sunlight symbol as in the earlier *Sunlight* and *Healing Light* art (Figures 12.7 and 12.8). I asked him if he noticed any changes. Jim spontaneously renamed the two images (12.7 *Trying to Be*; 12.11 *Is*). He said that in *Sunlight*, the source, the center, was fiery, and

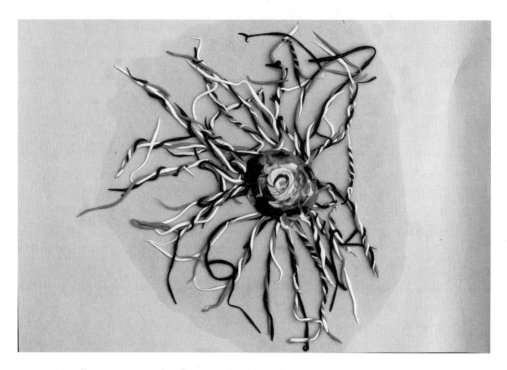

Figure 12.11 Illumination, *Jim's reflection, colored clay, four years after end of treatment.*

that *Illumination* was now more robust and powerful. His statement reflects on his felt experience of increased *dynamic, vivid, symbolic* and *coherent imagery* (Table 12.1).

Jim's journey with his art expressions had a profound impact on us. I believe his ability to embrace and enter a safe inwardly attuned state provided him with a heightened experience of mastery necessary to manipulate affect-laden images. The safe context of our work and the materials connected immune and relational brain functions adding a significant force in his overall dramatic healing. Our work reinforced my curiosity and respect for the intimate links between our body-mind and underscored how internal, external imagery, psychoeducation and a therapeutically secure environment can enhance therapeutic goals.

References

Achterberg, J. (1985). *Imagery in Healing, Shamanism and Modern Medicine*. Boston, MA: Shambala Publications.

Achterberg, J. (1999). Imagery, ceremony, and healing rituals. *Alternative Therapy Health Medicine, 5*(5), 76–83.

Achterberg, J., Dossey, B., and Kolkeimer, L. (1994). *Rituals of Healing: Using Imagery for Health and Wellness*. New York: Bantam Books.

Bach, S. (1990). *Life Paints Its Own Span*. Einsiedeln: Dainton Verlag.

Battino, R. (2000). *Guided Imagery and Other Approaches to Healing*. Camarthen: Crown House Publishing.

Beck, J. S. (1995). *Cognitive Therapy: Basics and Beyond*. New York: Guilford Press.

Cohen, S., Doyle, W. J., Skoner, D. P., Rabin, B. S., and Gwaltney, J. M. (1997). Social ties and susceptibility to the common cold in health adults. *Journal of the American Medical Association, 277*, 1940–1944.

Collins, M. P. and Dunn, L. F. (2005). The effects of meditation and visual imagery on an immune system disorder: Dermatomyositis. *The Journal of Alternative and Complementary Medicine, 11*(2), 275–284.

Conklin, C. A. and Tiffany, S. T. (2001). The impact of imagining personalized versus standardized urge scenarios on cigarette craving and autonomic reactivity. *Experimental and Clinical Psychopharmacology, 9*(4), 399–408.

Conway, M. A. (2001). Sensory perceptual episodic memory and its context: Autobiographical memory. *Philosophical Transactions of the Royal Society of London. Series B: Biological Sciences, 356*, 1375–1384.

Daruna, J. D. (2004). *Introduction to Psychoneuroimmunology*. Burlington, MA: Elsevier Academic Press.

Donaldson, V. W. (2000). A clinical study of visualization on depressed white blood cell count in medical patients. *Applied Psychophysiology and Feedback, 25*(2), 117–128.

Ganis, G., Thompson, W. L., and Kosslyn, S. M. (2004). Brain areas underlying visual mental imagery and visual perception: An fMRI study. *Brain Research Cognitive Brain Research, 20*(2), 226–241.

Giese-Davis, J., Koopman, C., Butler, L., Classen, C., Cordova, M., Fobair, P., *et al.* (2002). Change in emotion regulation strategy for women with metastatic breast cancer following supportive-expressive group therapy. *Journal of Consulting and Clinical Psychology, 70*(4), 914–925.

Gregg, M. and Hall, C. (2006). Measurement of motivational imagery abilities in sport. *Journal of Sports Sciences, 24*(9), 961–971.

Hass-Cohen, N. (2003). Art therapy mind body approaches. *Progress: Family Systems Research and Therapy, 12*, 24–38.

Hass-Cohen, N. (2005). *Phillips Graduate Institute Psychoneuroimmunology Applications 567 Syllabus*. Encino, CA: Phillips Graduate Institute.

Hass-Cohen, N. (2006). Personal Communication, September.

Holmes, E. A. and Matthews, A. M. (2005). Mental imagery and emotion: A special relationship? *Emotion, 5*(4), 489–497.

Irwin, M., Daniels, M., and Weiner, H. (1987). Immune and neuroendocrine changes during bereavement. *Psychiatry in Clinical North America, 10*, 449–465.

Jacobsen, E. (1929). Electrical measurement of neuromuscular states during mental activities: Imagination of movement involving skeletal muscle. *American Journal of Physiology, 91*, 597–608.

Kabat-Zinn, J. (1990). *Full Catastrophe Living*. New York: Delta.

Kemeny, M. E. (1994). Stressful events, psychological responses and progression of HIV infection. In R. Glaser and J. K. Keicolt-Glaser (eds) *Handbook of Human Stress and Immunity* (pp.245–266). San Diego, CA: Academic Press.

Kiecolt-Glaser, J. K., McGuire, L., Robles, T. F., and Glaser, R. (2002a). Emotions, morbidity and mortality: New perspectives from psychoneuroimmunology. *Annual Review of Psychology, 53*, 83–107.

Kiecolt-Glaser, J. K., McGuire, L., Robles, T. F., and Glaser, R. (2002b). Psychoneuroimmunology; psychological influences on immune function and health. *Journal of Consulting and Clinical Psychology, 70*(3), 537–547.

Kiecolt-Glaser, J. K., Robles, T. F., Heffner K. L., Loving, T. J., and Glaser, R. (2002c). Psycho-oncology and cancer: Psychoneuroimmunology and cancer. *European Society for Medical Oncology, 13*(4), 165–169.

Kosslyn, S. M., Ganis, G., and Thompson, W. L. (2001). Neural foundations of imagery. *Nature Review, Neuroscience, 2*, 635–642.

Lennart, N. (1973). *Behold Man: A Photographic Journey of Discovery Inside the Body*. Boston, MA: Little, Brown & Co.

Lekander, M. (2002). Ecological immunology: The role of the immune system in psychology and neuroscience. *European Psychologist, 7*(2), 98–115.

Malchiodi, C. A. (1999). *Medical Art Therapy with Adults*. London and Philadelphia, PA: Jessica Kingsley Publishers.

Martindale, C. (1990). Chapter 4: Creative imagination and neural activity. In R. G. Kunzendorf and A. A. Sheik (eds). *The Psychophysiology of Mental Imagery: Theory, Research and Application*. New York: Baywood Publishing, Inc.

Moshel, Y. A., Durkin, H. G., and Amassian, V. E. (2005). Lateralized neocortical control of T lymphocyte export from the thymus I. Increased export after left cortical stimulation in behaviorally active rats, mediated by sympathetic pathways in the upper spinal cord. *Journal of Neuroimmunology, 158*(1–2), 3–13.

Nainis, N., Paice, J. A., Ratner, J., Wirth, J. H., Lai, J., and Shott, S. (2006). Relieving pain symptoms in cancer: Innovative uses of art therapy. *Journal of Pain and Symptom Management, 31*(2), 162–169.

Naparstek, B. (1994). *Staying Well with Guided Imagery*. New York: Warner Books.

Nilsson, L. (1985). *The Body Victorious*. New York: Delacorte Press.

Pennebaker, J. W. (1997). *Opening Up: The Healing Power of Expressing Emotions*. New York: Guilford Press.

Pert, C. B. (1999). *Molecules of Emotion: The Science Behind Mind-body Medicine*. New York: Simon & Schuster.

Pillemer, D. B. (1998). *Momentous Events, Vivid Memories.* Cambridge, MA: Harvard University Press.

Rossman, M. (2002). Imagery: The body's natural language for healing. *Alternative Therapy Health Medicine, 8*(1): 80–89.

Ryff, C. D. and Singer, B. S. (1998). The contours of positive human health. *Psychological Inquiry, 9,* 1–28.

Sapolsky, R. M. (1998). *Why Zebras Don't Get Ulcers: An Updated Guide to Stress, Stress Related Diseases and Coping.* New York: W. H. Freeman and Company.

Siegel, B. S. (1986). *Love Medicine and Miracles.* New York: Harper and Row.

Shaw, W. A. (1940). The relaxation of muscular action potentials to imaginal weight lifting. *Archives of Psychology, 247,* 50.

Spiegel, D. (1999). Embodying the mind in psycho-oncology research. *Advances in Mind-Body Medicine, 15*(4), 267–273.

Spiegel, D. (2002). The effects of psychotherapy on cancer survival. *Nature Reviews Cancer, 2*(5), 383.

Spiegel, D., Bloom, J. R., Kraemer, H. C., and Gottheil, E. (1989). Effect of psychosocial treatment on survival of patients with metastatic breast cancer. *The Lancet, 2,* 888–891.

Spiegel, D. and Cordova, M. (2001). Supportive-expressive group therapy and life extension of breast cancer patients. *Advances in Mind-Body Medicine, 17*(1), 38–41.

Tuohy, V. K. (2005). Editorial: The neurocortical immune axis. *Journal of Neuroimmunology, 158,* 1–2.

Yaha, H. (2001). *The Miracle of the Immune System.* New Delhi: Goodword Books.

13

Art Therapy, Neuroscience and Complex PTSD

Erin King-West and Noah Hass-Cohen

Jo reported that when she broke her nose and saw blood on her hands she thought "Oh no, not blood on my hands again!" She had no memory of blood on her hands prior to this recollection in the first session with Erin, her art therapist. A 56-year-old Caucasian woman, Jo's waif-like presence belied the ferocity of her mental imagery. Flashbacks of bloody hands and knives, urges to cut and suicidal thoughts were the symbols of Jo's anxiety, depression, and rage (Figure 13.1).

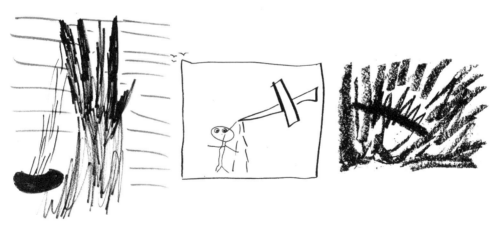

(a) Blood dripping off hand into a bowl (year 1).　(b) Flash of her death (year 2).　(c) Bloody hand holding a bloody knife (year 3).

Figure 13.1(a)–(c): Flashbacks of bloody hands and knives (years 1–3).

Self-hatred and other negative self-schemas also shielded Jo from the devastation of the violence perpetrated against her, and from the anger she felt towards her abusive family. Jo reported that her mother attempted to drown her when she was eight years old. She also reported multiple rapes by her father, uncle, cousin and aunt, as well as torture and sexual degradation. Jo was very thin, hated food, and had to force herself to eat (Figure 13.2).

The survival of childhood sexual abuse is frequently associated with compromised physical health (Briere and Scott 2006, review). Six years into treatment, Jo was diagnosed with breast cancer and underwent a mastectomy and chemotherapy. After seven years of remission, the cancer metastasized into bone cancer. Jo passed away 14 years after therapy began.

Following a memory of an uncle raping her in a graveyard, Jo recalled witnessing him kill another child, which created unbearable distress. Dissociating when feelings began to surface, Jo experienced episodes of lost time. She had memory loss pertaining to daily life events, and difficulties maintaining a train of thought when interacting with people. Mistrusting of most people, she preferred to have no contact for weeks at a time. Eye contact with Erin was infrequent. Jo spent much of the time looking at the floor, expressing her anxiety by tapping her temple with her fingers, possibly an intuitive action, which seemed to decrease the intensity of her traumatic mental imagery (Brewin and Holmes 2003; Brewin and Saunders 2001).

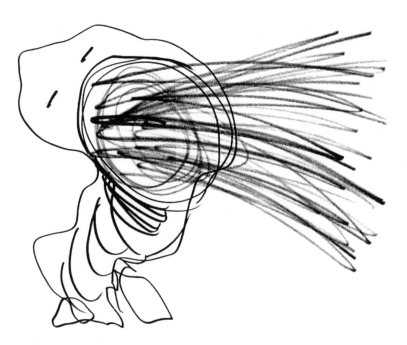

Figure 13.2 Food (year 9).

Jo's resources for coping with the effects of her traumatic childhood included writing. She reported feeling a sense of dread if she didn't write. She was an accomplished and frequently published poet, despite struggles with dyslexia. During treatment, she wrote one novel and was working on a second. Political activism supporting free speech; demonstrating against the war; a passion for nature; and hiking also provided her with a sense of purposefulness. Jo's love for her cats demonstrated her capacity for relational empathy.

Understanding Jo's traumatic story through a relational neurobiology lens is advantageous for: (1) explaining problems inherent in the original trauma and secondary re-traumatization; (2) redefining the interpretation of the art images to include non-symbolic sensory representations of fragmented memories; (3) amplifying the advantages of the visual motor activities associated with art-making; and (4) highlighting the significance of a here-and-now relationship with a caring and empathic therapist.

Complex post-traumatic stress disorder (C-PTSD)

The neuroscience of PTSD underscores the necessity in differentiating between PTSD and C-PTSD diagnoses for the setting of appropriate treatment goals (Briere and Scott 2006 review; Ogden, Minton, and Pain 2006). Jo's history and symptoms are consistent with the phenomena of C-PTSD and Disorders of Extreme Stress (DES). C-PTSD presents with complicated chronic symptoms that are resistant to change. Diagnosed clients have difficulty tolerating exposure and desensitization techniques (Ford 1999; Herman 1992; van der Kolk 2002; van der Kolk, McFarlane, and Weisaeth 1996). In comparison simple PTSD resolves more rapidly, and is more amendable to exposure and desensitization techniques (Briere and Scott 2006, review).

Jo was quick to resist cognitive behavioral approaches by dissociating and forgetting the various self-soothing activities discussed in the sessions. Her limited range of reactions and protective mechanisms required a slower treatment progression. Indeed, space is needed for a long stabilization period in which the client with C-PTSD can perceive, feel and experience emotional safety in the therapeutic setting (Briere and Scott 2006, review).

Art therapists have also emphasized that establishing a base line of control, safety and mastery precedes any treatment goals (Avrahami 2005; Chapman et al. 2001; Malchiodi 2001). Time must be permitted for grief and mourning, while communicating about trauma and receiving support for feelings of guilt, anger, self-blame, and depression. If the C-PTSD involves a fragmentation of the personhood, then a phase treatment approach is recommended in order to first decrease phobic responses, increase interpersonal trust, and carefully evaluate the possibility for integration (van der Hart, Nijenhuis, and Steele 2005).

C-PTSD usually involves more than one unresolved traumatic event; multiple trauma risk factors; and ongoing effects from pre-existing traumas (Brewin, Dalgleish, and Joseph 1996; McKenzie and Wright 1996; Resnick *et al.* 1995), ongoing chronic strains, and lack of social support (Ullman and Siegel 1995). Early childhood sexual and physical abuse puts women at high risk for multiple disorders (Putnam 1989; Ross 1997; Figure 13.3).

Jo's symptomalogy and history met criteria for Major Depression, Dysthemia, Generalized Anxiety Disorder NOS, Dissociative Identity Disorder (DID) and Schizoid Personality Disorder (DSM-IV-TR; American Psychiatric Association [APA] 2000). Clinicians have observed that more often than not, arousal, dissociation and avoidance symptoms are on a continuum of PTSD-related diagnoses (van der Hart *et al.* 2005).

The neurobiology of the stress response is of central interest in C-PTSD. Cortisol baseline responses and regulatory feedback loops are altered. The hypothalamus-pituitary-adrenal (HPA) axis synaptic connections may be permanently changed (Vermetten and Bremner 2002). Insufficient (hypo) cortisol levels have been implicated in hippocampal failure to contain fragmented memories (Schelling *et al.* 2006), and in dissociative symptoms. Decreased cortisol levels have been found for women with PTSD and a history of childhood sexual abuse (CSA) (de Kloet *et al.* 2006; Kaufman *et al.* 2000). Unremitting (hyper) cortisol levels were associated with constraints in

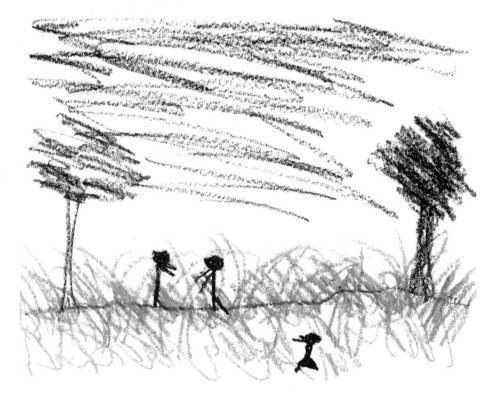

Figure 13.3 Illustration of the day Jo's brother lured her to be raped by a cousin (year 1).

immune system function (Sapolsky 2004), with difficulties in affect regulation (Briere and Scott 2006, review), as well as with memory problems related to decreased hippocampal volume. Cortisol feedback deficits may be either PTSD specific to situations and/or secondary to comorbid, pre-existing psychiatric conditions (Shin, Rauch, and Pitman 2006, review). Women with a history of CSA commonly have a smaller hippocampus (Newport *et al.* 2004; Teicher, Tomoda, and Andersen 2006). Hippocampal differences may be attributed to childhood trauma and/or depression, genetic vulnerability or cognitive constraints (Shea *et al.* 2005, review). Sequelae of stress and stressors sensitizes the stress response and compromises hippocampus function resulting in a loss of neuronal plasticity and long-term neurobiological deficits (Scaer 2001) that may negatively contribute to the ability to learn and change.

Expressions of affect dysregulation

C-PTSD is characterized by overwhelming anxiety, depression and anger accompanied by episodes of lack of feelings. Attempts at affect control result in increased self-destructive behaviors. Overriding fears (Yehuda 1999) also contribute to alterations in attentional systems and conscious states such as amnesia, depersonalization and dissociation. Trauma-based schemas organize sensory inputs as well as intrapersonal and interpersonal perceptual systems, resulting in sensory flashbacks, chronic guilt and shame, mistrust and intimacy issues. The experience of trauma organizes the person's emotional and meaning-making systems (Table 13.1).

Table 13.1 Trauma-based clusters.*

1. Dysregulated inhibition and exhibition of emotions

2. Affect dysregulation: anger, anxiety, depression and self-destructive behaviors

3. Attention/consciousness changes: amnesia, depersonalization, dissociation

4. Intra/interpersonal perceptual alterations: chronic guilt, trust-intimacy issues

5. Meaning-making alterations: trauma-based schemas organize self-world

* Adapted from Ford 1999, Herman 1992, van der Kolk 2002, van der Kolk, McFarlane, and Weisaeth 1996.)

In repeated attempts to regulate affect, Jo produced hundreds of intense color drawings representing what Spring (2001) considers a PTSD special artistic language. For C-PTSD survivors, this increased capacity to generate imagery is in itself a measure of therapeutic change (Brewin *et al.* 1996; Klorer 2001).

Jo used several visual schemas to represent affective and perceptual states. Disjointed stick figures illustrated Jo's tension and frustration. Spiral lines for the trunk and appendages spoke about her hypervigilant perceptual alterations. Gingerbread men outlines, at times left empty or filled with color, pointed to struggles with self-identity.

Along with her words, the images revealed her trauma-driven self-representations (Figure 13.4).

The color symbolism in Jo's drawings stayed consistent throughout treatment. Most frequently, she depicted herself in blue whereas the perpetrator was depicted in red. Rage was represented in red and black; depression was expressed in black, brown or blue. Jo used yellow and orange for hope, lightness and happiness. Anxiety was either depicted by frenetic jagged lines or shaky disintegrating body outlines.

A month into therapy, Jo's drawings began to express rage as a predominant theme. Jo stated that maybe her rage would subside if she could "scream for two years straight." The art imagery indicates that she "screamed" with color, line, shape and imagery for many of the years she was in therapy.

Imagery of bloody hands and daggers, caskets, a hangman's noose around her neck, or anxiety-filled stick figures scribbled out with dense red and black marker all indicated

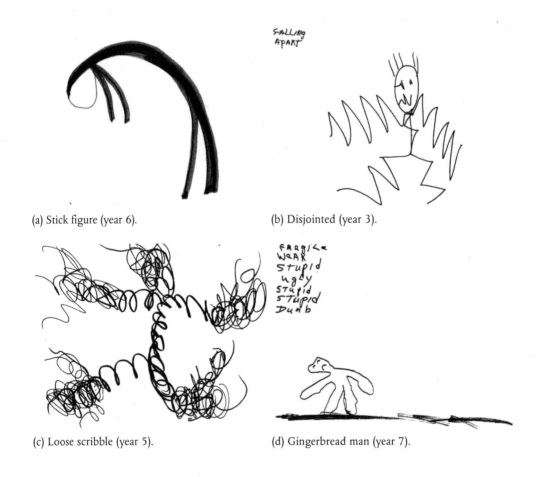

(a) Stick figure (year 6).   (b) Disjointed (year 3).

(c) Loose scribble (year 5).   (d) Gingerbread man (year 7).

Figure 13.4(a)-(d) Various self-representation images (years 3–7).

the intense rage and fear that Jo had experienced throughout her childhood and had re-experienced throughout her life. Repeated trauma associated with chronic fear conditioning through long-term potentiation (LTP) in the lateral nucleus of the amygdala (Rodrigues, Schafe, and LeDoux 2004) contributes to maladaptive re-experiencing of traumatic memories just as if they were occurring right now (Vermetten and Bremner 2002).

Heightened arousal and acute emotional processing, accompanied by attentional and memory problems, are chronically present in PTSD and C-PTSD. Secondary reactions such as depression, cognitive and behavioral avoidance, or anxiety and panic may also develop. Jo reported that her physiological experience of anxiety felt like electricity coursing through her body (Figure 13.5).

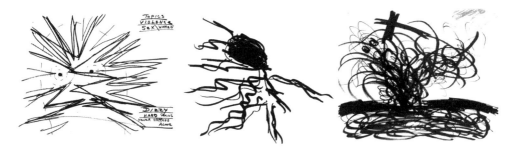

(a) Feelings of electricity (year 2). (b) Encroaching anxiety (year 7). (c) Anxiety coming up from underground overwhelming Jo (year 9).

Figure 13.5(a)–(c) Examples of Jo's anxiety (years 2–9).

Individuals with PTSD are hypervigilant for fearful threats. The metaphor mirrors the electric-like felt anxiety aroused by the hyperactivation of the sympathetic nervous system. The stress response to fear is experienced as increasing heart rate and an adrenaline rush which is released by the sympathetic adrenal medulla.

The amygdala is involved in PTSD assessment of threat-related stimuli (Shin *et al.* 2005, 2006). There is a strong potential for amygdala arousal in response and/or in anticipation of traumatic imagery and scripts (Frewen and Lanius 2006; Rauch *et al.* 2000; Shin *et al.* 2004, 2005). Neural connections between the amygdala and the social engagement system, the polyvagal vagus-system (Porges 2001), have also been associated with visceral symptoms related to anxiety (Lydiard *et al.* 1994). According to some of the research, the amygdala may remain inactivated in PTSD recall (Lanius *et al.* 2006, review). However, amygdala hyper-responsivity has been established for C-PTSD clients with a history of childhood sexual abuse (Bremner *et al.* 2005). Fear-amygdala C-PTSD response also activates the chronic stress HPA cortisol response described earlier. Decrease in serotonin production (Vermetten and Bremner 2002) and thalamic sensory processing problems (Lanius *et al.* 2006, review) are associated with chronic emotional processing deficits (Table 13.2).

Table 13.2 Neurobiology of C-PTSD-CSA.

1. Amygdala activation to specific threats associated with the trauma

2. Heightened sympathetic arousal associated with PTSD anticipatory response to dissociation and vagal numbing

3. Increased heart rate and adrenaline release

4. Dysregulated cortisol system:
   - hyper HPA cortisol response associated with anxiety and fear
   - hypo-cortisol response associated with dissociation responses

5. Sensory information-thalamic disruptions: Failure to screen out and/or relay sensory information

6. Decrease in serotonin production

7. Functional dysfunction and/or morphological changes to prefrontal cortex regions such as the anterior cingulate cortex responsible for modulating anxiety

8. Oscillation between PTSD over-expression and C-PTSD inhibition and dissociation:
   - over-expression: heightened right hemispheric (RH) response
   - inhibition: greater left hemispheric (LH) response

9. PTSD: RH autobiographical processing impairments

10. C-PTSD: LH and limbic emotional sensory processing deficits

The middle prefrontal cortex and surrounding regions help modulate and manage anxiety and fear aroused by traumatic stimuli and memories. C-PTSD symptoms have been associated with medial prefrontal cortex (MPFC) failures, related to the maintenance and extinction of fear conditioning in the amygdala (Shin *et al.* 2006). Therefore, MPFC activity is inversely related to the activity in the amygdala (Shin *et al.* 2004). Specifically, the anterior cingulate cortex's (ACC) failure to help dampen the limbic HPA responses during post-trauma recall (Lanius, Hopper, and Menon 2003) has been associated with chronic emotional processing of PTSD trauma. ACC function is changed in CSA-PTSD (Bremner *et al.* 1999). According to neuroimaging studies, ACC volumes appear to be smaller in abuse-related PTSD (Bremner 1999; Kitayama, Quinn, and Bremner 2006; Lanius *et al.* 2002), again underscoring childhood abuse PTSD risk factors (Brewin, Andrews, and Valentine 2000). Dysfunctions of the ACC have been implicated in numerous psychiatric disorders (Yücel *et al.* 2003, review), which may account for the correlation of PTSD with psychiatric problems.

Fearful and anxious responses are correlated significantly with decreased activation of the MPFC. Dissociation during traumatic narratives presents with greater activation in the MPFC (Lanius *et al.* 2004, 2005). Dissociation is therefore conceptualized as an extreme response of the MPFC attempting to regulate fear. These findings assist in understanding how simple PTSD presents with an over-expression of affect and how C-PTSD disassociation inhibits the expression of affect (Vermetten and Bremner 2002). Over-expression reflects right hemispheric (RH) functioning while inhibition is stronger in the left hemisphere (Shin *et al.* 2006, review).

Art directives may assist in recruiting ACC functions. Erin encouraged Jo to visualize and draw a container. The purpose of the directive was to help contain and master overwhelm from chronically re-experiencing the flashbacks and nightmares. Jo was asked to place the flashbacks in the container mentally and push it far away in her mind's eye. She was then asked to bring the container forward mentally, re-experience a small piece of the emotional contents, and then push it away again, until comfortable titrating the overwhelming affect. Jo, reluctant to do this exercise, believed that Erin was asking her to push the abuse memories back into denial. She was afraid that such regulating of the flow of the traumatic material would inhibit her recovery of memories.

In addition to anxiety and anger, Jo reported experiencing a chronic state of depression and isolation (Figure 13.6).

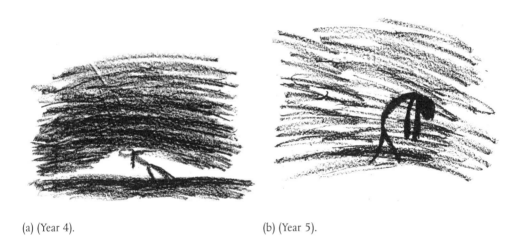

(a) (Year 4).   (b) (Year 5).

Figure 13.6(a)–(b) Depression (years 4–5).

Jo felt helpless to change her central feelings of mistrust towards people and her level of rage at the world. There are significant correlations between major depression and PTSD (Briere and Scott 2006, review; Kaufman *et al.* 2000). The dysregulation of serotonin production in PTSD (Table 13.2) has been implicated in symptoms of depression, irritability and aggression, but also in the re-experiencing of intrusive and avoidant symptoms associated with PTSD (Vermetten and Bremner 2002).

Attention/consciousness alterations: dreams and flashbacks

Not every person who has experienced trauma will go on to develop PTSD or C-PTSD. Fear and dissociative responses at the time of the trauma, such as a feeling that the experience is not happening in reality; time distortions; and out-of-body experiences, are risk factors (Engelhard *et al.* 2003; Murray, Ehlers, and Mayou 2002; Ozer *et al.* 2003).

Re-experiencing of the trauma in the form of flashbacks can alternate with avoidance, numbing, depersonalization, and dissociation (Briere and Scott 2006, review). The dissociative mental processes, often occurring after severe childhood sexual abuse (DSM-IV-TR), disrupt the integrated intrapersonal function (Figure 13.7).

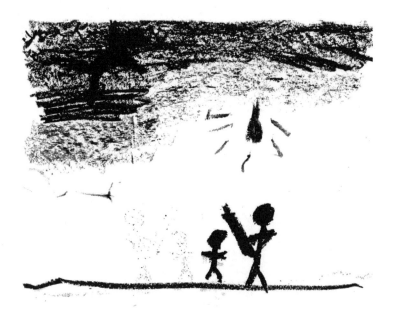

Figure 13.7 Watching the abuse from the ceiling (year 4). An out of body experience; note the dark floating figure in the upper left corner.

The re-experiencing of traumatic implicit, unconscious sensory and emotional memories is unintentional (van der Kolk and Fisler 1995). In the absence of awareness, implicit non-verbal memory strongly influences cognitions, behaviors, and emotions, which can be very alarming. The fear response intensifies the memory and enhances conditioned perceptual priming for traumatic stimuli (Ehlers and Clark 2000). The memory cues are often visual and spatially linked with the event. Clients may remember some insignificant detail from the surroundings (Ehlers and Clark 2000; van der Kolk and Fisler 1995; van der Kolk, Burbridge, and Suzuki 1997). Memory fragmentation results from thalamic sensory processing deficits in spatio-temporal stimuli. The relay of sensory stimuli to the limbic system and to the occipital lobe is also impacted, resulting in deficits in thalamo-cortical dialogues (Temporal Binding Theory; Lanius *et al.* 2006). Therefore, PTSD memory-triggering stimuli may not be semantically integrated into a cortical story. In contrast with art therapy reports (Avrahami 2005; review), it is more likely that many of the fragmented art expressions of C-PTSD flashbacks should not be interpreted as coherent autobiographical narratives or explicit stories.

Primary dissociation: fragmented sensory and emotional memories of traumatic elements

Primary dissociation is the fragmentation of traumatic sensory and emotional memories (Dietrich 2000; van der Kolk, van der Hart, and Marmar 1996). Dual Representation Theory (DRT) proposes two distinct memory systems, a verbally accessible memory system (VAM-DRT) and a situational accessible memory system (SAM-DRT) (Brewin 2001; Brewin *et al.* 1996). The SAM-DRT system is primarily non-verbal and represents fragmented visual-spatial sensory information encoded during trauma (Hellawell and Brewin 2002).

Jo reported hellish nightmares during the second year of treatment. Her images included: pushing a wagon with three dead babies; two girls sleeping in a bed full of rainwater; a small child being cooked for dinner with her tongue cut out and her mouth sewn shut; blood coming from a fan; ocean waves crashing into a house as the house crumbled around her while she tried to save her cats and cleaning her face with gasoline (Figure 13.8).

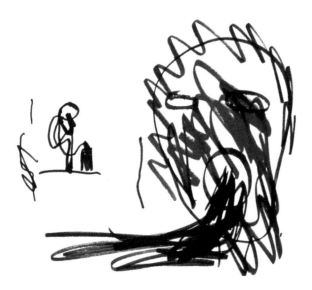

Figure 13.8 Nightmare, cleansing her face with gasoline (year 2).

Cortisol is thought to help integrate and contain traumatic memory (Schelling *et al.* 2006). Jo's fragmented imagery and verbal reports most likely reveal the influences of the dysregulated cortisol response linked to dissociation. Furthermore, the non-verbal anticipatory period of anxiety that precedes the dissociation probably ignites a sympa- thetic response that further conditions the ensuing fragmented memories (Frewen and Lanius 2006). It is therefore important for art therapists to help mitigate potential secondary traumatization by frequently checking in with their clients, avoiding the pre- sentation of ambiguous visual stimuli and introducing unfamiliar and unstructured media slowly (Chapman 2003).

During the first years of treatment, Jo experienced distressing, uncomfortable memories, most likely many SAM-DRT-based. Fragmented memories involve affect, vision, tactile, taste, smell, auditory, and motor systems (Hopper and van der Kolk 2001). By the second and third year, Jo reported having flashes that included hand or knife images dripping with blood and images of her death by murder or of seeing herself in a casket (Figures 13.1 and 13.9).

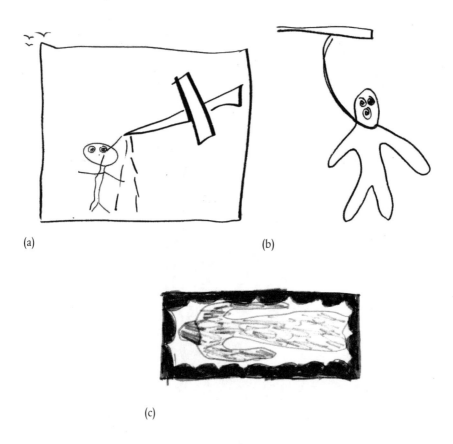

(a)

(b)

(c)

Figure 13.9(a)–(c) Visual flashes: Bloody knives and in the coffin (years 1–3).

Cognitive processes such as labeling, reasoning and narration activate inhibitory pathways, which connect the prefrontal cortex to the amygdala and regulate emotions (Hariri, Bookheimer, and Mazziotta 2000). The verbal narration of SAMS translates to increased thalamic-cortical connections (Holmes, Brewin, and Hennessy 2004). Verbalizations of the imagery processed by the hippocampus may also be able to inhibit lower level thalamic SAM-DRT representations (Holmes *et al.* 2004). Art-making and verbalization have also been linked to right and left hemispheric integration (McNamee 2003). Titling, and talking about the art, actively contribute to changes in the later stages of treatment. These, along with shifts in the DRT nature of imagery, could be considered measures of change.

The art therapist should be wary of expecting to see consistent imagery changes, especially as SAM-DRT processing may continue due to generalized traumatic triggers. For Jo, the Menendez brothers' shooting of their parents in 1989; the 1995 not-guilty verdict in the O. J. Simpson trial; the World Trade Center terrorist attacks in 1999 and on 9/11/2001; the subsequent war on terror; the U.S. bombing of children in Afghanistan in 2003; as well as the death of Jo's three beloved cats, all triggered further traumatic SAM responses in her art (not shown).

As treatment progressed, Jo reported that her dreams were more story-like and that she was able to take action in her dreams. For example, a man standing next to her was stabbed and she was able to call the police. In another, Jo and her ex-husband were walking chest-deep in a river. They met with some people at a cult gathering. Her ex-husband wanted to stay, but Jo wanted to leave, so she did, walking back through the water alone. According to Dual Representation Theory, VAM-DRT system is involved in the integration of trauma memories with autobiographical memories, which can be explicitly retrieved when needed. The contextual information during retrieval indicates that the memories are in the past.

In the later phase of treatment, the number of Jo's flashes and nightmares reduced; she only reported two or three a year and, occasionally, pleasant dreams replaced the violent dreams: a beautiful colorful plant image, and a dream of going for a pleasant drive with her ex-husband (Figure 13.10).

Increased positive affect is associated with a recovery stage where memories of the trauma are being more fully processed and integrated with other memories and a sense of self in the world (Hopper and van der Kolk 2001). The threat of recurrence in the future can then be assessed realistically, and experiences that induced guilt or shame are mitigated. Furthermore, reductions in negative affect may permit tolerance of residual situational memories, therefore allowing habituation and revaluation. Habituation is most often brought about by repeated exposure to the memories in states of gradually increasing calm and relaxation. Effective therapy therefore involves reductions in negative experiences and increases in positive ones.

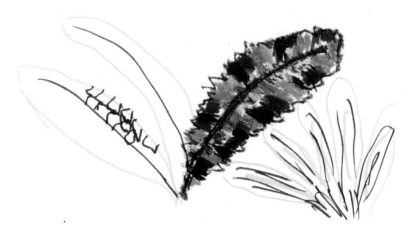

Figure 13.10 Pleasant dream (drawing unfinished, year 7).

> Reduction of affective intensity, the dampening of negative emotion also involves an amplification, an intensification of positive emotion, a condition necessary for more complex self-organization. Attachment is not just the reestablishment of security after a dysregulating experience and a stressful negative state, it is also the interactive amplification of positive affects, as in play states. (Schore 2001a, p.21)

Art therapy is a playful activity; the manipulation of the media simulates play states, which, in the presence of a supportive art therapist, can be a reparative emotional experience.

Secondary peritraumatic dissociation

Secondary dissociation involves a primary dissociation of cognition, depersonalization, confusion and bewilderment, along with the experience of leaving one's body and observing the trauma from a distance (Marmar *et al.* 1997; Figure 13.7). Secondary dissociation comes on the heels of the primary dissociation. It is a vicious PTSD cycle where at the time of the trauma, VAM-DRT processing is fragmented, which contributes to ongoing priming of the PTSD flashbacks (Holmes *et al.* 2004).

In the early years of treatment, Jo frequently experienced difficulties tracking conversations. She reported feeling unfocused. Many times, she asked to be reminded of the question or topic of conversation. The dissociated state was accompanied by a feeling of being in a fog much of the time, getting lost while driving, feeling like she was thrown down by a non-existent person, and hearing self-annihilating statements in her head.

Jo's drawings in the first month were amorphous scribbles depicting foggy disassociative experiences. During the first year of therapy, the fog imagery was prevalent, whereas representative imagery was uncommon. As treatment progressed, a figure appeared in the fog followed subsequently by other figures. By the end of Jo's treatment, fog images became non-existent.

The parts: tertiary level of dissociation

The third level of dissociation includes splitting into distinct ego states as in Dissociative Identity Disorder (DSM-IV-TR, APA 2000). In the first year of treatment, Jo reported experiencing split off parts of her self. *Baby, Punisher, Scars, Whimsy* and the *Twins* separately became present during sessions (Figure 13.11).

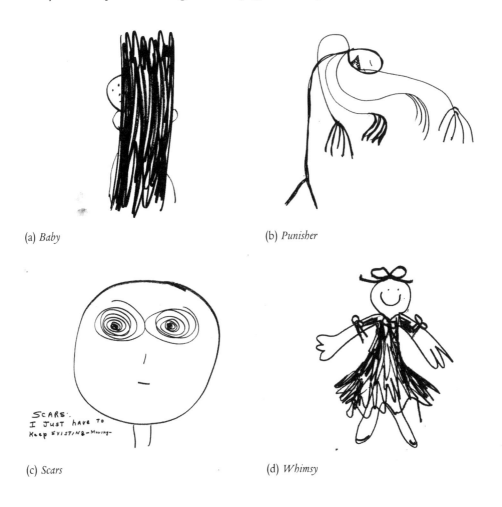

(a) *Baby*

(b) *Punisher*

(c) *Scars*

(d) *Whimsy*

Figure 13.11(a)–(d) Some of Jo's split off parts (year 1).

Baby expressed fear while Jo drew images of pain and violence. *Punisher* represented the split-off self of the introjected dangerous mother (Guntrip 1968; Ross 1997). When cutting desires, suicidal feelings, and flashes of the bloody hand surfaced, *Punisher* was active. Jo stated that when she was five, her father raped her. After the rape, as Jo looked into the bathroom mirror, *Scars* looked back. *Scars* carried the pain, fear, grief and isolation that Jo experienced. *Whimsy* was a four-year-old who liked to play and loved ruffled dresses and curly hair. The *Twins* were the two parts that expressed happiness (not drawn). One was a day person; the other a more seductive night person who liked cosmetics.

Working with the parts

From the first session, Jo stated emphatically that she did not want to integrate her parts (Figure 13.12). This phobic and avoidant response characterizes dissociation (van der Hart *et al.* 2005).

Erin, sensing Jo's distress, recommended that instead of focusing on integration they work on reducing amnestic barriers and encouraging communication between all the parts. Jo accepted these suggestions as to her they maintained the integrity of her personalities. Communication between the parts assists the therapist's and client's understanding of the internal structure of the dissociative defense (Putnam 1989; Ross 1997). The dissociative defense buffers the parts from knowing each other; each part holds different sensory, affective, and cognitive knowledge of the traumatic event.

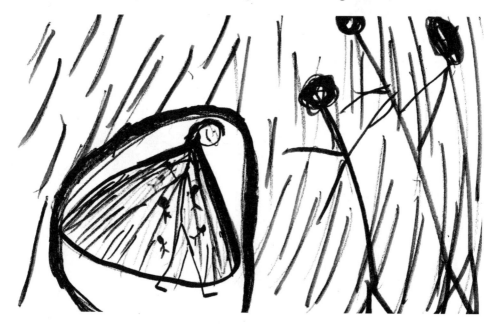

Figure 13.12 Protecting her parts from the outside world (year 3).

Sharing information about Jo's internal landscape, such as where each part lived in her body, the stringency of their boundaries, and the kind of environment in which each resided, helped soften dissociative barriers. In the art, there were less divided lines between the figures over time and the figures were able to share a common area with individualized space for each stick figure.

Inhibition is thought to be the result of sustained efforts to avoid the reactivation of unpleasant SAM or VAM-DRT representations. Trauma victims frequently describe strategies they use for avoiding thoughts about the trauma in order to escape the accompanying emotional arousal. Unfortunately, inhibition leaves unprocessed memories vulnerable to reactivation later in life. Furthermore, the physiological effects of inhibiting emotional expression appear to lead to impaired immune function (Pennebaker, Kiecolt-Glaser, and Glaser 1988) and poorer health status on a variety of indices (Brewin et al. 1996; van der Kolk 2002).

Early in treatment, Jo had a benign tumor lumpectomy. Jo shared that her surgery made her realize that no matter how small she had tried to make herself, she was not safe from the memory of her mother's sexualized behavior of rubbing cream on Jo's breasts (Figure 13.13).

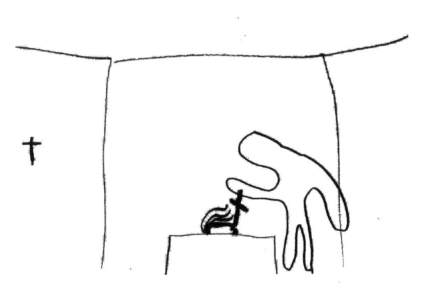

Figure 13.13 No safety. Mental image Jo had during lumpectomy resulted in this image of a small person on a table being stabbed, with a cross hanging on the wall in the background. She did not know if this image was a memory. Jo and Erin continued holding the "not knowing" if she was abused in this way.

Together with Erin, Jo began exploring this memory by asking each part to share its memories and feelings with the other parts. The parts that experienced the physical sensations reported that during the surgery, the body felt transparent and they felt outside of the body. Other parts believed that "touch hurts, people hurt, Jo must stay away from people." The part holding the feelings simultaneously reported revulsion and hunger for her mother's attention. Dissociated parts can be helped to share various aspects of the experience with each other in this kind of step-by-step exploration (Braun 1988a, 1988b). Thus, Jo was able to begin to link her current beliefs and actions regarding her isolation and fear of people with childhood events. Erin noted that over time Jo's needs to dissociate decreased.

Art therapy treatment opportunities

Erin noted that prolonged exposure to memories encoded in the art and/or desensitization approaches to treatment caused Jo great distress and intolerable emotional states. Exposure techniques may arouse very strong fear reactions, possibly dissociation and treatment failure (Chapman *et al.* 2001; deJong *et al.* 2005; McDonagh *et al.* 2005; van der Kolk 2002; van der Kolk *et al.* 2005). The hyper-responsivity to threat associated with C-PTSD/CSA women creates a risk for re-traumatizing and rekindling the amygdala (Allen 2001; Bremner *et al.* 2005). Research also suggested that the re-experiencing of traumatic memories competes for mental resources (Hellawell and Brewin 2002). Art therapy clients who experience intrusive images may find it hard to draw or talk, as the memories may take up most of their cognitive capacity.

When anxious, Jo had a habit of finger tapping on her temples. Finger tapping may help prevent the resurfacing of intense memories and the reconditioning of fear (Brewin and Holmes 2003; Brewin and Saunders, 2001). The motor activity blocks SAM-DRT formation as well as reduces and lessens vivid intrusions (Andrade, Kavanagh, and Baddeley 1997; Kavanagh *et al.* 2001; van den Hout *et al.* 2001). Jo's spontaneous tapping habit may have helped distract her from intrusive SAM-DRT imagery. Simple repetitive art therapy activities, such as kneading a piece of plasticine, cutting paper into shapes, or stringing beads together while talking about difficult memories may, in future research, be shown to help reduce the devastating influence of SAM-DRT intrusions.

Developing trust and intimacy: altering interpersonal perceptions

Art introduces experiences that differ from anything previously associated with the trauma. The novel process can help decrease implicit, automatic responses and increase flexible, adaptive, coherent, energized, and stable interpersonal mental states (FACES) (Siegel 2006). Jo's drawings demonstrated how clients could practice integrating bodily sensations, images, emotions, feelings and thoughts into one picture. With every drawing, Jo practiced engagement and disengagement with the art images. As the drawings were completed, they were viewed from a distance and then held in her art folder. Similar to titrating the exposure (Briere 2006), the art can be held at a distance, put away or taken out for discussion. The process increases interpersonal capacity through viewing of the art. Together with the art therapist, the art can be re-examined, discussed and titled in order to provide increased opportunities for mental flexibility and narrative coherency. Simple media, such as markers, helped Jo gain a sense of control as she adapted to a novel situation that decreased the possibility of automatic threat responses.

Jo often expressed a preference to be left alone. For weeks at a time, she wouldn't want to be with another human being. Early adverse experiences and prior relationship failures demanded a long stabilization period in order to develop the therapeutic alliance. This is common and, in fact, expected for C-PTSD survivors (Chapman *et al.* 2001; deJong *et al.* 2005; McDonagh *et al.* 2005; van der Kolk 2002; van der Kolk *et al.* 2005).

Exposure to childhood sexual abuse activates a pattern of unremitting amygdala fear-based responses to others. The ensuing neurochemical cascade can alter the child's developing brain, inhibit neurogenesis, and contribute to neurochemical alterations (as reviewed in Perry 2001; Schore 2001b). Child sexual abuse contributes to changed corpus callosum size, significant bi-lateral reduction in hippocampal volume, and greater than average non-verbal right hemispheric dominance (Teicher *et al.* 2006). Exposed to violence, the child, using a predominately hyperarousal response, will eventually become vulnerable to persistent hyperarousal-related symptoms and disorders within the spectrum of anxiety and fear disorders (Perry 2001; Perry *et al.* 1995). Prominent related symptoms include somatic complaints, dissociation, anxiety, helplessness, dependence and isolation.

The types of neurobiological changes and symptom severity depend on the child's adaptive response to the threat, the specific nature of the violence, as well as that of the family and community environment (Perry and Azad 1999). Jo's relationship with her parents provided a template forming her assumptions about relating to people. Her artwork indicated that her adaptive responses resulted in fears of either being consumed or annihilated. In order to ameliorate this hyperarousal around people, Jo preferred total isolation rather than attempt to handle the frightening confusion of defining boundaries between self and other. Fear of death or fusion strongly deterred her from developing emotionally intimate relationships.

Jo supplicated herself completely to her mother in order to survive her early years, hence developing an interpersonal perceptual alteration. The image of a dominating mother figure intimidating or attacking a weaker person remained consistent throughout the 14 years of therapy. In treatment, Jo processed the trauma, *Mother Forcing Jo to Eat Her Vomit*, and her internal critical voice, *Critical Self and Child Self*, and began to fight back and eventually own her power (Figure 13.14(a)–(c)).

The degree of menacing intimidation expressed in the dominating figure reduced over the years as Jo processed her fear, wrath and conflicts. She increased affect regulation in the safety of the graphic media and the therapeutic alliance.

At the beginning of therapy, Jo's father was still alive and time was spent exploring her conflicting memories about him. She reported memories of rape as well as memories of a kind and gentle father who taught her to love nature. Initially, Jo remembered and experienced either consuming rage or affectionate feelings. After several years, she was able to present both on one page, without needing to forget the other aspect (Figure 13.14(d)).

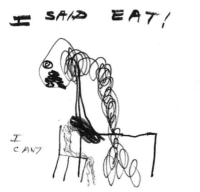
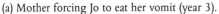

(a) Mother forcing Jo to eat her vomit (year 3).

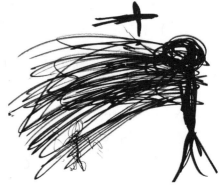

(b) Critical self and child self (year 11).

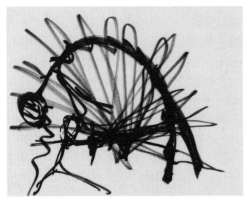

(c) Fighting back at mother (year 14).

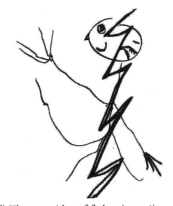

(d) The two sides of father (year 6).

Figure 13.14(a)–(d) The series of images reflects (a) the process of exposure to the trauma, (b) turning the anger upon herself, (c) owning the anger and directing it back towards mother, (d) the two sides of father (years 3–14).

Jo expressed a wish to develop more friendships, yet, as she spoke about it, she felt spacey and lost her train of thought and dissociated in the face of anticipatory fear. Jo's

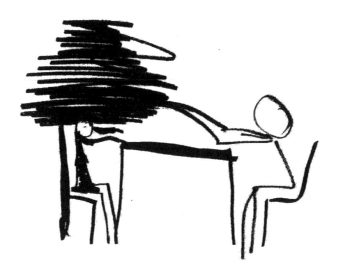

Figure 13.15 A friend pushing pills on her (year 2).

trauma-based schemas maintained her fear and distrust of people and relationships. Early on, her level of sensitivity to another person's emotional temperature was acute. Sensing any anger from an individual heightened her hyperarousal responses, increasing anxiety. She reported feeling an erosion of self-boundaries when a friend ignored her desires not to take herbal pills. Jo attempted to say no, but fearful of the friend's rage, dissociated, allowing a little part to acquiesce and take the pills (Figure 13.15).

Jo felt trapped by this friend's intrusiveness. She drew her friend, the larger dominating figure, and herself in a room (Figure 13.16(a)). In the second part of the drawing, Jo crossed out the friend, added a self-protective shield and a door. In the next image, she drew a teddy bear and a blanket providing safety for *Baby* (Figure 13.16(b)). Continuing to make *Baby*'s environment safer, Jo boarded up the window to block the angry friend's view. As the friend was still able to peek in through the boards, Jo scribbled out the window, obliterating his image, which provided relieving affect regulation. Several weeks later, continuing to process the feelings about providing safety for the little parts, Jo drew the last image, an internal safe place (Figure 13.16(c)).

As therapy progressed, Jo's trauma-based schemas started to change and she began to assert herself with friends and let them know what she wanted. The drawing of a friend rushing Jo through a store illustrates this change where she was able to tell the friend that this was not working for her (Figure 13.17).

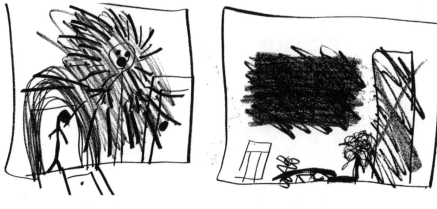

(a) Trapped/making it safe.   (b) Making it safe for Baby.

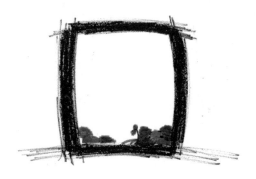

(c) A safe place for the little ones.

Figure 13.16(a)–(c) Processing safety in relationships (year 2).

Jo belonged to a writers' group during the entire time she and Erin worked together. Although she was a frequently published poet, interpersonal perceptual alterations continued to make her feel inferior to the other writers. Jo struggled to be in the group, at times saying nothing or leaving early due to intense fears of annihilation. Jo's fears of being in a group (Figure 13.18, left side) contrast with her wish to be included.

A few years before Jo's cancer reoccurred, she developed the confidence to organize a salon for about 40 writers, which included a catered dinner. The event went well and she expressed a beginning belief that she was developing some self-confidence and more comfort around people. Just prior to the diagnosis of bone cancer, she joined a 12-step group and found a sponsor. During chemotherapy and hospice care, she spoke to her sponsor daily. Jo withstood the vicissitudes of human relationships and stayed connected.

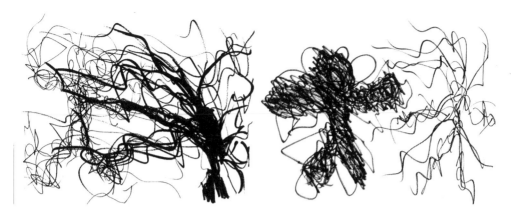

(a) A friend rushing her, Jo feeling invaded (Jo is the figure on the left).

(b) Stating what she wanted supported Jo's boundaries (Jo is the figure on the left).

Figure 13.17(a)–(b) Comparison of Jo's boundaries before and after she stated her desire to a friend (year 10).

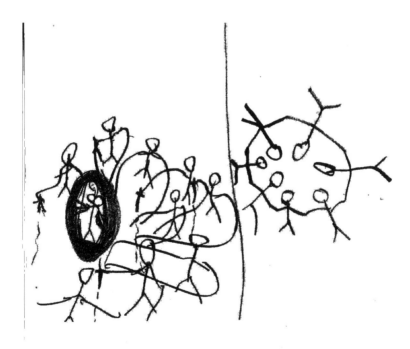

Figure 13.18 Processing fear experiences in groups. On the left group members holding bloody knives versus a fantasy group on the right (year 2).

The empathic art therapist

Empathy, from the Greek, means "to suffer with" (Walrond-Skinner 1986). Empathy is a form of emotional resonance (Siegel 2006) which involves the ability to put oneself into another's place, facilitating one's ability to recognize, perceive and directly experience the emotions and feelings, thoughts and beliefs of another. Despite a diversity of theoretical approaches, it is generally agreed upon that empathic responses involve several sequential conditions (Decety and Jackson 2004; Watt 2005). The first condition is an automatic contagious feeling of what someone is feeling or a conscious knowing what someone is feeling. This condition is not sufficient for an empathic response. If the therapist cannot explicitly differentiate between her *self* versus the client's *other*, she may respond with personal distress, which deters attention away from the client's needs and results in mis-attunement and circumvents a pro-social intent to alleviate suffering therapeutically.

Empathic social-emotional responses are thought to be involved in the activation of mirror-neuron regions previously associated only with the recognition of purposeful hand gestures (Iacoboni and Dapretto 2006, review). Observing the actions, sensations, emotions, and feelings of others activates the same brain areas that would be involved if the observer himself were performing/experiencing the actions, sensations and emotions (Keysers and Gazzola 2006; Wicker *et al.* 2003). The interpretation of this firing is made in the prefrontal cortex and involves the activation of a diffuse connection of subcortical and cortical regions (Watt 2005).

The client's anxious marker strokes, and severity of C-PTSD fragmented sensory memory images, challenge the art therapist's capacity for empathic responses. The distinct fragmented quality of C-PTSD imagery requires a therapist to tolerate seeing and experiencing the impact of these images, and their repeated elements encoded within difficult and painful autobiographical material. Because of the firing of the mirror neuron systems, the therapist may see and feel what the client says and makes, while the client's mirroring allows the experience of the therapist's actions and emotional messages to be registered (Hass-Cohen 2008; Siegel 2006). As images like Jo's display a lack of socially and personally evaluated meaning, the therapist may empathically find herself experiencing a similar lack of meaning internally. Activation of mirror systems put Erin and Jo on the same page on the same emotional matrix. The therapist gets a tremendous sense of helplessness, which feels like fatigue, and results in a lack of concentration. For example, Erin reported feelings of sleepiness in the early years of therapy as a result of the empathic resonance to the dissociative states. Empathic responses challenge both parties to integrate aspects of the self that would otherwise be unknown. The sensory, motor and tactile quality of the SAM-DRT art representations may further tax the art therapist's capacity for empathic responses. The art therapist may have a hard time separating his or her internally generated affect and implicit sensations from those of his or her client's. Consultation with another therapist, one who is outside of the therapy shared neuro-circuitry mirror neurons systems, may help clarify the therapist's subjective experience. Erin found that consultation provided needed support and insight to compensate for this effect.

Erin allowed Jo's vision, sound, and art-making to excite her own brain circuitry, facilitating intuitive insights into, and empathy for, Jo's inner life. Erin's empathic responses involved juggling the art interventions so that Jo could experience some recollection and integration, but without too much overwhelming emotions that may have triggered more avoidance behaviors and dissociation, according to Briere and Scott (2006, review). The therapist's empathic response to images of shame and pain can provide an intuitive understanding about when therapeutic exploration of the traumatic memories encoded in the imagery may be supportive, or contraindicated. Erin used the art to adapt to Jo's tolerance of therapy and accommodate Jo's goals while affording her the experience of memories and allowing for a tolerable level of emotional engagement. Erin's empathic use of the art facilitated affect regulation in the here and now, which most likely titrated Jo's re-exposure to traumatic memories. How art therapy processes activate empathic resonance holds fascinating implications (Hass-Cohen 2007) and remains to be researched.

Over time, the empathic art therapy resonances reinforced a positive working relationship. Several years into therapy, Jo expressed anger at Erin for not attuning to her needs in the session. She expressed that Erin was not taking her dreams seriously. Jo felt Erin was denying Jo's reality, belittling her for her beliefs and judging her artwork. Erin interpreted this reaction as a positive change, compared to Jo's shy withdrawn first year responses (Figure 13.19).

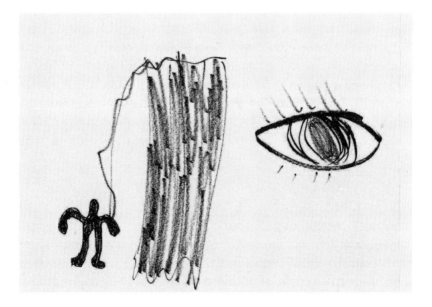

Figure 13.19 Hiding from Erin (year 2).

Erin warmly supported Jo while gently exploring these feelings. Art therapists are vulnerable to countertransference and secondary traumatic responses to the art (Riley 1997) and to traumatic verbal scripts (Shin *et al.* 2006). The receptivity of the mirror neurons to meaning-making in action may account for this sensitivity. It is likely that Jo's depictions of pain inflicted on her by others evoked a strong affective response in Erin. Brain imaging has shown that inter-subjective representation of pain registers both the presence of observed pain and its intensity (Saarela *et al.* 2007) in the observer's brain. For example, Jo asked Erin to watch the movie *Bastard out of Carolina*, directed by Angelica Huston, about a young girl who is beaten and raped by her mother's boyfriend. Erin reported struggling with watching the rape scene and turned the video off. Neuroimaging suggests that this countertransference response associates more with Erin's affective response than with any actual pain sensations. The

> neural response in AI and rostral ACC, activated in common for "self" and "other" conditions, suggests that the neural substrate for empathic experience does not involve the entire "pain matrix"... We conclude that only that part of the pain network associated with affective qualities, not sensory qualities, mediate empathy. (Singer *et al.* 2004, p.1157).

Additional neuroimaging findings also show that empathy and self-other perspectives do not involve a full neurological merge with the other (reviewed in Decety and Lamm 2006).

Empathic responses support clients' improvement with identifying dangerous signs and safe cues, as well as identifying positive experiences capable of counter-conditioning avoidance responses (Briere and Scott 2006, review). For example, when Erin reported to Jo that she was unable to watch the rape scene in the movie, Jo felt safe enough with Erin to tell her that if she, Jo, could live through such abuse in real life, then the least Erin could do was watch a movie about it. She spoke with Erin about perceived mis-attunements, despite worrying that Erin would abandon her as three previous therapists had. Learning from each other through empathic and motor mirror-neuron systems perhaps facilitated Jo's realization that her expectation was a source attribution error (Briere and Scott 2006, review) stemming from her relationship with her mother. Thus, her anger was substantially reduced, altering a trauma-based schema in the therapeutic relationship.

Epilogue

Before undergoing chemotherapy for her bone cancer, Jo reviewed the gains she had made in therapy. She drew her life at the beginning of therapy, and now as well as her goals for the future (Figure 13.20).

The first image reflected the affect dysregulation including anger, depression and the disassociative fog Jo lived with daily. The second image shows some remaining anxiety, but she added green for nature and the yellow for positive hope, which was

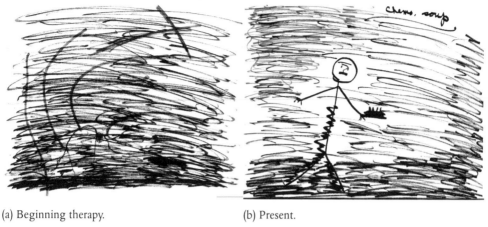

(a) Beginning therapy.   (b) Present.

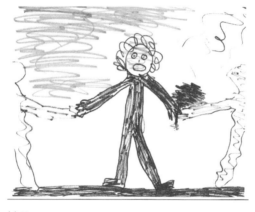

(c) Future.

Figure 13.20(a)–(c) Jo's internal experience at the beginning of treatment, at termination and her fantasized future (year 14).

more present in her life. The future depicted a whole body making contact with others, with none of the disassociative fog or anxiety in the background.

Jo passed away within the year. About 18 to 20 people came to Jo's memorial service. Many shared how deeply she had touched their lives with her passion, spirit, and adamant insistence on facing her past and present as honestly as possible. Her sponsor remarked on Jo's perception of herself as a loner, and yet she died with many friends around her, which was her dying wish to be at home surrounded by friends.

References

Allen, J. G. (2001). *Traumatic Relationships and Serious Mental Disorders*. Chichester, NY: John Wiley.

American Psychiatric Association. (2000). *Diagnostic and Statistical Manual of Mental Disorders* (4th edition). Washington, DC: Author.

American Psychiatric Association. (2000). *Diagnostic and Statistical Manual of Mental Disorders* (4th edition, text revision). Washington, DC: Author.

Andrade, J., Kavanagh, D., and Baddeley, A. (1997). Eye-movements and visual imagery: A working memory approach to the treatment of post-traumatic stress disorder. *British Journal of Clinical Psychology, 36*(2), 209–223.

Avrahami, D. (2005). Visual art therapy's unique contribution in the treatment of post-traumatic stress disorders. *Journal of Trauma and Dissociation, 6*(4), 5–38.

Braun, B. (1988a). The BASK (behavior, affect, sensation, knowledge) model of dissociation. *Dissociation, 1*(1), 4–23.

Braun, B. (1988b). The BASK model of dissociation: Clinical applications. *Dissociation, 1*(2), 16–23.

Bremner, J. D. (1999). Does stress damage the brain? *Biological Psychiatry, 45*(7), 797–805.

Bremner, J. D., Narayan, M., Staib, L. H., Southwick, S. M., McGlashan, T., and Charney, D. S. (1999). Neural correlates of memories of childhood sexual abuse in women with and without posttraumatic stress disorder. *The American Journal of Psychiatry, 156*(11), 1787–1795.

Bremner, J. D., Vermetten, E., Schmahl, C., Vaccarino, V., Vythilingam, M., Afzal, N., *et al.* (2005). Positron emission tomographic imaging of neural correlates of a fear acquisition and extinction paradigm in women with childhood sexual-abuse-related post-traumatic stress disorder. *Psychological Medicine, 35*(6), 791–806.

Brewin, C. R. (2001). A cognitive neuroscience account of posttraumatic stress disorder and its treatment. *Behaviour Research and Therapy, 39*(4), 373–393.

Brewin, C. R., Andrews, B., and Valentine, J. D. (2000). Meta-analysis of risk factors for posttraumatic stress disorder in trauma-exposed adults. *Journal of Consulting and Clinical Psychology, 68*(5), 748–766.

Brewin, C. R., Dalgleish, T., and Joseph, S. (1996). A dual representation theory of posttraumatic stress disorder. *Psychological Review, 103*(4), 670–686.

Brewin, C. R. and Holmes, E. A. (2003). Psychological theories of posttraumatic stress disorder. *Clinical Psychology Review, 23*(3), 339–376.

Brewin, C. R. and Saunders, J. (2001). The effect of dissociation at encoding on intrusive memories for a stressful film. *The British Journal of Medical Psychology, 74*(4), 467–472.

Briere, J. (2006). Dissociative symptoms and trauma exposure: Specificity, affect dysregulation, and posttraumatic stress. *The Journal of Nervous and Mental Disease, 194*(2), 78–82.

Briere, J. and Scott, C. (2006). *Principles of Trauma Therapy: A Guide to Symptoms, Evaluation, and Treatment*. Thousand Oaks, CA: Sage Publications.

Chapman, L. (2003). Neuro-developmental art therapy: Treating acute and chronic post-traumatic stress disorder and symptoms. Paper presented at the annual meeting of the American Art Therapy Association, Chicago, IL.

Chapman, L., Morabito, D., Ladakakos, C., Schrier, H., and Knudson, M. M. (2001). The effectiveness of art therapy intervention in reducing posttraumatic stress disorder (PTSD) symptoms in pediatric trauma patients. *Art Therapy, 18*(2), 100–104.

Decety, J. and Jackson, P. L. (2004). The functional architecture of human empathy. *Behavioral and Cognitive Neuroscience Reviews, 3*(2), 71–100.

Decety, J. and Lamm, C. (2006). Human empathy through the lens of social neuroscience. *The Scientific World Journal, 6*, 1146–1163.

de Jong, J. T., Komproe, I. H., Spinazzola, J., van der Kolk, B. A., and Van Ommeren, M. H. (2005). DESNOS in three postconflict settings: Assessing cross-cultural construct equivalence. *Journal of Traumatic Stress, 18*(1), 13–21.

de Kloet, C. S., Vermetten, E., Geuze, E., Kavelaars, A., Heijnen, C. J. and Westenberg, H. G. M. (2006). Assessment of HPA-axis function in posttraumatic stress disorder: Pharmacological and non-pharmacological challenge tests, a review. *Journal of Psychiatric Research, 40*(6), 550–567.

Dietrich, A. M. (2000). A review of visual/kinesthetic disassociation in the treatment of posttraumatic disorders: Theory, efficacy and practice recommendations. *Traumatology, 6*(2), 85–107.

Ehlers, A. and Clark, D. M. (2000). A cognitive model of posttraumatic stress disorder. *Behaviour Research and Therapy, 38*(4), 319–345.

Engelhard, I. M., van den Hout, M. A., Kindt, M., Arntz, A., and Schouten, E. (2003). Peritraumatic dissociation and posttraumatic stress after pregnancy loss: A prospective study. *Behaviour Research and Therapy, 41*(1), 67–78.

Ford, J. D. (1999). Disorders of extreme stress following war-zone military trauma: Associated features of posttraumatic stress disorder or comorbid but distinct syndromes? *Journal of Consulting and Clinical Psychology, 67*(1), 3–12.

Frewen, P. A. and Lanius, R. A. (2006). Toward a psychobiology of posttraumatic self-dysregulation: Reexperiencing, hyperarousal, dissociation, and emotional numbing. *Annals of the New York Academy of Sciences, 1071,* 110–124.

Guntrip, H. J. S. (1968). *Schizoid Phenomena, Object-relations, and the Self.* New York: International Universities Press, Inc.

Hariri, A. R., Bookheimer, S. Y., and Mazziotta, J. C. (2000). Modulating emotional responses: Effects of a neocortical network on the limbic system. *Neuroreport, 11*(1), 43–48.

Hass-Cohen, N. (2007, in press). Cultural Arts in Action: Musings on Empathy. GAINS *Community Newsletter: Connections and Reflections.*

Hass-Cohen, N. (2008). *CREATE*: Art Therapy Relational Neuroscience Principles. In N. Hass-Cohen and R. Carr (eds) *Art Therapy and Clinical Neuroscience.* London: Jessica Kingsley Publishers.

Hellawell, S. J. and Brewin, C. R. (2002). A comparison of flashbacks and ordinary autobiographical memories of trauma: Cognitive resources and behavioural observations. *Behaviour Research and Therapy, 40*(10), 1143–1156.

Herman, J. L. (1992). *Trauma and Recovery.* New York: Basic Books.

Holmes, E. A., Brewin, C. R., and Hennessy, R. G. (2004). Trauma films, information processing, and intrusive memory development. *Journal of Experimental Psychology. General, 133*(1), 3–22.

Hopper, J. W. and van der Kolk, B. A. (2001). Retrieving, assessing, and classifying traumatic memories: A preliminary report on three case studies of a new standardized method. *Journal of Aggression, Maltreatment and Trauma, 4*(2), 33–71.

Iacoboni, M. and Dapretto, M. (2006). The mirror neuron system and the consequences of its dysfunction. *Nature Reviews. Neuroscience, 7*(12), 942–951.

Kaufman, J., Plotsky, P. M., Nemeroff, C. B., and Charney, D. S. (2000). Effects of early adverse experiences on brain structure and function: Clinical implications. *Biological Psychiatry, 48*(8), 778–790.

Kavanagh, D. J., Freese, S., Andrade, J., and May, J. (2001). Effects of visuospatial tasks on desensitization to emotive memories. *The British Journal of Clinical Psychology, 40*(3), 267–280.

Keysers, C. and Gazzola, V. (2006). Towards a unifying neural theory of social cognition. *Progress in Brain Research, 156,* 379–401.

Kitayama, N., Quinn, S., and Bremner, J. D. (2006). Smaller volume of anterior cingulate cortex in abuse-related posttraumatic stress disorder. *Journal of Affective Disorders, 90*(2–3), 171–174.

Klorer, G. P. (2001). *Expressive Therapy with Troubled Children.* Lanham, MD: Jason Aronson, Inc.

Lanius, R, A., Hopper, J. W., and Menon, R. S. (2003) Individual differences in a husband and wife who developed PTSD after a motor vehicle accident: A functional MRI case study. *American Journal of Psychiatry, 160,* 667–669.

Lanius, R., Lanius, U., Fisher, J., and Ogden, P. (2006). Psychological trauma and the brain: Toward a neurobiological treatment model. In P. Ogden, K. Minton, and C. Pain (eds) *Trauma and the Body.* New York and London: W.W. Norton & Company.

Lanius, R. A., Williamson, P. C., Bluhr, R. L., Densmore, M., Boksman, K., Neufeld, R. W., *et al.* (2005). Functional connectivity of dissociative responses in posttraumatic stress disorder: A functional magnetic resonance imaging investigation. *Biological Psychiatry, 57*(8), 873–884.

Lanius, R. A., Williamson, P. C., Boksman, K., Densmore, M., Gupta, M., Neufeld, R. W., *et al.* (2002). Brain activation during script-driven imagery induced dissociative responses in PTSD: A functional magnetic resonance imaging investigation. *Biological Psychiatry, 52*(4), 305–311.

Lanius, R. A., Williamson, P. C., Densmore, M., Boksman, K., Neufeld, R. W., Gati, J. S., *et al.* (2004). The nature of traumatic memories: A 4-T fMRI functional connectivity analysis. *The American Journal of Psychiatry, 160*(1), 1–9.

Lydiard, R. B., Greenwald, S., Weissman, M. M., Johnson, J., Drossman, D. A., and Ballenger, J. C. (1994). Panic disorder and gastrointestinal symptoms: Findings from the NIMH Epidemiologic Catchment Area project. *The American Journal of Psychiatry, 151*(1), 64–70.

Malchiodi, C. A. (2001). Using drawings as interventions with traumatized children. *Trauma and Loss: Research and Interventions, 1*(1), 21–28.

Marmar, C. R., Weiss, D. S., and Metzler, T. (1997). Peritraumatic dissociation and posttraumatic stress disorder. In J. D. Bremner and C. R. Marmar (eds) *Trauma, Memory, and Dissociation.* Washington, DC: American Psychiatric Press.

McDonagh, A., Friedman, M., McHugo, G., Ford, J., Sengupta, A., Mueser, K., *et al.* (2005). Randomized trial of cognitive-behavioral therapy for chronic posttraumatic stress disorder in adult female survivors of childhood sexual abuse. *Journal of Consulting and Clinical Psychology, 73*(3), 515–524.

McKenzie, C. D. and Wright, L. S. (1996). *Delayed Posttraumatic Stress Disorder from Infancy: The Two Trauma Mechanisms.* Amsterdam: Harwood Academic Publishers.

McNamee, C. (2003). *Bilateral Art: A Creative Response to Advances in Neuroscience.* Paper presented at the annual meeting of the American Art Therapy Association, Chicago, IL.

Murray, J., Ehlers, A., and Mayou, R. A. (2002). Dissociation and post-traumatic stress disorder: Two prospective studies of road traffic accident survivors. *The British Journal of Psychiatry, 180,* 363–368.

Newport, D. J., Heim, C., Bonsall, R., Miller, A. H., and Nemeroff, C. B. (2004). Pituitary-adrenal responses to standard and low-dose dexamethasone suppression tests in adult survivors of child abuse. *Biological Psychiatry, 55*(1), 10–20.

Ogden, P., Minton, K., and Pain, C. (2006). *Trauma and the Body: A Sensorimotor Approach to Psychotherapy.* New York: W. W. Norton.

Ozer, E. J., Best, S. R., Lipsey, T. L., and Weiss, D. S. (2003). Predictors of posttraumatic stress disorder and symptoms in adults: A meta-analysis. *Psychological Bulletin, 129*(1), 52–73.

Pennebaker, J. W., Kiecolt-Glaser, J. K., and Glaser, R. (1988). Disclosure of traumas and immune function: Health implications for psychotherapy. *Journal of Consulting and Clinical Psychology, 56*(2), 239–245.

Perry, B. D. (2001). The neurodevelopmental impact of violence in childhood. In D. Schetky and E. Benedek (eds) *Textbook of Child and Adolescent Forensic Psychiatry* (pp.221–238). Washington, DC: American Psychiatric Press.

Perry, B. D. and Azad, I. (1999). Posttraumatic stress disorders in children and adolescents. *Current Opinion in Pediatrics, 11*(4), 310–316.

Perry, B. D., Pollard, R. A., Blakley, T. L., Baker, W. L., and Vigilante, D. (1995). Childhood trauma, the neurobiology of adaptation and "use-dependent" development of the brain: How "states" become "traits." *Infant Mental Health Journal, 16*(4), 271–291.

Porges, S. W. (2001). The polyvagal theory: Phylogenetic substrates of a social nervous system. *International Journal of Psychophysiology, 42*(2), 123–146.

Putnam, F. (1989). *Diagnosis and Treatment of Multiple Personality Disorder.* New York: Guilford Press.

Rauch, S. L., Whalen, P. J., Shin, L. M., McInerney, S. C., Macklin, M. L., Lasko, N. B., *et al.* (2000). Exaggerated amygdala response to masked facial stimuli in posttraumatic stress disorder: A functional MRI study. *Biological Psychiatry, 47*(9), 769–776.

Resnick, H. S., Yehuda, R., Pitman, R. K., and Foy, D. W. (1995). Effect of previous trauma on acute plasma cortisol level following rape. *The American Journal of Psychiatry, 152*(11), 1675–1677.

Riley, S. (1997). An art psychotherapy stress reduction group: For therapists dealing with a severely abused client population. *The Arts in Psychotherapy, 23*(5), 407–415.

Rodrigues, S. M., Schafe, G. E., and LeDoux, J. E. (2004). Molecular mechanisms underlying emotional learning and memory in the lateral amygdala. *Neuron, 44*(1), 75–91.

Ross, C. (1997). *Dissociative Identity Disorder: Diagnosis, Clinical Features and Treatment of Multiple Personality.* New York: John Wiley & Sons, Inc.

Saarela, M. V., Hlushchuk, Y., Williams, A. C., Schurmann, M., Kalso, E., and Hari, R. (2007). The compassionate brain: Humans detect intensity of pain from another's face. *Cerebral Cortex, 17*(1), 230–237.

Sapolsky, R. M. (2004). *Why Zebras Don't Get Ulcers.* New York: Henry Holt and Co.

Scaer, R. C. (2001). *The Body Bears the Burden.* New York: Haworth Press.

Schelling, G., Roozendaal, B., Krauseneck, T., Schmoelz, M., de Quervain, D., and Briegel, J. (2006). Efficacy of hydrocortisone in preventing posttraumatic stress disorder following critical illness and major surgery. *Annals of the New York Academy of Sciences, 1071,* 46–53.

Schore, A. N. (2001a). The effects of a secure attachment relationship on right brain development, affect regulation, and infant mental health. *Infant Mental Health Journal, 22*(1–2), 7–66.

Schore, A. N. (2001b). The effects of early relational trauma on right brain development, affect regulation, and infant mental health. *Infant Mental Health Journal, 22*(1–2), 201–269.

Shea, A., Walsh, C., MacMillan, H., and Steiner, M. (2005). Child maltreatment and HPA axis dysregulation: Relationship to major depressive disorder and post traumatic stress disorder in females. *Psychoneuroendocrinology, 30*(2), 162–178.

Shin, L. M., Orr, S. P., Carson, M. A., Rauch, S. L., Macklin, M. L., Lasko, N. B., *et al.* (2004). Regional cerebral blood flow in the amygdala and medial prefrontal cortex during traumatic imagery in male and female Vietnam veterans with PTSD. *Archives of General Psychiatry, 61*(2), 168–176.

Shin, L. M., Rauch, S. L., and Pitman, R. K. (2006). Amygdala, medial prefrontal cortex, and hippocampal function in PTSD. *Annals of the New York Academy of Sciences, 1071,* 67–79.

Shin, L. M., Wright, C. I., Cannistraro, P. A., Wedig, M. M., McMullin, K., Martis, B., *et al.* (2005). A functional magnetic resonance imaging study of amygdala and medial prefrontal cortex responses to overtly presented fearful faces in posttraumatic stress disorder. *Archives of General Psychiatry, 62*(3), 273–281.

Siegel, D. J. (2006). An interpersonal neurobiology approach to psychotherapy: Awareness, mirror neurons, and neural plasticity in the development of well-being. *Psychiatric Annals, 36*(4), 248–258.

Singer, T., Seymour, B., O'Doherty, J., Kaube, H., Dolan, R. J., and Frith, C. D. (2004). Empathy for pain involves the affective but not sensory components of pain. *Science, 303*(5661), 1157–1162.

Spring, D. (2001). Image and Mirage, Art Therapy with Dissociative Clients. Springfield, IL: Charles C. Thomas.

Teicher, M. H., Tomoda, A., and Andersen, S. L. (2006). Neurobiological consequences of early stress and childhood maltreatment: Are results from human and animal studies comparable? *Annals of the New York Academy of Sciences, 1071*, 313–323.

Ullman, S. E. and Siegel, J. M. (1995). Sexual assault, social reactions, and physical health. *Women's Health, 1*(4), 289–308.

van den Hout, M., Muris, P., Salemink, E., and Kindt, M. (2001). Autobiographical memories become less vivid and emotional after eye movements. *The British Journal of Clinical Psychology, 40*(2), 121–130.

van der Hart, O., Nijenhuis, E. R., and Steele, K. (2005). Dissociation: An insufficiently recognized major feature of complex posttraumatic stress disorder. *Journal of Traumatic Stress, 18*(5), 413–423.

van der Kolk, B. A. (2002). Assessment and treatment of complex PTSD. In R. Yehuda (ed.) *Treating Trauma Survivors with PTSD*. Washington, DC: American Psychiatric Publishing.

van der Kolk, B. A., Burbridge, J. A., and Suzuki, J. (1997). The psychobiology of traumatic memory. Clinical implications of neuroimaging studies. *Annals of the New York Academy of Sciences, 821*, 99–113.

van der Kolk, B. A. and Fisler, R. (1995). Dissociation and the fragmentary nature of traumatic memories: Overview and exploratory study. *Journal of Traumatic Stress, 8*(4), 505–525.

van der Kolk, B. A., McFarlane, A. C., and Weisaeth, L. (eds) (1996). *Traumatic Stress: The Effects of Overwhelming Experience on Mind, Body and Society*. New York: Guilford Press.

van der Kolk, B. A., van der Hart, O., and Marmar, C. R. (1996). In B. A. van der Kolk, A. C. McFarlane and L. Weisaeth (eds). Dissociation and information processing in Posttraumatic Stress Disorder in *Traumatic Stress: The Effects of Overwhelming Experience on Mind, Body and Society* (pp.303–330). New York: Guilford Press.

van der Kolk, B. A., Roth, S., Pelcovitz, D., Sunday, S., and Spinazzola, J. (2005). Disorders of extreme stress: The empirical foundation of a complex adaptation to trauma. *Journal of Traumatic Stress, 18*(5), 389–399.

Vermetten, E. and Bremner, J. D. (2002). Circuits and systems in stress. II. Applications to neurobiology and treatment in posttraumatic stress disorder. *Depression and Anxiety, 16*(1), 14–38.

Walrond-Skinner, S. (1986). *A Dictionary of Psychotherapy*. London and New York: Routledge and Kegan Paul, Inc.

Watt, D. (2005). Social bonds and the nature of empathy. *Journal of Consciousness Studies, 12*(8–10), 185–209.

Wicker, B., Keysers, C., Plailly, J., Royet, J.-P., Gallese, V., and Rizzolatti, G. (2003). Both of us disgusted in my insula: The common neural basis of seeing and feeling disgust. *Neuron, 40*, 655–664.

Yehuda, R. (ed.) (1999). *Risk Factors for Posttraumatic Stress Disorder*. Progress in Psychiatry series. Washington, DC: American Psychiatric Association.

Yücel, M., Wood, S. J., Fornito, A., Riffkin, J., Velakoulis, D., and Pantelis, C. (2003). Anterior cingulate dysfunction: Implications for psychiatric disorders? *Journal of Psychiatry and Neuroscience, 28*(5), 350–354.

14

Alzheimer's Disease:
Art, Creativity and the Brain

Anne Galbraith, Ruth Subrin, and Drew Ross

Early stages of Alzheimer's disease (AD), conceptualized as Mild Cognitive Impairment (MCI), present with subtle neurocognitive and biochemical changes (Petersen *et al.* 1999, 2006). These changes can occur a few years to decades before the onset of AD (Albert and Drachman 2000; Collie and Maruff 2000; Morris *et al.* 2001; Small, Herlitz and Backman 2004). The boundaries between normal aging, MCI and AD blur due to the heterogeneity of age-related changes (Galvin *et al.* 2005; Morris and Becker 2004, Small *et al.* 2004). MCI is a pathologic condition where there is some cognitive impairment, with a slight degree of functional impairment, which is not severe enough to interrupt activities of daily living (Petersen 2004).

Anne Galbraith, Ruth Subrin, Drew Ross, and Shirley Riley (1921–2004) are art therapists who have worked collaboratively at an adult day center. Taking the approach that neuroscience can inform creative arts interventions for early stages of AD/MCI (Riley 2001), we linked sensory stimulation with social-emotional connections to improve the overall sense of well-being and quality of life for our MCI/AD group.

Much of the learning and work stretched our vision of what is therapeutic. For instance, we found a sub-group ratio of one art therapist to two group members better serves effective communication than the traditional one or two co-therapist model for a group of six to eight participants. In order to activate and motivate brain pathways and bodily systems, we included music (Ross 2005), movement and dramatic gestures (Malchiodi 1998; Riley 2001). Being mindful not to infantilize, we used the art to stimulate memory banks, and provided opportunities for emotional regulation and cognitive stimulation through repetition, cueing, playfulness, and a sense of humor (Riley 2001). Incorporating psycho-educational efforts, this expressive arts clinical neuroscience approach helps MCI/AD clients and their families better understand and cope with the disease's progression. The ideas are to mitigate psychosocial impacts (Riley 2004, 2006) and open the possibility for preserving cognitive abilities (Galvin *et al.* 2005; Goldberg 2005; Rivas-Vazquez *et al.* 2004).

Mild Cognitive Impairment (MCI) and early Alzheimer's disease (AD)

Mild Cognitive Impairment (MCI) has been defined in the last decade as a pathological syndrome apart from normal aging (Rivas-Vazquez *et al.* 2004). Early AD symptoms include memory loss, language difficulties (aphasia), perceptual impairment (agnosia), and a decline in thinking abilities (DSM-IV-TR, American Psychiatric Association [APA] 2000). Most frequently, impairments reflect an inability to carry out complex instrumental daily living activities such as balancing a checkbook, while the ability to perform simple activities of daily living remains intact (Rivas-Vazquez *et al.* 2004).

A person with MCI/early AD may notice prominent memory impairments, primarily short-term memory (STM) loss as well as impairments in reasoning, planning, and organizing (Snowdon 2001). In order to meet the diagnosis of MCI, the patient's subjective memory complaints must be corroborated by an additional significant other, as well as by objective neuropsychological testing. Only one age/education-matched impairment is allowed for the diagnosis of MCI. The person must otherwise demonstrate an average ability on intelligence testing. Additional early signs include difficulty with attention, fatigue, apathy and mood changes including irritability, anger and depression (Cummings 2004). The care-partner, friends or family usually notice these early signs first, since people with MCI/AD may often be unaware due to impaired self-awareness (Morris and Hannesdottir. 2004).

The MCI/AD experience

Imagine reading a book, watching a movie, or being engaged in a conversation with friends, yet experiencing difficulty holding on to the thread of conversation, or the names of the other people talking. During the art therapy group, short-term memory (STM) problems, fear, embarrassment, sadness, and concern for the future are shared by members. Neural brain networks are so highly interconnected and interdependent that problems in one domain, such as memory, impact other cognitive domains; group members often complain of additional associated symptoms, such as perceptual difficulties and word finding problems. Mood and emotion also have a global impact on all cognitive domains, as frustration, fear, fatigue and depression associated with the diagnosis can exacerbate cognitive deficits.

Understanding the bi-directionality of affective and cognitive domains and their impact on daily life informs any therapist working with the MCI/AD population. Using imagery provides art therapists with background material from which to create opportunities that encourage social and/or cognitive stimulation rather than brain passivity (Riley 2001). Art activates visual pathways, stimulating self-narratives and emotional expressions while reinforcing existing language, memory, socialization, and visuospatial abilities. The novelty of art-making, an enjoyable new activity, stimulates the senses, supporting brain reserve (Satz 1993; Stern 2002; Wolf *et al.* 2004), brain plasticity (Goldberg 2005; Scarmeas *et al.* 2001; Snowdon 2001), the growth of new neurons in the hippocampus (Goldberg 2005; Kozorovitskiy and Gould 2003), and activates alternate or adaptive connections in the brain, potentially alleviating stress or depression (Riley 2006).

Riley introduced a unique approach using art directives with large white sheets of banner paper intended to maximize cognitive stimulation by creating a shared physical and mental workspace (2006). Oftentimes, our theme for discussion was predetermined. An image or symbol representing the topic was drawn beforehand as a visual stimulus in the center of the paper. In order to help members bypass apathy and fatigue, the art therapist may begin the group by focusing members' attention on the stimulus, asking, "What does it remind you of?" The ensuing discussion and art-making allows members to execute their thoughts, feelings and emotions conjointly on paper.

The art therapy studio space: cognitive functions in action

Executive function, attributed to the prefrontal cortex and the conductor of all cognitive domains (Goldberg 2005), plays an important part in decision-making, thoughtful planning and action (Collette and Van der Linden 2004; Wischik, Theuring, and Harrington 2001). Executive function is linked to working memory (WM), which is considered the workspace for juggling and manipulating executive function along with long- and short-term memories (LeDoux 2002). Brain areas associated with executive function and working memory are impacted early on in the course of AD and MCI, primarily in the hippocampus, entorhinal cortex, and prefrontal cortex. People with MCI/AD experience loss of some executive abilities and demonstrate STM and WM deficits (Overman and Becker 2004; Raz 2005; Small *et al.* 2004; Wischik *et al.* 2001; Figure 14.1).

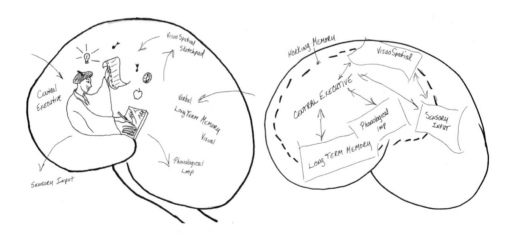

Figure 14.1 Psychoeducational drawing of working memory space. Two versions of a visual stimulus drawing created by the art therapist, Anne, for the purpose of educating the group.

To explain WM, we suggest to the group the metaphor of an artist working in his studio. Following a brief discussion, we help members generate and retrieve memories, stimulate executive function, and exercise a sense of control by asking group members to make WM boxes. Members place inside the boxes objects or symbols of their thoughts, concerns and memories that they want to keep and/or release (Figure 14.2).

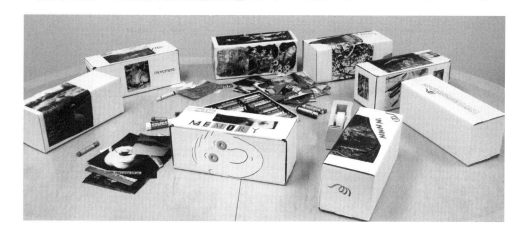

Figure 14.2 Working memory boxes (boxes, mixed media).

Chasm is another directive we designed to stimulate planning and problem-solving. This banner paper directive begins with a pre-drawn stimulus of two land masses, with a *Chasm* in the middle. In response, some groups have drawn a tightrope between the two land masses with a figure gingerly walking across the open space. Difficult crossings are symbolic of navigating the thin line of living with memory loss and maintaining hope. Sometimes a safety net is added to save the person should they fall. The net is covered with a piece of paper and the question "What would happen without a safety net?" is posed. The social interaction and support this directive stimulates reinforces long-term memory and a sense of accomplishment from past successes (Figure 14.3).

Old and new memory storages

Short-term memory and working memory are activated whenever clients engage with new information, such as that generated by the art-making. Clients with MCI find that moving information from short- to long-term memory becomes increasingly challenging. Sometimes more time is needed, sometimes more stimuli, and sometimes it takes novel stimuli to catch memory's attention. Saliency and working memory processing over time increases the likelihood that new information becomes stored (Cozolino

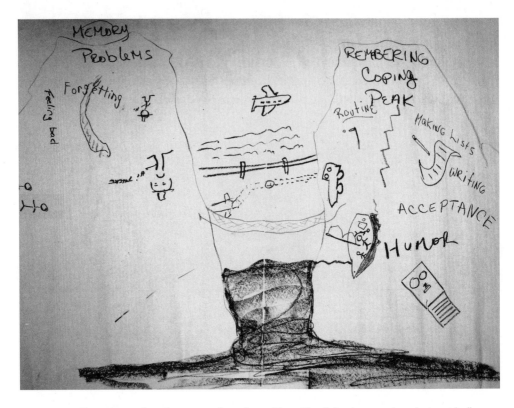

Figure 14.3 Chasm. *Members draw away from the problem side of the chasm to the solution side (banner paper, tape, markers or oil pastels). Group drawing by Alzheimer's patients.*

2002). Brain regions most closely associated with memory, primarily the hippocampus, entorhinal cortex, and amygdala, are located in the temporal lobes.

Long-term memory is categorized as explicit or declarative memory versus implicit or procedural memory. MCI clients find explicit/declarative conscious memory more difficult. Conscious explicit learning and remembering breaks down into two sub-groups: (1) semantic memory, memory for facts independent of context; and (2) episodic, personal memory, the ability to store and retrieve facts in context, recollections of the day's events and the awareness of oneself in time (LeDoux 2002; Siegel 1999). Making self-portraits activates and reinforces episodic memories as participants recall and retrieve autobiographical memories.

For members who need more help reinforcing semantic memory, breaking the directive down into steps may be necessary: (1) draw a head; (2) eyes; (3) a nose, etc. Transforming abstract concepts into concrete steps should decrease cognitive overload, difficulties with retrieval, feelings of being overwhelmed, and lead to increased enjoyment and self-esteem while validating lived stories.

Implicit/procedural memory is encoded pre-verbally, and is shaped by information absorbed through the senses. Implicit knowing is pertinent to skills and procedures learned early on and used frequently in daily activities: brushing teeth, dressing, riding a bike or playing an instrument. Procedural memory can be more resilient to the effects of AD. The repetition of rituals supports procedural memory, helping both short- and long-term memory. The rituals used in the opening and closing of the group include stretching, guided visualizations, drama, hand holding, giving a round of applause for work well done, and/or music and songs. Creating consistent environments is also important, such as events held at the same time and place. We also found that the meaningful content of the group discussion/art activity maximized the level of engagement, attention, and positively affected group members' ability to remember their group experience for a variable period of time, a few hours to a week (Kazui *et al.* 2003).

Out of sight, out of mind: attention

The ability to attend is a key factor in making memories and maintaining social interaction. Therefore, the art therapy group includes a combination of physical, visual, verbal or auditory stimuli to help members maintain attention. Celebrations are good attention grabbers, triggering a variety of memories. On banner paper in the middle of the table, a cake with candles and a face blowing out the candles is predrawn by the art therapists. To activate attention processes, we ask participants what they see. A discussion of celebratory events follows as words and drawings are added to the paper. The session ends with a closing ritual. Each member holds a lighted candle, makes a wish, blows the candle out and gives it to the person on their left or right. As each member makes a wish, hope and a sense of control are ignited.

Moving in space and time: the visuospatial sketch pad

The visuospatial domain in the parietal lobe pertains to visual and spatial perception, such as the ability to remember or recognize shapes, colors, textures, and identify the location and/or speed of objects in space, including one's own body. Damage to this area can create problems such as bumping into objects, sitting in a chair without falling, and, more basically, the ability to dress and feed oneself.

Working with pre-cut shapes supports visuospatial functioning for all levels of impairment. Each person is given a handful of construction paper shapes (squares, circles, lines, arrows, etc.). Sometimes the art therapist assists by showing where a shape could be placed on the paper. Pleasing Matisse-style designs may begin to emerge (Figure 14.4).

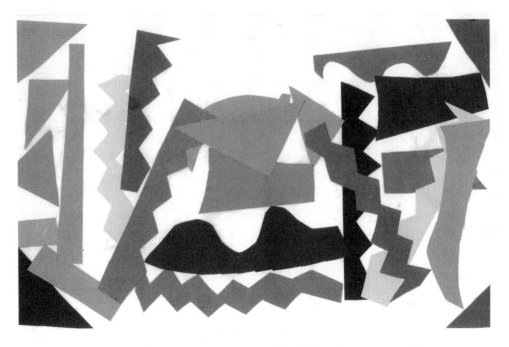

Figure 14.4 Using pre-cut shapes to support visuospatial functioning (11" × 17" paper).

Language and the art of communication

Language problems include difficulty with word-finding, naming, and fluency. In the early stages, clients report knowing what they want to say, yet they cannot find the words—a retrieval problem, rather than forgetting (Morris and Hannesdottir 2004). Language problems are associated with neuronal death in the left temporal language centers. Language is broadly defined as a system of sounds, gestures, or written symbols communicating thoughts and/or feelings. Visuals can complement verbal exchanges. In a narrative activity, participants are encouraged to tell a group or individual story. While gluing pictures on paper, stories are created with words, gestures, and sounds; alternate modes of communication are stimulated and explored. The art therapist can also randomly hand out pictures from the collage box for each client asking each to free associate, pantomime, or describe what the image looks, sounds or feels like.

Emotion

Mood changes and apathy commonly reported by care partners are associated with progression of MCI to AD (Cummings 2004; Morris and Hannesdottir 2004; Norris, MacNeill, and Haines 2003). Differentiating between depression and apathy is necessary as changes in personality and behavior are 61 to 92 percent more attributable to apathy than to depression (Landes , Sperry and Strauss 2005). Common to MCI/AD is the loss of interest or pleasure, most likely caused by the loss of motivation and the ability to initiate (Landes *et al.* 2005). Further complicating the issue, people in earlier stages of AD may be more prone to depression due to intact awareness of self and how their losses impact their families. During more advanced stages, people tend to be less aware of cognitive losses and are therefore less depressed (Morris and Hannesdottir 2004; Spitznagel, Tremont, and Gunstad 2006).

The pathophysiology of apathy and depression differs. Depression often accompanies decreased levels of serotonin, which is generally observed in the aging process (Lichtenberg and Mast 2003), while apathy involves cholinergic deficits (Landes *et al.* 2005).

In consideration of cognitive impairment, apathy, and depression, we may include other expressive arts modalities, like drama or music, to stimulate neural pathways that help regulate emotions (Riley 2006). Utilizing music at the start of a group provides immediate gratification, helping to override the apathy or depression. The contours and spacing, varied intensities, and modulations in sound take the listener on an emotional journey, tapping into long imprinted memories and well-established brain circuitry (Siegel 1999). Studies on music processing in the brain have generally concluded that no one single music processing center exists; rather, a network of specialized areas work simultaneously to process music (Aldridge 2000; Hodges 2000).

The right hemisphere, more than the left, strongly recognizes music instrument timbre and the right auditory cortex is more retentive of rhythmic patterns (Hodges 2000; Levitin 2006). However, tonal memory, melody recognition, and intensity do not appear to be stronger in the right. For AD and MCI clients, music has the capability to stimulate the entire brain, facilitating memory retention.

Using music in concert with art therapy creates truly outstanding benefits for AD and MCI clients; even if a song's words are lost, the tune is often retained, allowing all to join in. Indeed, memories evoked by familiar songs frequently spark story telling by some members, exercising another form of memory. Musical stimulation also provides emotional soothing, increased participation, and group cohesiveness through shared musical memories.

Family members may find it very difficult to cope with relational challenges related to apathy, depression and loss of the loved one's personality. Social isolation becomes problematic as social contact becomes more infrequent; family get-togethers or outings begin to dissolve, reducing stimulation and further contributing to the progression of AD while increasing potential depression.

The art therapy group offers social support and safety. Expressing positive and negative feelings is encouraged. Families may minimize the distress experienced by the diagnosed in the beginning AD/MCI stages, and in later stages, may patronize with cheery remarks, discouraging expression of a full range of emotion. The art therapist emphasizes that no one is going to be judged or graded on his or her art (Ross 2005). Individuals often show relief when they are able to talk about their sadness, loss, and other emotions that seem too traumatic to discuss outside the group. Utilizing creative visual expression, a non-verbal form of communication, adds other pathways, connecting individuals on emotional and psychosocial levels. Being part of a community is an important factor in maintaining social function (Snowdon 2001). The study on nuns described the positive effects that community, positive outlook, social belonging, and engagement can have on body and mind (Snowdon 2001).

The *Creating a Community* banner directive facilitates new connections, helping decrease isolation. After a short warm up, we begin discussing what would be needed for our community. As participants respond, they work together with the art materials to create their community. The directive indirectly invites participants to meet their emotional and physical needs (Figure 14.5).

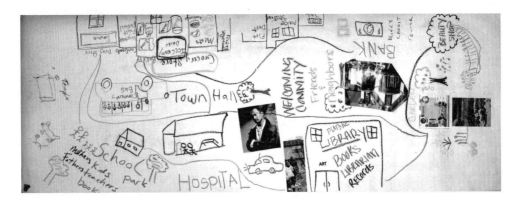

Figure 14.5 Creating a community (banner paper, oil pastels, collage).

Brain reserve: use it or lose it

Brain reserve capacity (BRC) means increased density of synaptic connections established postmortem by weight measures (Staff *et al.* 2004). Cognitive reserve (CR) is the malleable ability to compensate for brain insults. CR reveals the brain's ability to compensate or efficiently utilize alternate cognitive strategies by recruiting alternate brain networks (Satz 1993; Stern 2002). Genetics, brain size, synaptic count, and intellectual challenges found in education, occupation and life-long social activities contribute to both (Goldberg 2005; Scarmeas *et al.* 2001; Staff *et al.* 2004; Stern 2002). BRC and CR may forestall AD's onset or progression (Satz 1993). Therefore, some individual brains may be clinically diagnosed later than others, and sustained creative challenges can positively contribute to maintaining mental functioning supporting the brain reserve hypothesis (Goldberg 2005; Staff *et al.* 2004; Stern 2002).

Art directives help concretize abstractions and redirect focus to current strengths and abilities. We ask the group to outline their hands on paper or we provide schematic stimuli of a pre-drawn hand followed by the directive: "What have these hands done and what can they do for the future?" (Figure 14.6).

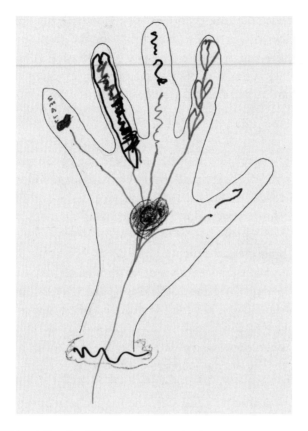

Figure 14.6 BRC-CR hand directive (9" × 12" paper, markers).

The directive and the discussion reinforce a sense of accomplishment, identity, and self-worth, increasing an appreciation for how life activities and experiences contribute to their protective cognitive abilities. We also encourage group members to select collage pictures or to draw image representations of these activities and place them in their hand images.

The concept of reserve came out of the discrepancy or lack of a direct relationship between pathology and clinical symptoms (Stern 2002). BRC is linked to a passive threshold model; once AD pathology reaches a critical mass in terms of neuronal and synaptic loss, brain atrophy and clinical symptoms become apparent. CR connects to an active threshold model where the brain actively compensates by working around damaged areas of the brain until reaching a threshold where compensation is no longer possible (Gracon and Emmerling 2001; Staff *et al.* 2004; Stern 2002). Combining these two models may best help clients and therapists understand and explain differences in clinical manifestations (Stern 2002).

Although inconclusive, research on brain/cognitive reserve theories, brain plasticity, and neurogenesis support the importance of continued brain stimulation in the face of pathology, whether through music, visual art, and/or physical exercise (Goldberg 2005). These activities may stimulate the brain by increasing or maintaining synaptic connections or density in the neocortical association cortex (Stern 2002), which brings hope for clients, families and therapists alike.

Neurogenesis

As the brain changes in relation to experience and the environment throughout the lifespan (plasticity), the discovery that certain brain regions produce new neurons has broadened the old adage "use it or lose it" to include "use it and get more" (Goldberg 2005). This wonderful reframe helps when visualizing the possible effects and complexities involved in the phenomena of neurogenesis. Neurogenesis associates with the capacity of specific brain areas, the hippocampal dentate gyrus and the olfactory bulb, to produce new neurons and enhances this process through cognitive stimulation, aerobic exercise and new learning (Cozolino 2002; Horner and Gage 2002; Kozorovitskiy and Gould 2003; Snowdon 2001). The long-term effects of chronic stress associated with chronic diseases like AD and social isolation (Snowdon 2001), as well as elevated cortisol, inhibits neurogenesis by damaging the hippocampus and long-term potentiation (LTP). The neural damage leads to repression, reduced dendritic branching, and deficits in episodic and spatial memory. Enriched environments create opportunities for physical activity, learning, and social interaction, producing structural and functional brain changes along with new neuron production and survival (Scarmeas *et al.* 2001).

The discussion of neurogenesis in the group stimulates curiosity and supports a sense of control and hope, decreasing resistance to experimenting with art materials. Often, group members have not used art materials since childhood. Participation in group art therapy can be a novel and enriching experience. Experiences range from scribbled drawings and non-verbal conversations on paper to more complicated directives that stimulate executive function through collaboration, planning, and creativity, like the banner directives. Sometimes, an art directive and guided visualization follow a discussion about what neurons do, how they communicate and what happens if they cannot connect with other neurons. Group members are encouraged to imagine the neuron as a healthy tree growing new branches and passing messages from one neuron to another. After drawing their own neurons, they are challenged with figuring out how to connect theirs with others.

The neuropathology of MCI/AD

The shared neuropathologic features between MCI and AD are less severe in MCI patients. They include medial temporal lobe atrophy, reduced entorhinal cortex (EC) glucose metabolism and increased neurofibrillary distribution (De Leon *et al.* 2004). With respect to amyloid plaque formation, MCI patients and healthy elderly share common features (Petersen 2004).

The art directive enhancing the dialogues about how the brain works and what AD neuropathology is usually begins with a stimulus drawing of the brain or a neuron. Members are asked what they see on the page and to free-associate to the stimulus drawings, activating the visuo-spatial, executive, and language domains during a discussion followed by an art directive. The approach is repeated over the course of three to four sessions and/or is reintroduced throughout treatment. Sometimes it is followed by guided imagery where members take an internal scan of their brain or body and follow up by drawing or sculpting what they noticed during the guided imagery and what they imagine to be happening inside their brains. In one instance, a group member made a concise drawing of two disconnected lines symbolizing what was happening in his brain.

Plaques and tangles

The most common AD feature is the abundance of plaques and neurofibrillary tangles (NFTs). Plaques are external to the neurons; NFTs happen in the neurons. NFTs and plaques are not specific to AD, also occurring in aging brains with no clinical signs. Autopsies, however, reveal increased plaque and NFT formation in MCI and AD brains (Esiri 2001; Morris 2004).

Plaques are circular structures developing outside the neuron (0.2 millimeters in diameter). Three main types or stages of plaque development have been identified: diffuse, neuritic, and burnt out. Neuritic plaques occur from the breakdown of amyloid precursor protein that supports the neuron (Figure 14.7).

Enzymes attack the amyloid precursor protein (APP), breaking it down into fragments. One of the fragments, Beta-Amyloid, clumps together outside the neuron, forming insoluble plaques (Figure 14.7; NIH 2002). Consequently, neurons are cut off from necessary support. Plaque formation stimulates free radical production, causing oxidative stress and cell death by choking neurons (Yan *et al.* 2001; Gracon and Emmerling 2001). It is unclear if plaques contribute to AD development or are a byproduct (NIH 2002).

Tangles are created by a breakdown of the TAU protein. Normally this protein stabilizes the internal structure of the neuron, but for some reason, the TAU changes chemically, forming threads and paired helical filaments, thereby disintegrating the infrastructure of microtubules collapsing the neuron and electrical transmission processes (Esiri 2001; Figure 14.8).

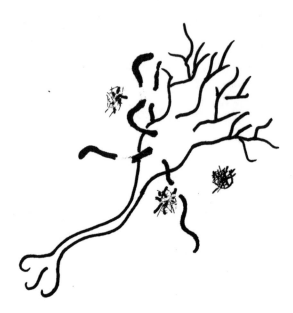

Figure 14.7 Psychoeducational drawing of plaque formation. Drawn by Anne Galbraith, therapist, to show clients how plaques form (9 "× 12" paper, markers).

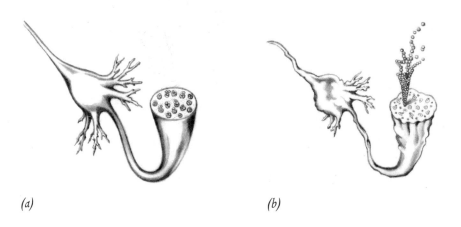

(a)   (b)

Figure 14.8(a)–(b) Healthy neuron (left). Breakdown of tau protein collapsing the neuron (right). Illustrations by Jennifer Kirk.

As a result of tangle formation and plaques, neurons don't communicate, become more isolated, and die off (NIH 2002). It is unclear why tangles and plaques develop. Inflammation, oxidation, genetic and environmental contributions are being considered (Lopez and Bell 2004).

For individuals with MCI amnestic type and early AD, the plaques and NFTs contribute to losses of cholinergic neurons in the basal forebrain that project widely into the hippocampus and neocortex. This loss impairs the function of acetylcholine, a neurotransmitter important in memory and thinking (Morris 2004; Esiri 2001; Gracon and Emmerling 2001). They may also have low concentrations of serotonin and a reduced sensitivity to serotonin imipramine binding, creating serious disturbances in serotonin-based metabolism and therefore depression. Thus, emotional disturbances and behavioral symptoms in AD patients may manifest as increased anxiety, confusion, irritability, and restlessness. Other contributing factors to depression include neuronal damage from over-stimulation of N-methyl-D-aspartate receptors by glutamate, a principal excitatory brain neurotransmitter. Glutamatergic over-stimulation results in neuronal calcium overload and brain cell death, creating memory loss and dementia (Lopez and Bell 2004).

Summary

Therapeutic stimulation through art therapy and music provides an affective antidote to the isolation and other debilitating effects of Mild Cognitive Impairment and Alzheimer's disease. On the shared ground of the art therapy paper, group members create imagery related to their lived stories, coming to terms with the diagnosis and looking at what is happening in their here and now experience. The discussion of the art further helps to decrease the sense of isolation that group members often feel; they experience a sense of control by supporting and reflecting on the new connections they make and what they can do to help each other and themselves live meaningful lives in the here and now. Evocative art therapy experiences coupled with the understanding from clinical neuroscience can provide a powerful visual memory bank of a shared journey.

References

Albert, M. S. and Drachman, D. A. (2000). Alzheimer's Disease: What is it, how many people have it, and why do we need to know? *Neurology Music Educators Journal, 87*(2), 166–168.

Aldridge, D. (2000). *Music Therapy in Dementia Care.* London: Jessica Kingsley Publishers.

Allen, J. S. (2001). Alzheimer's Disease: Past, present, and future themes. In D. Dawbarn and A. J. Shelley (eds) *Neurobiology of Alzheimer's Disease* (pp.1–32). New York: Oxford University Press.

American Psychiatric Association (2000). *Diagnostic and Statistical Manual of Mental Disorders* (4th edition—TR). Washington, DC: American Psychiatric Association.

Collie, A. and Maruff, P. (2000). The neuropsychology of preclinical Alzheimer's disease and mild cognitive impairment. *Neuroscience Biobehavioral Review, 24,* 365–374.

Collette, F. and Van der Linden, M. (2004). Executive functions in Alzheimer's disease. In R. Morris and J. Becker (eds) *Cognitive Neuropsychology of Alzheimer's Disease* (pp.103–120). New York: Oxford University Press.

Cozolino, L. (2002). *The Neuroscience of Psychotherapy: Building and Rebuilding the Human Brain*. New York: W. W. Norton and Company.

Cummings, J. L. (2004). Alzheimer's disease. *The New England Journal of Medicine, 351*, 56–67.

De Leon, M. J., Desanti, S., Zinkowski, R., Mehta, P. D., Pratico, D., Segal, S., *et al.* (2004). MRI and CSF studies in the early diagnosis of Alzheimer's Disease. *Journal of Internal Medicine, 256*, 205–223.

Esiri, M. M. (2001). The neuropathology of Alzheimer's Disease. In D. Dawbarn and J. Shelley (eds) *Neurobiology of Alzheimer's Disease* (pp.33–53). New York: Oxford University Press.

Galvin, J. E., Powlishta, K. K., Wilkins, K., McKeel, D. W., Xiong, C., Grant, E., *et al.* (2005). Predictors of preclinical Alzheimer's disease and dementia. *Archives of Neurology, 62*, 758–765.

Gracon, S. I. and Emmerling, M. (2001). Current perspectives, future directions. In D. Dawbarn and J. Shelley (eds) *Neurobiology of Alzheimer's Disease* (pp.369–387). New York: Oxford University Press.

Goldberg, E. (2005). *The Wisdom Paradox*. New York: Gotham Books.

Hodges, D. A. (2000). Implications of music and brain research. Special Focus: Music and the Brain. *Music Educators Journal, 87*(2), 17–22.

Horner, P. J. and Gage, F. H. (2002). Regeneration in the adult and aging brain. *Archives of Neurology, 59*, 1717–1720.

Kazui, H., Mori, E., Hashimoto, M., and Hirono, N. (2003). Enhancement of declarative memory by emotional arousal and visual memory function in Alzheimer's disease. *Journal of Neuropsychiatry and Clinical Neuroscience, 15*, 221–226.

Kozorovitskiy, Y. and Gould, E. (2003). Adult neurogenesis: A mechanism for brain repair? *Journal of Clinical and Experimental Neuropsychology, 25*, 721–732.

Landes, A. M., Sperry, S. D., and Strauss, M. E. (2005). Prevalence of apathy, dysphoria, and depression in relation to dementia severity in Alzheimer's disease. *Journal of Neuropsychiatry and Clinical Neuroscience, 17*, 342–349.

LeDoux, J. (2002). *Synaptic Self*. Harmondsworth: Penguin Books.

Levitin, D. J. (2006). *This is Your Brain on Music: The Science of a Human Obsession*. Boston, MA: Dutton.

Lichtenberg, P. A. and Mast, B. T. (2003). Psychological and nonpharmacological aspects of depression in dementia. In P. A. Lichtenberg, D. L. Murman, and A. M. Mellow (eds) *Handbook of Dementia* (pp.309–334). Hoboken, NJ: John Wiley & Sons, Inc.

Lopez, O. L. and Bell, S. (2004). Neurobiological approaches to the treatment of Alzheimer's Disease. In R. Morris and J. Becker (eds) *Cognitive Neuropsychology of Alzheimer's Disease* (pp.391–414). New York: Oxford University Press.

Malchiodi, C. (1998). *The Art Therapy Sourcebook*. Los Angeles, CA: Lowell House.

Morris, R. G. (2004). Neurobiological abnormalities in Alzheimer's disease: Structural, genetic, and functional correlates of cognitive dysfunction. In R. Morris and J. Becker (eds) *Cognitive Neuropsychology of Alzheimer's Disease* (pp.299–319). New York: Oxford University Press.

Morris, J. C., Storandt, M., Miller, J. P., McKeel, D. W., Price, J. L., Rubin, E. H., *et al.* (2001). Mild cognitive impairment represents early-stage Alzheimer's Disease. *Archives of Neurology, 58*, 397–405.

Morris, R. G. and Becker, J. T. (2004). A cognitive neuropsychology of Alzheimer's disease. In R. Morris and J. Becker (eds) *Cognitive Neuropsychology of Alzheimer's Disease* (pp.3–10). New York: Oxford University Press.

Morris, R. G. and Hannesdottir, K. (2004). Loss of "awareness" in Alzheimer's disease. In R. Morris and J. Becker (eds) *Cognitive Neuropsychology of Alzheimer's Disease* (pp.275–298). New York: Oxford University Press.

National Institutes of Health (NIH) (2002). *The Changing Brain in Alzheimer's Disease*. U. S. Department of Health and Human Services NIH, 02–3782.

Norris, M. P., MacNeill, S. E., and Haines, M. E. (2003). Psychological and neuropsychological aspects of vascular and mixed dementia. In P. A. Lichtenberg, D. L. Murman, and A. M. Mellow (eds) *Handbook of Dementia* (pp.173–196). Hoboken, NJ: John Wiley & Sons, Inc.

Overman, A. A. and Becker, J. T. (2004). Information processing defects in episodic memory in Alzheimer's disease. In R. Morris and J. Becker (eds) *Cognitive Neuropsychology of Alzheimer's Disease* (pp.275–298). New York: Oxford University Press.

Petersen, R. C. (2004). Mild cognitive impairment as a diagnostic entity. *Journal of Internal Medicine, 256*, 183–194.

Petersen, R. C. and O'Brien, J. (2006). Mild cognitive impairment should be considered for DSM-V. *Journal of Geriatric Psychiatry and Neurology, 19*, 147–154.

Petersen, R. C., Parisi, J. E., Dickson, D. W., Johnson, K. A., Knopman, D. S., Boeve, B. F., *et al.* (2006). Neuropathologic features of amnestic mild cognitive impairment. *Archives of Neurology, 63*, 665–672.

Petersen, R. C., Smith, G. E., Waring, S. C., Ivnik, R. J., Tangalos, E. G., and Kokman, E. (1999). Mild cognitive impairment: Clinical characterization and outcome. *Archives of Neurology, 56*, 303–308.

Raz, N. (2005). The aging brain observed in vivo: Differential changes and their modifiers. In R. Cabeza, L. Nyberg, and D. Park (eds) *Cognitive Neuroscience of Aging* (pp.19–57). New York: Oxford University Press.

Riley, S. (2004). The creative mind. Art therapy: *Journal of the American Art Therapy Association, 21*(4), 184–190.

Riley, S. E. (2001). *Group Process Made Visible: The Use of Art in Group Therapy.* Ann Arbor, MI: Sheridan Books.

Riley, S. E. (2006). Why bother? Art therapy integrated with neuroscience for persons with Alzheimer's Disease. *Progress Journal, 13,* 37–48.

Rivas-Vazquez, R. A., Mendez, C., Rey G. J., and Carrazana, E. J. (2004). Mild cognitive impairment: new psychological and pharmacological target. *Archives of Clinical Neuropsychology, 19,* 11–27.

Ross, D. (2005). Therapeutic stimulation: A creative arts therapy approach to working with Alzheimer's and other memory loss clients. *The Therapist,* Redwood Empire CAMFT, November.

Satz, P. (1993). Brain reserve capacity on symptom onset after brain injury: A formulation and review of evidence for threshold theory. *Neuropsychology, 7,* 273–295.

Scarmeas, N., Levy, G., Tang, M.-X., Manly, J., and Stern, Y. (2001). Influence of leisure activity on the incidence of Alzheimer's disease. *Neurology, 57,* 2236–2242.

Siegel, D. J. (1999). *The Developing Mind.* New York: Guilford Press.

Small, B. J., Herlitz, A., and Backman, L. (2004). In R. Morris and J. Becker (eds) Preclinical Alzheimer's disease: Cognitive and memory functioning. *Cognitive Neuropsychology of Alzheimer's Disease* (pp.63–80). New York: Oxford University Press.

Smith, G. and Rush, B. (2006). Normal aging and mild cognitive impairment. In L. Sperry (1992). Aging: A developmental perspective. *Individual Psychology, 49*(4), 387–401.

Snowdon, D. (2001). *Aging with Grace.* New York: Bantam Books.

Spitznagel, M, B., Tremont, G., and Gunstad, J. (2006). Cognitive reserve and the relationship between depressive symptoms and awareness of deficits in dementia. *The Journal of Neuropsychiatry and Clinical Neurosciences, 18,* 186–190.

Staff, R. T., Murray, A. D., Deary, I. J., and Whalley, L. J. (2004). What provides cerebral reserve? *Brain, 127,* 1191–1199.

Stern, Y. (2002). What is cognitive reserve? Theory and research application of the reserve concept. *Journal of the Neuropsychological Society, 8,* 448–460.

Wischik, C. M., Theuring, F., and Harrington, C. R. (2001). The molecular basis of tau protein pathology in Alzheimer's disease and related neurodegenerative dementias. In D. Dawbarn and S. J. Allen (eds) *Neurobiology of Alzheimer's Disease* (pp.103–206). New York: Oxford University Press.

Wolf, H., Julin, P., Gertz, H.-J., Winblad, B., and Wahlund, L.-O. (2004). Intracranial volume in mild cognitive impairment, Alzheimer's disease and vascular dementia: Evidence for brain reserve? *International Journal of Geriatric Psychiatry,19,* 995–1007.

Yan, S. D., Roher, A., Soto, C., Futwan, A.-M., Collison, K., Schmidt, A. M., and Stern, D. (2001). Cellular targets of amyloid beta peptide: Potential roles of neuronal cell stress and toxicity. In D. Dawbarn and S. J. Allen (eds) *Neurobiology of Alzheimer's Disease* (pp.252–269). New York: Oxford University Press.

15

Art Therapy and Acquired Immune Deficiency Syndrome (AIDS): A Relational Neuroscience Case Conceptualization

Terre Bridgham and Noah Hass-Cohen

Feelings, thoughts, and memories are experienced as spoken and unspoken words as well as mental pictures (Beck 1995). Experiencing sad, fearful, or aggressive affect activates neurotransmitters, such as dopamine and adrenaline, that form vivid image-based memories (Achterberg, Dossey, and Kolkmeier 1994; Daruna 2004). Failure to identify and reconcile emotionally upsetting images over time contributes to stressful felt experiences, which correlate with severe medical problems and associate with a sense of a loss of control over one's life (Henry and Wang 1998).

At the time of this narrative Dillon, a 37-year-old Caucasian homosexual male, lived alone and had no current partner. He was self-employed and attended a full-time graduate college program. Dillon was diagnosed with human immunodeficiency virus (HIV) at age 24; the disease progressed to AIDS ten years later. Dillon's medical arts therapy protocol is conceptualized as an art therapy relational neuroscience approach (Hass-Cohen 2008; Figure 15.1). We explore ideas about how relational impacts of the stress response, trauma, memory, developmental history, and affect regulation are expressed in the imagery. Understanding how neurobiological structures and functions are involved in the client's stress response, and reflected in their expression of affect, informs therapeutic goals and promotes meaningful interactions about the evolving art imagery.

Metaphors, symbolism, vividness, clarity of color and line quality reveal the *affective language of the limbic system* expressing inner emotional experiences, memories and thoughts. The strength of a line, color choices, and movement correspond with identity and sense of control over problems (Landgarten 1981). Choices in these areas, while personal in nature, are also rooted in culture and experience.

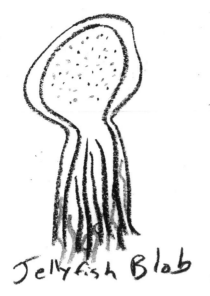

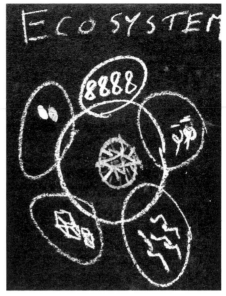

Jellyfish Blob
If you were to draw the problem, what would it look like? (Art request #1)

Ecosystem
Draw an image or a symbol for external and internal resources that help with the problem. (Art request #3)

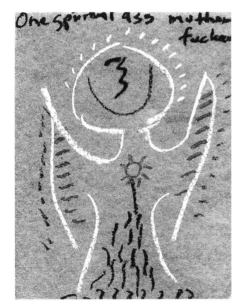

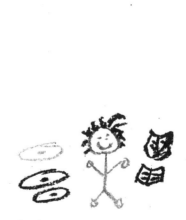

One Spiritual Ass Muther Fucker!
Draw an image of yourself. (Art request #2)

Nana's Baby
Draw yourself as you see yourself now. (Art request #4)

Figure 15.1 (#1–4) Dillon's art therapy clinical neuroscience art therapy protocol.

Vying for control

People living with AIDS are prone to developing secondary medical problems (Herek 1990). Dillon had a case of shingles that led to a severe secondary infection that his body was unable to fend off. Because of this opportunistic infection, he developed a facial disfigurement, impacting his social relationships and his self-image. Dillon also experienced minor discomfort from hypertension, which, in his opinion, was a side effect of his medication regiment.

Stress, dysphoric mood, and limited social support have been correlated with the rapid clinical progression of HIV infection and raised cortisol levels accelerated the disease (Leserman *et al.* 2002). Psychological distress, impacting a person's ability to adjust to the illness, often affects the prognosis more than physical symptoms, which may not significantly affect their feelings about the quality of life (Siegel, Karus, and Dean 2004). Increased social support and coping skills can replace depressive symptoms with hope, connectedness and attachment, and improve the quality of life (Jia *et al.* 2004). These findings underscored that psychosocial stressors experienced by people living with HIV/AIDS are not solely related to physical symptoms. Both psychosocial stressors and physical symptoms were captured in Dillon's images.

Dillon described himself as an optimist. He considers service to the community a mainstay of his optimism and his spiritual foundation. He reported that he enjoys spending time with his family members and characterized his relationships with them as close. Due to Dillon's facial disfigurement, he reported struggling with feeling unattractive, and described his biggest challenge as dating. Dillon's detailed and cohesive verbal narratives suggested a person in control of his life and capable of resolving social conflicts as they arise. The truthful quality and succinct quantity of his pertinent verbal expressions (Grice 1975, 1989) positively contributed to the coherence of his report. His organized linear discourse suggested that left hemisphere functions organized his self-view, reflecting a finely tuned and high functioning prefrontal cortex. Imagery making provided an additional worldview by activating predominately non-verbal limbic system and right hemispheric expressiveness (Kane 2004). Dillon's mindful interactions with the therapist and his art images reflected relationship challenges, chronic stress and expressive strengths.

Art therapy protocol

The art therapy protocol includes four specific requests (adapted from Achterberg *et al.* 1994). The art requests *do not* exclusively focus on the biomedical condition, but allow for the expression of both psychosocial and medical concerns. The artwork characteristics provide clues about how the client regulates his interpersonal stress response, and expression of affect and are analyzed according to: (1) vividness versus faintness; (2) symbolism versus concrete representations; (3) cohesiveness of narrative versus fragmentation; 4) dynamic versus static imagery, and 5) resources versus isolation (Achterberg *et al.* 1994; Clyde Findlay 2008; Hass Cohen 2006; Table 15.1).

Table 15.1 Analysis of drawing characteristics.

Drawing characteristics (I–V)	Affect expression[1]	Stress response[2]
I. Vividness/Faintness (1–4)		
II. Symbolic/Concrete Representations (1–4)		
III. Cohesiveness of Narrative/Fragmentized Details (1–4)		
IV. Dynamic/Static Imagery (1–4)		
V. Resources/Isolation (1–4)		

1 self expressive/regulation; striving for regulation/expression; dysregulation/expressive;

2 control; striving for control; loss of control.

The drawing characteristics provide clues to how affect and stress are expressed, regulated and managed. The first level of analysis is rated from one to four (1–4): one (1) indicates the least expression; while four (4) represents highly expressive. Symbolic imagery tends to be rich in right hemispheric poetry, often representing the preferred or implicit self, and can be the entrance to deep emotional content (Kane 2004; Schore 1994). The analysis must integrate ratings for all five areas. The first level of consideration looks at how fear, anger and motivation are expressed in the artwork. These are usually tied into crisis issues and the client's state of mind. Arousal and/or dampened affect contribute to attention, concentration and executive function. In other words, affect expression seen from a clinical neuroscience domain delineates where the client's limbic reactions interface with cortical function and action in the moment and in the world.

Next, we consider each of the characteristics of the four drawings in light of the stress response (Table 15.1). Are the hurried marks on the page reflective of an acute sympathetic nervous system stress response and efforts at control? Are they reflective of an HPA (hypothalamus-pituitary-adrenal) axis endocrine response to trauma and/or grief threatening a loss of control? Or are they stylistic and intentional? The client's explanations and titles during the protocol's progression support the therapeutic dialogue about these questions. Insights into the relational self are furthered by exploring the correspondences between drawing characteristics and the neurocorrelates of the stress response, affect regulation and memory function (Table 15.2).

Table 15.2 Neurocorrelate correspondences in broad strokes.

Domain	Neurocorrelates
Affect expressions	Limbic subcortical structures (thalamus, amygdala, anterior cingulate cortex), right hemisphere and catecholamine/arousal (dopamine, noradrenaline, and adrenaline—subcortical neurotransmitters) functions predominate over dorsolateral prefrontal
	or
	Prefrontal cortical structures; left hemisphere lateralized biases and monoaminergic (cortical neurotransmitters) functions predominate over limbic structures.
Stress response	SAM (control), SAM and HPA (striving for control), HPA (lack of control); noradrenergic-locus coeruleus system (control); serotonergic-raphe nuclei system (lack of control)
Memory	Enhanced, aroused, or hypo function of hippocampus/amygdala; prefrontal and temporal lobe functioning, implicit/explicit regulation and representation
Attachment*	Visual system vigilance (eye movements); right hemisphere and limbic brain activation-insula, anterior cingulate, amygdala, OFC

* Involved in both affect expression and memory function.

While no brain scans are available to support our linking between neurobiology and art therapy practices, our ideas are drawn from current known research and are presented for future verification. For example, we think that expressive coherency and clear art protocols, with relevant titles, are suggestive of integrated hemispheric function, prefrontal cortex regulated functioning, and hippocampal explicit memory functions. Faint, fragmented or isolated images may indicate a failure in the anterior cingulate cortex (ACC).

ACC is the connection that allows for communication between the limbic system and prefrontal lobe (Allman *et al.* 2001). We think that evoking implicit memories through image-making commands the limbic system to re-imprint the cerebral cortex. The results of re-imprinting the cerebral cortex generate hemispheric lateralization activating the immune system and supporting personal growth (Meador *et al.* 2004). Art therapy directly activates right hemispheric functioning, attempting to convince the limbic system of alternate possibilities (Hariri, Bookheimer, and Mazziotta 2000). ATR-N (art therapy relational neuroscience) approaches can help desensitize stress responses and support a sense of mastery and control. Visually exposing implicit memories can provide a blueprint for further directives that explore relationship systems, thinking, personal belief systems and self-narratives that support empowerment. The idea is that making affect, phobias, and vulnerabilities tangible provides the opportunity to create new narratives, to capitalize on brain plasticity and to strengthen new neural networks in different sections of the brain. An enriched therapeutic environment may reduce depression by stimulating new neuron growth in the hippocampus (Gabrieli 1998; Southwick *et al.* 2005). The relational interaction between the art therapist, client, and art contributes to affect regulation and increases the client's sense of limbic mastery to solidify implicit and explicit changes. Clinical neuroscience psycho-educational efforts further the therapeutic collaboration and help establish how ATR-N novel art directives and interpretations can assist in building coherency, relevancy and flexibility (Siegel 2006).

If you were to draw the problem, what would it look like? (art request #1)

Dillon drew a large jellyfish and said, "I think of it as a blob, like a jellyfish. It's kind of beautiful, but if you get too close, it will sting you" (Figure 15.1 #1: *Jellyfish Blob*).

The symbolic lone jellyfish image is an emotionally vivid response. The centrality of the figure, bright colors and dynamic lines correspond with Dillon's desires to be in control. The outside contour and the title are drawn in blue, which Dillon called "peaceful." In contrast, the inside contour is in black and contains black dots, which Dillon called "shitty." The blue attempts to hold the black, and there are a few lines in green, his favorite color, at the bottom of the image that assist in effortful control.

Dillon accesses limbic emotion, recruiting right hemispheric cortical symbolism and left hemispheric words to describe the problem coherently. Dillon stated, "Though graceful and depicting a kind of beauty, jellyfish are mysterious and deadly. Their sting may be painful." The mind operates by finding likenesses; the use of a symbolic metaphor seems to be the language of the higher right hemisphere (Kane 2004). Similar to the deadly virus swimming within Dillon's body, jellyfish often exist unseen. The beauty of the colors and the strong affect reveal unspoken limbic impulses. To the art therapist, this image is a metaphor connecting Dillon's struggle with striving and losing control. There are often elements in the art that are implicit representations of disease (Bach 1990). It is plausible that the black dots in the upper part of the image reflect shingles and represent a visible imprint of the metaphoric jellyfish sting. The jellyfish danger symbolically conveys a duality in possible symbolic meanings: AIDS as an endangerment to self and others.

Dillon's symbolism, felt subcortically, is registered in the prefrontal. AIDS poses a dilemma about closeness and being solitary. The solitary jellyfish image replaces a human symbol, perhaps avoiding and reflecting anxiety about relationships imposed upon Dillon by his medical conditions. Dillon's relationship needs conflict with the deadly disease that makes him a danger to others. The black, "shitty" dots may also symbolize contagion. Despite cooler green and blue colors representing some emotional control, the line pattern shows agitation.

This rather large *Jellyfish Blob* image, centrally placed and filling the page, leaves no room for resources or for changes. Its fixed position suggests that Dillon felt no place to move on the page. The non-human symbolism represents a need to distance from the severity of the problem. It implies a limbic amygdala-based fear or freeze state, or, conversely, an increased norepinephrine-locus coeruleus reaction, creating a vigilant attentive response. The image, while quite static, shows possible movement represented by green squiggles in the tentacles of the jellyfish. Their squiggly line quality at the bottom of the image may signal the onset of anxiety connected with his narrative. Comparing Dillon's regulated discourse in the interview with his emotional reaction to "Draw the problem" suggests that left hemispheric dominance over right hemisphere and limbic arousal is problematic. This attempt to move away symbolically and verbally may be causing emotional conflict and stimulating the medial prefrontal cortex, known for detecting conflict. The jellyfish may represent his anxiously controlling underlying conflicts through the sympathetic adrenal medulla stress response system (SAM). This image demonstrated one of the ways Dillon copes with the difficult, life-threatening, interpersonal implications of AIDS. A protective strategy is sometimes necessary and can be a strength. This time, the strategy created stress. As Dillon was motivated to work with the art therapist, he worked to find new solutions and reconcile the demands of the art request with his habituated responses.

Draw an image of yourself (art request #2)

Dillon drew an angel with a yellow crayon on a purple background. The art therapist noticed that he was visibly surprised by this affectively expressive image. The mouth was red. The squiggle representing a nose, and an eye, were dark blue, with yellow sparks flying off his head. He said:

> Wow, that just came out. That's the angel from the top of our Christmas tree. My mom still has it. The yellow is me, living in my head, full of ideas, connecting with the universe, the *OHM* sign. The light in my heart [the orange flower] is centered and connected with the [brown] roots in the earth. I'm grounded. It isn't a death angel, so it has a shit-eating grin.

He titled this image *One Spiritual Ass Muther Fucker!* (Figure 15.1, #2). He went on to discuss the closeness between his mother, sister and stepfather, and how supportive they had always been. The art therapist wondered if the title of the image also conveyed anger and irritation experienced as he rejected the death interpretation. While it is reasonable to associate the angel with death given the context of AIDS, the immediate rejection of this possibility may again reflect struggles with incorporating limbic affects.

The second art request, "Draw an image of yourself," prompted Dillon to connect to an episodic, affect-laden, autobiographical memory. Retrieving affect-laden personal memories has been found predominantly to involve activation in the right temporal lobe, the right posterior cingulate areas, the right insula, and the right prefrontal areas (Fink *et al.* 1996). When specific personal memories are retrieved, right temporal activation includes the amygdala and increased activity in the hippocampus (Eldridge *et al.* 2000).

Dillon's reaction to the angel image seemed to express an amygdala-based startle reaction. To self-soothe, he verbally drew upon earlier memories of familial closeness, answering a strongly felt need for support. Perhaps the right hippocampal/dorsolateral functions of working memory recruited the frontal-temporal pathway to provide this cortical image (Tomita *et al.* 1999). The art therapist thought that the art activated an affect-laden episodic memory associated with pleasure. Dillon's attempts to manage fear, stigma and isolation utilizing the left hemisphere led to a surprising novel right hemisphere image which Dillon found a way to embrace.

The image of *One Spiritual Ass Muther Fucker!* is similar to *Jellyfish Blob* in shape, size, vividness, and coherency, supporting the hypothesis that right hemispheric subcortical limbic responses activated during the first directive. Dillon's emotion emerging into consciousness surprised him. The emerging affect perhaps provided relief from the discomfort portrayed in *Jellyfish Blob*. Both images suggest conscious reliance upon personal strength and resources, while the emergence of the seriousness of the problem, and attachment longings, attempt to enter consciousness. The angel image has a human-like form and embodies a longing for connection. Spirituality seems to be the vehicle that allows a safe attachment to be remembered and re-experienced despite feelings of isolation. The angel connects feeling-based implicit memory to autobiographical explicit experience. The radiating broken line quality and the falling droplets are seen as representations of disturbing conflicts. It is as if limbic emotional reactions and sympathetic nervous system responses are leaking onto the page: drops or tears fall from the left side of the image from what would be the left wing or hand of the angel. Meanwhile, the right wing seems to be radiating exclamation marks. This visual representation is similar to the emotional/non-verbal and verbal dichotomy noted in Dillon's presentation of himself. The right emotional hemisphere regulates the left side of the body, and the left verbal hemisphere regulates the right, just as in the drawing: tears on the left side counterpoint exclamation points on the right. There are similar visual phenomena around the head in yellow in a parallel direction. A closer examination of the angel's facial features mirrors a correlation to Dillon's own facial distortion.

From an ATR-N perspective, Dillon's imagery is seen as striving for maintenance of control, as well as for connectedness. The drawings embody implicit autobiographical and somatic memories, which may have triggered an anxious ambivalent attachment style response. The jellyfish and the angel represent an ambivalent state, neither human, both incapable of reaching out for contact. This response may reflect both current medical and psychosocial issues as well as Dillon's past relational history.

Draw an image or a symbol for external and internal resources that help with the problem (art request #3)

The third art request represents a somewhat different direction of inquiry. It asks for a reflection on the person's resources and support system. On a second level of meaning (Bateson 1972), the directive implies that change can be discovered (i.e. help is available within the person as well as from outside sources). Exploring the perceived quality and quantity of internal and external resources allows the art therapist to gain a sense of the degree of allostatic burden that the person might be experiencing.

Ecosystem is the first drawing displaying multiple interrelated images (Figure 15.1, #3). Dillon stated that each of the outer circles represented an external resource surrounding an internal resource image:

> My internal resource is my spiritual, divine connection with God. I got that from a 12-step program, which is one of the external resources [see the 1 o'clock position]. My spirituality had to be ferreted out and the program made that possible. I chose black paper because I haven't used it yet and the infinity sign represents external resources I can't really put my finger on [12 o'clock position]. I have a lot of support. The boxes represent the agencies and social support [7 o'clock position] and the squiggles are my mom, stepfather, and sister [5 o'clock position]. The last circle is my meds and the new doctor I'm working with. He's great [10 o'clock position].

Dillon attributed his recent facial distortion to medical neglect.

Each image within this diagram contains autobiographical material. Together, they tell Dillon's life story of connectedness. The effort to connect resources and integrate memories results in scribbled, vague marks. Faint colors, lines, and fragmented cohesiveness seem to indicate that emotional overload is replacing arousal. There is a sense of loss of control and increasing allostatic load. Art expression parallels experience; the chronicity of AIDS reflects allostatic overload as the HPA stress response depletes resources over time. The art therapist noticed visual similarity between *Ecosystems'* drawn structure and microscopic slides of how the HIV virus enters cells and restructures them for its own benefit. Similar to the representation of the facial distortion in the angel image, this may be an implicit limbic portrayal of biologically appropriate cell images (Bach 1990).

Dillon drew a meaningful and familiar portrait of his resources on unfamiliar black background. He said he had not previously drawn on black. Meaning-making functionally engages the visual ventral system in the temporal cortex. The black page, chosen for its novelty, engages the amygdala, a key responder to new experiences. Combining the primary meaning of his supportive resources, and the secondary meaning of the black paper, seem to represent the unknown accurately: It is unknown if his resources will hold up, which contributes to his stress levels. The squiggles representing Dillon's family do not match his narrative. Apparently dissociation from meaningful metaphorical symbolism is characteristic during a right subcortical stress response (Cozolino 2002). The squiggles do not seem to be the kind of conscious mental representations of his family that would be expected from a consciousness-guiding left hemisphere. Given the unusual nature of this family picture, it occurs to the art therapist that the squiggles may contain fleeting implicit feelings. They suggest a private unconscious innate symbolism that may represent psychosocial challenges within his relational systems.

Draw yourself as you see yourself now and protocol summary (art request #4)

The last art therapy request examines the possibility of changes that may have been stimulated by participating in the protocol. Dillon drew himself as a little boy. Laughing, he stated that he was a 37-year-old grandson. He said:

> My grandmother is dead, but she is another internal resource. She always said I was Nana's baby and sometimes I feel that way. I knew she would always be there for me no matter what. When AIDS gets overwhelming, I think of Nana and read a lot.

Dillon titled this last image *Nana's Baby* (Figure 15.1, #4).

In *Nana's Baby*, there is a notable change—an emergence of a human image. *Nana's Baby* is a concrete representation; a family member is evoked for comfort, and the ethereal symbolism is gone. It is a prognostic refection on Dillon's ability to move towards remembered support despite the social stigma and isolation expressed by the jellyfish/angel desperation.

Dillon chose to put on paper an image of an autobiographical memory where he felt connected and safe. The picture title is cohesive, revealing the desire to be connected. The drawing's characteristics suggest a reduction in his stress response. There is a dampening of the highs and the lows seen in the second and third image, as well as a leveling of the allostatic load experienced in the third request. This thinking is based upon the shift to naturalistic colors, as well as the clear, non-sarcastic titling of the art. Colors are represented more realistically and less dramatically.

In the first and second drawings, the titles seem to represent left hemispheric thought processes, overriding felt right hemispheric limbic art experiences, while in the third drawing, the metaphorical title, *Ecosystems*, more closely resembles the floating experience. It is with the titling of the fourth drawing that Dillon is able simply to state his need for relationships, bringing about coherent awareness and thus further reducing some of his stress.

There is a chronic stress response expressed through the art that is characteristic of all four drawings: Dillon's initial response to participating in the protocol (*Jellyfish Blob*) and the emerging autobiographical information (*One Spiritual Ass Muther Fucker!*) is that of alarm. Drawing the first two images, and inviting the active participation of the right hemisphere, may have excited the amygdala, activating the sympathetic nervous system and creating his stress response. The small anxious marks and large images constrained by the boundaries of the page in these two drawings illustrate these ideas. This quick stress response appears to subside in *Ecosystem*, revealing an underlying chronic long-term stress response that erodes his resources and invades all the psychosocial systems in which Dillon participates.

In each image, the stress response is indicated through line quality and subsequent fading of coherency resulting in disintegration of the images. Despite the *cortex's* attempt to maintain control, the *limbic system* continues to inform Dillon quietly of emotional and relational needs. Chronic stress responses possibly aggravate and contribute to the hypertension reported as a side effect to the medication. It is important to educate Dillon about this finding and discuss with him stress reduction techniques. The analysis of affect expression and emotion provides additional support for this concern. The startling titles, along with vivid and coherent drawings of animal/metaphoric images, suggest a hypervigilant prefrontal cortex and right hemisphere contributions to the left hemisphere's language. As the protocol continued, in drawings three and four, the art seems to have provided the right hemisphere with an emergent voice, activating limbic memories and revealing emotional content to Dillon's narrative left hemisphere. Coherent, new, and more integrated meaning emerged from the continuous interaction of right and left hemispheres. The last drawing shows that participating in the art-making clearly decreased Dillon's anxiety, and seems to have afforded a more balanced expression of his emotions and attachment needs.

The differences between the fourth drawing *Nana's Baby*, and the second drawing *One Spiritual Ass Muther Fucker!*, are startling. In both drawings, the client is asked to draw a self-portrait. The first self-portrait request invites implicit responses (Hammer 1997) and, as in Dillon's case, often includes somatic aspects of the self. The second self-portrait request invites attention to a more aware and explicit sense of self: "Draw yourself as you see yourself now." *Nana's Baby* directly represents the vulnerability that Dillon may experience as he faces the ongoing struggle for quality of life, past, present and future. *Nana's Baby* reveals a gap between Dillon and his relational connectivity. Nana is not included in the picture and there is a relatively large space between her name and the child in the drawing. The pattern of attachment that emerges in the face of a possible connection continues to include extreme anxiety (Sroufe 1996), which is expressed as a connection held at a distance without direct contact to the figure. In the Adult Attainment Interview (AAI) protocol (Main and Goldwyn 1998), the interviewer records the time the interviewee takes to respond to questions about love. Can the pauses in the AAI be seen as space in art? The AAI measures time and pauses. Relevance is gained by a long pause. It's interesting to compare pauses in the narration of love and loving to visuospatial gaps of love and loving. When faced with the possibility of connection, a fear of rejection and/or implicit memories of rejection are evoked for Dillon.

As therapy commences, the art therapist may want to invite Dillon to participate in dual drawings, bridge the space, and experience successful interpersonal connections.

Dillon's mind/body journey is sensitively coded in each image produced through the art therapy protocol. The art embodies the research that suggests that stress, negative mood, and isolation undermine living with AIDS (Leserman *et al.* 2002). The ability of ATR-N approaches to ignite *implicit memory and trigger integrated right and left hemispheric functioning* may be uniquely posed to decrease the stress response, regulate disturbing emotions, increase a sense of mastery and control, and expand relational interconnectedness.

References

Achterberg, J., Dossey, B., and Kolkmeier, L. (1994). *Rituals of Healing: Using Imagery for Health and Wellness.* New York: Bantam Books.

Allman, J. M., Hakeem, A., Erwin, J. M., Nimchinsky, E., and Hof, P. (2001). The anterior cingulated cortex: The evolution of an interface between emotion and cognition. *Annals of the New York Academy of Sciences, 935,* 107–117.

Bach, S. (1990). *Life Paints Its Own Span: On the Significance of Spontaneous Paintings by Severely Ill Children.* Einsiedeln: Daimon Verlag.

Bateson, G. (1972). *Steps to an Ecology of Mind: Collected Essays in Anthropology, Psychiatry, Evolution, and Epistemology.* San Francisco: Chandler.

Beck, J. S. (1995). *Cognitive Therapy: Basics and Beyond.* New York: Guilford Press.

Clyde Findlay, J. (2008). Immunity at risk and art therapy. In N. Hass-Cohen and R. Carr (eds), *Art Therapy and Clinical Neuroscience.* London and Philadelphia, PA: Jessica Kingsley Publishers.

Cozolino, L. J. (2002). The Neuroscience of Psychotherapy: Building and Rebuilding the Human Brain. New York: W. W. Norton and Company.

Daruna, J. H. (2004). *Introduction to Psychoneuroimmunology.* Boston, MA: Elsevier Academic Press.

Eldridge, L. L., Knowlton, B. J., Furmanski, C. S., Bookheimer, S. Y., and Engel, S. A. (2000). Remembering episodes: A selective role for the hippocampus during retrieval. *Nature Neuroscience, 3*(11), 1149–1152.

Fink, G. R., Markowitsch, H. J., Reinkemeier, M., Bruckbauer, T., Kessler, J., and Heiss, W. D. (1996). Cerebral representation of one's own past: Neural networks involved in autobiographical memory. *The Journal of Neuroscience, 16*(13), 4275–4282.

Gabrieli, J. D. (1998). Cognitive neuroscience of human memory. *Annual Review of Psychology, 49,* 87–115.

Grice, H. P. (1975). Logic and conversation. In P. Cole and J. L. Moran (eds) *Syntax and Semantics: Speech Acts* (pp.41–58). New York: Academic Press.

Grice, H. P. (1989). *Studies in the Way of Words.* Cambridge, MA: Harvard University Press.

Hariri, A. R., Bookheimer, S. Y., and Mazziotta, J. C. (2000). Modulating emotional responses: Effects of a neocortical network on the limbic system. *Neuroreport, 11*(1), 43–48.

Hass-Cohen, N. (2006). PSY567: Psychoneurobiology Applications syllabus. Unpublished manuscript, Phillips Graduate Institute, Encino, CA.

Hass-Cohen, N. (2008). *CREATE: Art Therapy Relational Neuroscience Principles.* In N. Hass-Cohen and R. Carr (eds) *Art Therapy and Clinical Neuroscience.* London, Philadelphia, PA: Jessica Kingsley Publishers.

Hammer, E. F. (ed) (1997). *Advances in Projective Drawing Interpretation.* Springfield, IL: Charles C. Thomas Pub Ltd.

Henry, J. P., and Wang, S. (1998). Effects of early stress on adult affiliative behavior. *Psychoneuroendocrinology, 23*(8), 863–875.

Herek, G. (1990). Illness, stigma, and aids. In P. T. Costa and G. R. VandenBos (eds), *Psychological Aspects of Serious Illness: Chronic Conditions, Fatal Diseases, and Clinical Care* (pp. 107–150). Washington, DC: American Psychological Association.

Jia, H., Uphold, C. R., Wu, S., Reid, K., Findley, K., and Duncan, P. W. (2004). Health-related quality of life among men with HIV infection: Effects of social support, coping, and depression. *AIDS Patient Care and STDs, 18*(10), 594–603.

Kane, J. (2004). Poetry as right-hemispheric language. *Journal of Consciousness Studies, 11*(5–6), 21–59.

Landgarten, H. B. (1981). *Clinical Art Therapy: A Comprehensive Guide.* New York: Brunner-Routledge.

Leserman, J., Petitto, J. M., Gu, H., Gaynes, B. N., Barroso, J., Golden, R. N., *et al.* (2002). Progression to AIDS, a clinical AIDS condition and mortality: Psychosocial and physiological predictors. *Psychological Medicine, 32*(6), 1059–1073.

Main, M. and Goldwyn, R. (1998). Adult attachment classification system. Unpublished manuscript, University of California, Berkeley, CA.

Meador, K. J., Loring, D. W., Ray, P. G., Helman, S. W., Vazquez, B. R., and Neveu, P. J. (2004). Role of lateralization in control of immune processes in humans. *Annals of Neurology, 55*(6), 840–844.

Siegel, D. J. (2006). An interpersonal neurobiology approach to psychotherapy: Awareness, mirror neurons, and neural plasticity in the development of well-being. *Psychiatric Annals, 36*(4), 248–256.

Siegel, K., Karus, D., and Dean, L. (2004). Psychosocial characteristics of New York City HIV-infected women before and after the advent of HAART. *American Journal of Public Health, 94*(7), 1127–1132.

Schore, A. N. (1994). *Affect Regulation and the Origin of the Self: The Neurobiology of Emotional Development.* Hillsdale, NJ: Lawrence Erlbaum Associates, Inc.

Sroufe, L. A. (1996). *Emotional Development: The Organization of Emotional Life in the Early Years.* New York: Cambridge University Press.

Southwick, S. M., Rasmusson, A., Barron, J., and Arnsten, A. (2005). Neurobiological and neurocognitive alterations in PTSD: A focus on norepinephrine, serotonin, and the hypothalamic-pituitary-adrenal axis. In J. J. Vasterling and C. R. Brewin (eds) *Neuropsychology of PTSD: Biological, Cognitive, and Clinical Perspectives* (pp.27–58). New York: Guilford Press.

Tomita, H., Ohbayashi, M., Nakahara, K., Hasegawa, I., and Miyashita, Y. (1999). Top-down signal from prefrontal cortex in executive control of memory retrieval. *Nature, 401*(6754), 699–703.

CREATE: Art Therapy Relational Neuroscience Principles (ATR-N)

Noah Hass-Cohen

The unique contributions of art therapy approaches can be better understood and appreciated by utilizing findings from neuroscience research. From this linking of art therapy practices with clinical neuroscience, six proposed art therapy relational neuroscience (ATR-N) principles emerge: Creativity in action; Relational resonance; Expressive communication; Adaptive responses: Transformation; and Empathy (*CREATE*).

The *CREATE* framework makes available to art therapy valuable information from the interpersonal neurobiology of emotion, cognition and action that are expressed in the dynamic interplay of bodily systems during art therapy. *CREATE* principles can help art therapists understand the neurological underpinnings of psychopathology and allows for the fine-tuning of art therapy interventions and theories of change.

CREATE emerged from the search for an understanding of how the functional entrainment and synchronization of the bodily systems—the nervous, immune, endocrine, sensory, visual and motor systems—express in art therapy processes. Each *CREATE* principle is connected with the function of specific brain structures yet is also associated with more than one bodily region or system. For example, motor system functions, as delineated in the Creativity in action principle, require cortical feedback and are more often associated with cognitive function than previously thought (MacLeod *et al.* 2003, review). Cortical thoughts and feelings are motivated by basic emotions associated with the limbic central regions of the brain (Damasio 1994). The amygdala, which triggers the fear response, and the hippocampus that holds emotional experiences in short-term memory are involved (Figure 16.1).

Adding to this dynamic complexity, limbic structures in the central brain area also link to immune and endocrine system functions through hormonal feedback loops. Therefore, a systems perspective helps place the association of structures and functions in context (Kandel 1998). For example, the attraction to pleasure, dictated by the biological reward system, can be functional, as in art-making, or it can be dysfunctional, as in chemical abuse. Within a context, neurological structures express themselves along a

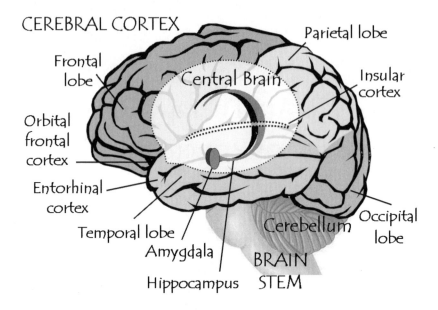

CEREBRAL CORTEX

Parietal lobe

Frontal lobe

Central Brain

Insular cortex

Orbital frontal cortex

Entorhinal cortex

Temporal lobe

Occipital lobe

Cerebellum

Amygdala

BRAIN

Hippocampus   STEM

Figure 16.1 The cerebral cortex, central brain and brainstem. The brainstem and the cerebellum are important for motor reactions and basic body processes. Limbic system structures located in the center region of the brain are considered responsible for social-emotional processing. The amygdala triggers the fear response and the hippocampus holds emotional experiences in memory. The cortex responsible for more sophisticated social cognitive function includes the occipital lobe, the parietal lobe, the temporal lobe, the frontal lobes and the insular cortex, located within the sulcus, which separates the temporal lobe and inferior parietal cortex. The insular cortex conveys bodily states to the cortex. The entorhinal cortex (EC) located at the caudal (tail) of the temporal lobe is a brain memory center. Both the insular and the EC are discussed later in the chapter. Also see Figure 1.5.

continuum from functional chaos to regulation to rigidity. Repeated positive feedback influences recurrent responses and reinforces sensitivity, sameness and rigidity. For most people, art therapy provides a novel context, which can supply them with new information to process. Flexible states may therefore result from this negative feedback when it conveys unpredictable yet helpful information. Visual artwork and the kinesthetic activity associated with art therapy can do just that. Art therapy practices potentially generate a new perspective on the client's problem by jumpstarting a mind-body negative feedback loop. The hypothesis is that as clients put art into action within a defined space, a different entrainment occurs, synchronizing psychosocial function, and bodily structures. The advantage of negative mind-body feedback loops, and thus art therapy as well, is that they diminish or interrupt the continuation of pre-existing functions.

To better understand the utilization of the *CREATE* principles they can be likened to self-similar fractals. Fractals are pieces of the whole. M. C. Escher's symmetry art is a wonderful example of self-similar images (Fish & Frogs, 1949, wood engraving), or alternatively, think about natural forms such as the bark of a tree or broccoli heads. Many natural forms such as a cauliflower are self-similar in that they represent a slightly different picture of the whole (Briggs 2001). Similarly, every ATR-N principle provides a perspective on the innate human tendency to take in salient information and organize it to our advantage. Each self-similar ATR-N principle also recursively underscores how feelings of well-being, safety and mastery are supported by interpersonal art exchanges and intrapersonal art expressivity. Self-similarity can be found at all systemic levels of human function: cellular, structural, functional and in the relational self. The *CREATE* systemic framework assists in understanding the complexities of human existence and can stimulate ongoing conceptualizations of art therapy relational neurobiology principles and practices (Hass-Cohen 2008).

CREATE: Creativity in Action

The expressive arts therapies–art therapy, drama therapy and play therapy—are characterized by the inclusion of movement and action, from deliberately large movements to fine motor actions. Understanding of stress responses supports the significance of including action and movement in a therapeutic environment. People are compelled to resolve fears by moving away or moving towards stressors (Sapolsky 1998). The idea that movement is indicative of coping attempts is also supported by the literature on projection drawings. For example, the examinee's projection of human movement onto Rorschach inkblots represents internal resources that may help in coping with stressors (Weiner 2003). The physical dimensions of art-making directly contribute to the therapeutic value. Art therapy provides an opportunity to reduce defensive avoidant states and instead engage adaptive action systems as suggested by Ogden, Minton, and Pain (2006). We encourage clients to take action by creating tangible art that expresses their inner state (Hass-Cohen 2006; Riley 2004). The exploration of emotions through the manipulation of art media (simple forms, colors or cut-outs) within a therapeutic relationship results in concrete art (Camic 1999; Naparstek 1994) that can successfully match the client's internal experiences.

Survival-based responses result from the inability to match expectations with appropriate actions and are accompanied by a rush of emotions and physical urges (Llinás 2001). Similarly, when clients are unable to match expectations of creating realistic and representative art with appropriate art-making actions, they may also feel overwhelmed by a rush of self-judgment and frustration. Art therapy facilitates the expression and regulation of these urgent emotions and corporeal surges in a therapeutic and controlled environment, which allows clients to experience and symbolically interpret expressive endeavors. For example, one of my clients was trying to show her relationships with her abusive male partner. Maya, quickly frustrated by what she perceived as her lack of ability to render a realistic figure, tore the page up. I suggested she use abstract shapes instead and she decided to use black squares to represent her husband. Dotted by black squares with pointed edges, the page looked like it had been stabbed. Doing so, Maya was able to match her feelings of anger and rage successfully with her expressions and talk about corresponding life events. Consequently, the experience of matching inner states with external manifestations of art provided her with the therapeutic opportunity to practice higher tolerance for mismatches of experiences with internal expectations creating different outcomes that can be predicted. As judgmental feelings are explored, the art therapist can act as a third hand that shows how to take advantage of the media in such a way as to overcome obstacles to visual expression (Kramer 1972). This process can contribute to increased feelings of resiliency.

Resiliency is the ability to respond to traumatic events by initiating appropriate seeking actions (Birmes *et al.* 2003; Lanius, Hopper, and Menon 2003; Voges and Romney 2003). In the face of perceived danger, higher risk for post-traumatic stress disorder (PTSD) is signaled by peritraumatic feelings of helplessness and certain death and physiological experiences of freezing and dissociation (Beck *et al.* 2006; Brewin, Andrews, and Valentine 2000). Post-trauma avoidant responses pose further risks to recovery (Briere, Scott, and Weathers 2005). In a safe therapeutic context, conscious physical actions can be an antidote to the unconscious responses associated with traumatic events (Ogden and Minton 2000). Perhaps, in a similar way, art therapy provides an outlet for unspoken feelings through non-verbal action, bringing about a felt sense of control and mastery (Malchiodi 1998) that assists in calming the body. While talking about trauma may be re-stimulating for people with PTSD, creating a sense of action and the ability to control that action may engender increased energy, a felt sense of accomplishment and personal creative agency.

Motor system functions of the cortex, the brainstem and the spinal cord contribute to taking action. Inputs to the motor control system depend on the thalamic processing of sensory stimuli, such as those found in art-making and on the cerebellum's coordination of motions that are required for making art. The thalamus is the gateway of sensory processing, and it shuttles impulses from the cerebellum and the basal ganglia to cortical prefrontal motor areas (Carr 2008; Kalat 2004; Figure 16.2).

The cerebellum, also called the little brain, significantly contributes to the coordination of voluntary movements, analyzing the timing of visual signals that correspond to self and/or others' movements. It does so by balancing the excitation and the inhibition of impulses. The output of the cerebellum is excitatory, while the basal ganglia outputs are inhibitory and refine movements. Utilizing sensory input from the body, the balance between these two systems results in coordinated movements required for matching actions, such as touching your nose with your forefinger. The cerebellum is linked to cortical motor regions that activate the muscles. Linked to the brainstem, the cerebellum assists in calculating anticipated positions of movement and in compensating when

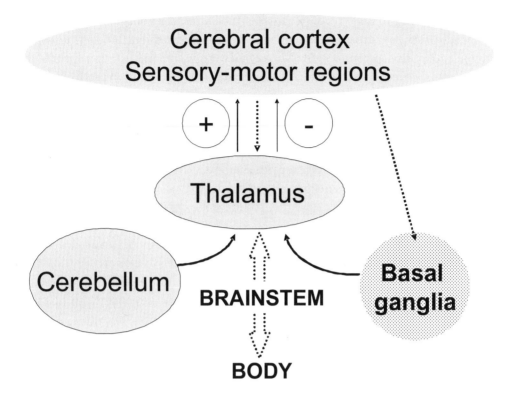

Figure 16.2 Motor control system involves the cerebellum at the back of the brain, the basal ganglia, the thalamus in limbic-central brain structures and the motor strip in the cortex. The cerebellum and the basal ganglia inform the thalamus, which in turn informs the cerebral cortex. Information from the cerebral cortex then doubles back providing feedback that facilitate basal ganglia functions. The cerebellum also directly informs the brainstem, involved in the actual control of movement (Kalat 2004).

movements do not occur as intended. Cerebellum dysfunction is implicated in neuro-psychiatric disorders, such as autism, Attention Deficit/Hyperactivity Disorder, mood disorders, obsessive-compulsive disorder and schizophrenia (Allen and Courchesne 2003, review; Schmahmann and Sherman 1998). The role of the cerebellum has been expanded and it is now thought that it is involved in directing movement as well as in influencing cognition and directing emotions. It most likely activates to not only actual movement, but also to sensory stimuli that might direct movement (Kalat 2004). Because art therapy practices routinely include a range of motions, the cerebellum's function is of high interest.

There are three parts to the cerebellum: the vestibulocerebellum, the spino-cerebellum and the newest part, which is of interest for this discussion, the neocerebellum. The neocerebellum has two hemispheres and is larger in humans. Its activation is fundamental to cognitive processing (MacLeod *et al.* 2003, review) and contributes to the coordination of visual-spatial skills, planning of complex movements, procedural learning, attention switching and sensory discrimination during digital manipulation (Schmahmann 1996). With regard to cognition and learning, areas of the cerebellum have been implicated in classical conditioning, in attention processes and in sequencing.

In addition to aiding movement and cognition, the cerebellum-thalamic-cortical circuitry provides important connections during emotional functioning (Konarski *et al.* 2005, review). There are cerebellum connections to non-motor, central brain circuitry that are associated with affect processing (the raphe nucleus, the locus coeruleus and the ventral tegmental area). This circuitry, also called the reward circuitry, is responsible for producing neurotransmitters that contribute to positive emotions. The main neurotransmitters involved are serotonin, associated with a sense of well-being; norepinephrine, associated with a sense of arousal; and dopamine, associated with a sense of reward and pleasure and enhanced positive mood. No wonder we feel better when we move. As clients create the art with their hands, it is therefore a good idea to encourage them to draw by standing up and or adding body movements. For example, Robin Vance, art therapist and artist, describes how she dances while creating mixed media collages of her implicit and explicit memories (Vance and Wahlin 2008).

Movements and gestures also have a relational role. We recognize someone else's action as one that we can do and learn. In my art therapy practice, I may quickly scribble on scratch paper to show clients the advantages of soft versus harder oil pastels. As they try out the media, they imitate my purposeful hand actions. Neural representations of learning through imitation occur in motor-mirror neurons and parietal circuitry (Buccino *et al.* 2001; Rizzolatti *et al.* 1996). Macque monkeys' mirror neurons also fired in response to observed, or intended but hidden, purposeful actions, such as successful grasping, tearing, holding or manipulating of objects, but not to non-purposeful movements (Keysers and Gazzola 2006, review). In humans, a corresponding mirror-motor system is found close to Broca's speech area in the frontal lobes (Buccino *et al.* 2001; Buccino, Binkofski, and Riggio 2004). From this research, we can extrapolate that people interact with each others' purposes through mimicry, imitation and simulation. The imitation of gestures and actions contributes to shared visceral-emotional meaning-making (Gallese 2003).

Many of the therapeutic exchanges in the expressive arts happen through mirrored actions between the client-artist and artist-therapist. Within a couple of sessions, most clients will associate the therapist's reaching out for the art media with a purpose. The client's mirror neurons will fire in response to the therapist's purposeful gestures and actions. Likewise, the therapist's neurons will most likely fire in response to the client's drawing gestures. Both brains activate in response to actual movements, or in response to implied bodily movement such as in an image (Kourtzi and Kanwisher 2000). The proximity of mirror neurons to Broca's area suggests an evolutionary link between non-verbal gestures and language development (Binkofski and Buccino 2004) with media manipulation as a suggested non-verbal language. The empirical research reviewed suggests that inviting purposeful action into therapy may be an identifiable therapeutic factor.

The expressive arts therapies rely upon a full spectrum of purposeful actions. In the face of adversity, simple purposeful activities, such as reaching out for media, washing brushes and hands and moving between media centers, may be shown to have relieving effects. For this reason, Shirley Riley, a pioneering and influential systems art therapist, was fond of asking group participants to walk around the room with their art. She instructed them to look for a similar art piece. Nevertheless, further study is necessary to understand more fully the positive effects of the therapeutic arts in action on cognition, emotion, learning and well-being.

CREATE: Relational Resonance

Attachment theory and applied clinical neuroscience research have created an evolutionary paradigm for psychologists. Empirical findings on how interpersonal relationships affect people's lives help explain this paradigmatic evolution. Conceptual-ized by John Bowlby (1988) and empirically tested and refined by Mary Ainsworth (Ainsworth *et al.* 1978), Mary Main (Main and Solomon 1990), and Eric Hesse (1999), attachment theory emphasizes how the security of early attachments, and relational patterns built from these attachments, resonate and recur throughout the lifespan.

Processes involved in art-making assist therapist-client interpersonal resonance and can positively impact attachment. Art-making and art products can act as regulatory mechanisms that mimic the reiterative dynamics of approach and avoidance observed by Mead (2001) in mother-child play. In such play, the child divides his or her attention between the mother and the play object, providing the child with the opportunity to self-regulate emotions. The attuned mother resonates with her infant and intuitively understands the infant's need to gaze at her as well as look away and take a break from the mutual interaction (Tronick 2007). Art therapy provides client and art therapist with similar opportunities for mutually dependent communication that builds contingent attachment. Paying attention to the art helps facilitate attunement as it allows for contained pauses that assist in self-regulation. If eye contact becomes overwhelming, the client and the art therapist can focus on the art-making and look at the messages in the art. Similar to a transitional object the inanimate objects, the art and the art-making, afford an opportunity to modify how client and therapist resonate and individuate, yet stay connected (Robbins 1999). Layers of resonance allow the art therapist to be inter-personally sensitive during art directives and interpretive moments (Hass-Cohen 2003; Riley and Malchiodi 1994). The clear and consistent therapeutic relationship builds coherent attachment as the client can count on the art therapist and the media to be there for him or her.

Purposeful art-making, intended to explore clients' issues, can evolve over time into a coherent mental narrative. Safety and the therapeutic alliance are increased when art therapists encourage the expression of vivid and dynamic imagery (Naparstek 1994) that is congruent with a person's existing mental imagery (Anderson 1997). In other words, allowing the clients' own imagery and understanding to surface rather than imposing prescribed directives contributes to better attunement. For example, asking a female client to draw "a bridge" between conflicting emotions may not fit with her mental representations of connectivity. Instead, asking her to "bridge" between her conflicts may allow for her internal, idiosyncratic representations to come forward; a hand, a path and/or even an abstract shape or color.

Asking the client to make art in the presence of the art therapist is an invitation to take a relational risk as art-making is culturally more associated with privacy. It is more common for the artist to share a final product than it is to share the art-making process. Similarly, asking the client to shift direction (or media) in session is an invitation to trust that the art therapist will refrain from judgment and provide support. Such interactions have the potential to promote connectivity and increase attachment. Ideally, re-attachment to another human results in a reordered neural organization of perceptual and attentional systems (Johnson and Hirst 1993; Johnson et al. 2005; Schore 1999). A higher order of reflective, supervisory psychosocial functions can emerge from shared experiences of art-making that involve mutual trust and bonds of hope. Sharing intimate moments helps clients experience and regain a felt sense of coherent and contingent attachment. Art therapy provides clients and therapists with unique opportunities for intimate resonance.

The art directive, the shared art-making and the discussion of the art product, offers an opportunity for the expression of the person's life story. The sharing of life stories with a significant other is self-informative, develops relational connectivity and elicits further resonances (Alea and Bluck 2003, review). Processing the social and self-aspects in the art therapy experience enhances autobiographical memory multifold, both verbally and visually. As I ask the client to draw a series of symbols to depict meaningful events along a timeline, I observe the process of drawing and I listen to the client's description of each meaningful episode. Episodes of meaningful memory help connect a sense of one's self to his or her past, present and future. The art therapist encourages the use of rich symbolic imagery to help present a coherent life story, as well as stories that fill in the gaps between episodic memories.

Non-verbal and symbolic visual expressions are a right-hemispheric language that directly stimulate the right orbitofrontal cortex (OFC) (Petrides, Alivisatos, and Frey 2002; Figure 16.1). Much of unconscious processing also happens in the right OFC, where autobiographical memories, including traumatic experiences, are stored (Neborsky 2006). These memories help identify which emotions are familiar and/or expected (Hass-Cohen 2008). The art therapy timeline directive can aid in finding out what kinds of autobiographical memories the OFC holds, and whether or not they are present in an expected or unexpected form. Revisiting the timeline can increase familiarity and thus help mitigate negative reactions to the visual expression of difficult times.

It is not uncommon for clients to develop a personal style of expressive art designs that are repeated over and over again in different variations. For example, Penny, who was dealing with hormonal problems, repeatedly used the symbols of a spiral to self-soothe and make sense of her condition (Hass-Cohen 2003). Such repetition of self-similar abstract lines and colors helps create a cohesive story that makes sense. Visual processes can then resonate with internal representations of connectivity and attachment (Alea and Bluck 2003, review). I encourage clients to delineate their new experiences and life story because vivid and meaningful details within art help concretize the relational experience. On a meta-level, clients associate the detailed telling of their life story vividly with a felt sense of trust. Thus, a "self-referential" personal memory (Macrae *et al.* 2004, p.647) can be immediately created in the room.

Repeated experiences of perceptual details contribute to short- and long-term consolidation of new memories (Gonsalves and Paller 2000; Macrae *et al.* 2004). Furthermore, research has shown increased consolidation of memory when dealing with a familiar other (Alea and Bluck 2003, review). Over time the art therapist becomes such a familiar figure. Memory consolidation involves bi-directional interactions between the hippocampus, a limbic system structure associated with the processing of short-term memories, the entorhinal cortex, linked with long-term memories (Eichenbaum 2001), and cerebral cortex regions. The entorhinal cortex is a main memory center and is located at the front end of the temporal lobe (Figures 16.3 and 16.1).

short-term consolidation (hippocampal) & **long-term consolidation** (entorhinal cortex)

cued by detailed vivid imagery of self (medial prefrontal activation) lead to

long-term storage (in widespread cerebral cortex regions)

Figure 16.3 How art therapy supports the consolidation of self-memories.

There is a positive correlation between the sense of security in an individual's attachment style and his or her capacity to access and share autobiographical memories (Hesse 1999). Consequently, adults with an insecure attachment style do not access the past easily. They describe autobiographical memories incoherently and usually have trouble accessing the positive aspects of their lives (Hesse 1999). Drawing the art therapy timeline may be difficult for certain clients. However, completing the experience may contribute to their cache of successful and more positive experiences, facilitating the development of a cohesive life story.

Before I explored neuroscience, I used the art therapy timeline exclusively during the "beginning stages" of therapy. Now, I include the timeline directive at the "mid-stage" of therapy when the social attachment between my client and me assists in revisiting memories. By asking clients to manifest vivid life imagery, we call forth auto-biographical sorting, selection of salient life memories and an update of life stories. Updating one's life story in the presence of a trusted therapist is advantageous. The "mid-therapy" autobiographical art therapy timeline helps clients and therapists string together meaningful memories that visually reveal the "life story schema" (Bluck and Habermas 2000, p.122). In comparison, the "beginning" art therapy timeline clarifies information related to the person's chronological history and/or symptomatology.

The significance of autobiographical art-making and man-made ritualized objects, such as altars, religious artifacts and community artwork, stems from their relational resonance (Hass-Cohen 2007). These transitional objects are reminiscent of familial relationships and early childhood upbringing. Memories triggered by such artifacts may facilitate an organized calm, normally activated by the parasympathetic nervous system, or, alternately, cause an urgent, disorganized, internal chaos associated with sympathetic stress responses, depending on the nature of the memories. On an interpersonal level, the art therapy studio (Hass-Cohen 2007), artwork and transitional, familiar objects

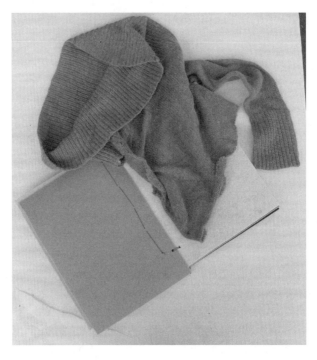

Figure 16.4 Lee Recalled the Nature of a Transitional Object. *The green woolly sweater is soft and soothing to touch (Lee Ignacio, attachment cloth album, 2006).*

(Winnicott 1971) function as relational objects that facilitate an understanding of the autobiographical self. The understanding of the autobiographical self is crucial for art therapy's curative value and overall significance (Figure 16.4).

CREATE: Expressive Communication and Emotional Processing

Emotional processing in a safe-enough relational context is a pivotal curative factor (Bridges 2006, review). *Emotional processing* involves *arousal, regulation, transformation, awareness* and *meaning-making* (Greenberg and Pascual-Leone 2006). Likened to a vertical ladder within the brain, *emotional processing* ascends and descends through the brainstem, basal ganglia, the limbic system and the right cerebral cortex. *Arousal* corresponds with firing in the amygdala, the autonomic nervous system and the basal ganglia. *Regulation* recruits the orbitofrontal cortex (OFC) and the anterior cingulate cortex (ACC); both areas lie above the limbic brain in the ventral areas of the prefrontal cortex. *Transformation, awareness* and *meaning* are associated with frontal lobe cortical integration (Figure 16.1).

Art therapy calls emotions into the room by asking clients to make art about difficult life circumstances in the presence of another. The novel situation invites arousal as well as curiosity, which can balance emotional reactivity. Emotions are heightened by less structured media, such as paint and clay (Riley 2004), whereas pencils and markers, which are more structured media, modulate arousal. The use of chromatic or achromatic color also puts emotional processing in the center of art therapy practices. Across all media, the meaning of chromatic color is less defined than shape (Kellogg 1992). Color invites the expression of basic core emotions. Basic emotions are namely happiness, surprise, fear, anger, disgust and sadness (Tamietto *et al.* 2007).

Emotional processing engages the superior temporal sulcus (STS), a cerebral cortex function associated (amongst other functions) with the processing of salient polymodal sensory stimuli (Wright *et al.* 2003). The STS is a connective boundary between the frontal lobe, the temporal lobe and the parietal lobe. Affective processing is aroused by STS sensitivity to human movement or implied human movement symbols, which can be found in collages or art imagery. Figure 16.5 shows the location of the STS in relationship to other brain structures explained later on in the chapter.

The processing of positive and negative emotions has been associated with left and right hemispheric function. Theoretical models claim that right hemisphere activation is more associated with automatic emotions, such as anger, whereas left hemisphere activation reflects conscious analysis of emotions and control (Gainotti 2005). However, a meta-analysis of 65 neuroimaging studies demonstrates that right/left lateralization more precisely follows an approach/withdrawal, motivational model (Wager *et al.* 2003). In the frontal cortex, emotions associated with approach are left-lateralized, while emotions associated with avoidant behaviors are right-lateralized. For example, anger that propels "towards" action is associated with a left lateralization; whereas anger

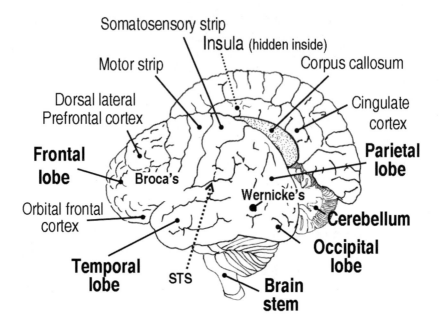

Figure 16.5 The superior temporal sulcus (STS) facilitates polymodal sensory information integration between frontal lobe willful actions, the temporal lobe emotional and the parietal visual-spatial processing. Other cortical structures and functions: The left prefrontal lobe includes Broca's expressive language center. Corpus callosum: bridges left and right hemispheres. The left temporal cortex includes Wernicke's area responsible for language comprehension. Somatosensory strip: holds a map of the body. Motor strip: association of motor activity with visual-spatial. Insular cortex: located within the sulcus, which separates the temporal lobe and inferior parietal cortex. The insular cortex conveys bodily states to the cortex.

that results in avoidance is associated with a right hemispheric activation (Harmon-Jones 2007). More recently, a review of the approaches to brain lateralization of emotional processing (Demaree, Everhart and Youngstrom 2005) suggests that approach emotions be classified as high dominance, and that avoidance or submission emotions be classified as low dominance. Pending neuroimaging studies, the dominance theory may help quantify approach and avoidance (Demaree *et al.* 2005). Split-brain research exemplifies right-left brain lateralization and dominance (Gazzaniga 2002). After split-brain surgery, patients were observed engaging in discordant avoidant-approach behaviors (Carter 1998). The right hand, representing the left hemisphere, wants to pick up an object and the left hand (representing the right hemisphere) intervenes pulling the right hand away (Parkin 1996). The phenomena is called the alien hand: when the corpus callosum is severed the connection between the two hemispheres is split. The dominant hemisphere, which for most people is the left hemisphere, loses control over the non-dominant hemisphere, which for most people is the right hemisphere, and the left hand becomes alien and disobedient.

Both right and left hemispheric activation most likely work with the art. In the future, neuroimaging research may show that as the fearful, right hemisphere-activated client is encouraged to approach art-making, the left hemisphere is engaged to modulate emotional avoidance. The artwork may also provide clues to hemispheric lateralization of emotion. Similar to the lateralized processing of visual stimuli, drawing on the right side of the page most likely represents left hemispheric function, whereas the opposite is true for drawing on the left side of the page (McNamee 2003). Richard Carr (2007) notes that this argument assumes that the paper is centered and that the person maintains a central focus. Otherwise, in every drawing, the emotions would be read in the left side of an image rather than the left side of the page. Or perhaps avoidant emotions would show on the left side, and approach emotions would show on the right side of every image (or page).

Clients may spontaneously select to represent hemispheric lateralization of affect by dividing the page and/or an image. For example, when asked to draw "the problem," Claire drew a large heart that filled up an entire page. She divided the heart into two parts. On the heart's right side, perhaps representing the left hemisphere, she drew herself on a sunny day. On the left side, representing the right brain, she drew herself on a foggy day covered with black and grey marks. She then quickly drew a fog over her sunny day. It seemed as if right hemispheric avoidant reactions hijacked the left hemisphere's sunny art expression. She directly represented the problem of depression, which is more associated with right hemispheric dominance (Lezak *et al.* 2004) and with decreased left frontal arousal (Demaree *et al.* 2005). Dividing the page into two and inviting opposites on each side is a common art therapy directive, an activity that may encourage inter-hemispheric engagement (McNamee 2003).

It is necessary to reduce the intensity of fears that may be controlling the client's life and may even threaten to take over the art therapy sessions. *Emotional regulation* allows for tolerable levels of affect, so that meaning can motivate the prefrontal cortex rather than shut it down (Briere and Scott 2006). The cingulate cortex, located between the higher cortical areas and limbic structures, plays an instrumental role in affect regulation. It bridges body and limbic information with cortical processing (Carter 1998; Figure 16.5).

The anterior part of the cingulate cortex (ACC) is involved in the development of emotional cognition, self-control, social awareness, and conflict resolution (Rueda, Posner, and Rothbart 2004; Turken and Swick 1999). Lianna was terminating her therapy and wanted to review her art-making. When she saw her art folder, her face reddened and she said: "I cannot look at that. Put it away and staple it shut." The folder contained too many conflicted memories that she was unsure she could regulate and she became frightened. She seemed to be exercising self-control over anticipated conflicts, which is an ACC function. However, without the support of neuroimaging, Lianna's response cannot be attributed solely to the function of one structure, the ACC. Her avoidant reaction was probably also mediated by the right hemisphere (RH), the amygdala and the autonomic nervous system acting in concert.

Key to understanding *emotional arousal* is the almond-shaped amygdala. Linked to fear responses and specific emotion circuitry (LeDoux 2000, 2002), it is also associated with anxious and depressed reactions (Sapolsky 2003). The amygdala is the self's lookout. Upon detecting a potentially threatening stimulus, the lookout immediately sounds bodily and emotional alarms. LeDoux's beautiful description of how the amygdala fires in response to a visual of a stick mistaken for a snake (LeDoux 2002; Briere and Scott 2006) demonstrates how the amygdala can easily be triggered even when the visual is less well-defined. Vague art imagery may stimulate a stronger amygdala than a cortical response. Cortical processing utilizes more detail to interpret the stimuli within a known context. Until clarified by cortical processing, vague art imagery may stir unrecognized fears in the client. Art therapy helps clients discover the nature of hidden or unconscious feelings through working with their reactions to vague stimuli. In response to undefined collage images or lumpy media, for example, clients are unlikely to flee the room. However, they may have a strong internally felt sense of wanting to escape due to evoked fears and memories.

Fear can be paired and conditioned with seemingly unrelated events, possibly forming the foundation for phobias or anxiety disorders. The fear response is linked to a passive coping response, which inhibits active coping (Blair *et al.* 2003; Miller and McEwen 2006). Conditioned passive responses involve specialized amygdala areas. The middle (or central) amygdala area, associated with passive coping, fires with the top part (the dorsal), which is also most sensitive to new fears as well as the reconditioning of old fears (LeDoux 2000; Figure 16.6).

If the amygdala becomes desensitized to the disturbing and/or vague image, the individual may calm down and amygdala functioning can be reconditioned. Extinction, reconsolidation and coping strategies are processes that regulate fear responses. Extinction, the elimination of fear responses, happens through conscious and unconscious conditioning and is mediated by the release of the neurotransmitter serotonin (Vasterling and Brewin 2005). Art therapy may help pair the experience of a new benign image with the memory of old fearful images. Thus, providing positive experiences associated with serotonin release can mediate fear. Altering amygdala reactions helps generate more active cortically driven coping responses (Phelps *et al.* 2004). Safe, repeated visiting with the image of a feared memory can weaken the memory's ability to produce fear. I try to assist clients in realizing that there are no here-and-now negative consequences to the black-and-blue marks of their abuse on paper. "It's my mother shouting at me, but only on paper, and there will not be a negative consequence." Uniting old memories with a different quality of emotions consolidates a new experience. The explicitly benign perception of the art product can further stimulate an inwardly attuned, alert state that supports improved hippocampal and cortical process-

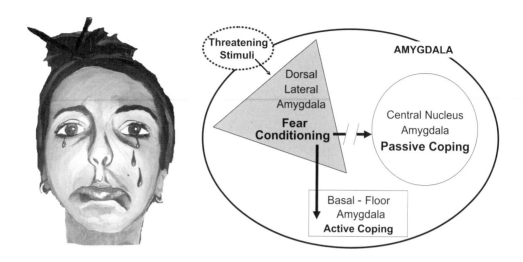

Figure 16.6 Conditioned amygdala responses. The amygdala has three specialized areas. The top (dorsal lateral) is most sensitive to new fears and the reconditioning of old fears. The mid section (mid-central nucleus) is associated with passive coping, and the bottom (basal lateral) amygdala is associated with active coping with fear. The goal is to inhibit the dorsal lateral amygdala (DLA) firing to the central nucleus (CE) and to excite connections to the basal amygdala (LeDoux 2000). Art by Juli Ann Martinez.

ing of new memories. Safe symbolic sensory experiences within a therapeutic relationship can bring a heightened sense of perceived control and well-being (Malchiodi 1999).

Emotion regulation skills increase a person's ability to tolerate arousal from negative emotions, such as anger, and experience more of the positive kinds of emotions. Counterbalancing negative or more reactive emotions with positive emotions reduces the impact of those negative emotions. Emotional awareness via labeling, contextualizing and/or self-soothing and distraction, have all been found to help in regulating high distress (Greenberg and Pascual-Leone 2006, review; Linehan 1993a, 1993b).

Emotion regulation skills engage the right OFC (Schore 1999, 2007), which is located just above and behind the eyes, at the bottom of the prefrontal cortex. The OFC is the pinnacle of non-verbal vertically integrated and regulated emotional processing. The back and side portion of the OFC is strongly associated with sensory limbic processing of negative emotions and unexpected stimuli (Petrides *et al.* 2002; Figures 16.1 and 16.5). Lesions in the OFC result in impulsivity, along with interpersonal and personality changes (Beer 2007, review). The front portion fires in response to positive emotions, as well as to familiar and expected stimuli.

Developmentally, the OFC is linked to the quality of early dyadic relationships (Schore 1999). OFC functions play a vital role in one's ability to evaluate others' emotional states (Damasio 1994). Early attachment experiences, body language, gazes, facial expressions, and gestures inform right OFC function. Non-verbal communication is needed for the reparative work in relational therapies (Schore 2007). In light of this understanding, the creation of art in the presence of a supportive art therapist provides a context for reparative attachment work. The creation of art in the room greatly increases the amount of shared non-verbal communication. Subtle exchanges of gestures and eye contact characterize much of the communication that occurs while the client makes art. Bringing in works of art created elsewhere and then talking about them in art therapy sessions may be less effective than in-session art approaches.

Emotional processing must include positive emotional expressions (Bridges 2006). Experiences of joy demonstrate faster cardiovascular recovery from negative emotions than do neutral experiences (Tugade, Frederickson, and Barrett 2004). It is likely that meaningful change happens by inviting positive experiences and integrating them with older, avoidant responses. The transformation of a negative response into a positive or assertive response can result in a shift from neuroendocrine-mediated feeling of *loss of* control, to a sympathetic nervous system-based feeling of being *in* control (Henry and Wang 1999). Positive emotions broaden perceptions and increase the range of action and social options (Fredrickson and Branigan 2005, review). The pleasures of art-making in the face of adverse emotions may very well assist in this transformation.

Expressive communication includes *transformation, awareness* and *meaning-making.* Many clients report that the sense of well-being, pleasure and reward felt during and after the creation of art is profound and fundamental to their change processes. Therefore, rather than reasoning or assigning a new cognitive meaning to an emotion, one can use the art to transform one emotion directly into another. Art-making results in positive and joyful responses facilitated by the brain's natural reward systems. Positive emotions have been found to facilitate physical well-being and mental health changes (Fredrickson 2001; Fredrickson and Levenson 1998). Therapeutic positive emotions have been associated with self-mastery, pride (Bridges 2006), gratitude, and love (Fosha 2005).

Making meaning from emotional experiences is the essence of *emotional awareness.* "It is important to make a distinction between the intensity of emotion and the depth of processing of the emotion. It is not the former but the latter that is curative in therapy" (Greenberg and Pascual-Leone 2006, review, p.616). Once emotions are expressed, people are able to reflect on what they are feeling, create new meanings, evaluate their own emotional experience and share it verbally with others (Pennebaker 1997; Rimé *et al.* 1998). People also reflect on what they are feeling in order to find words, and the words cement the experience if they match the non-verbal awareness. The felt meaning attributed to words is a right hemisphere function, not left. In trauma, it is activating and integrating the right that dispels PTSD. Through left hemispheric verbalization and symbols, individuals are able to organize, structure and ultimately include their emotional reactions. Being able to symbolize and explain emotional trauma in words helps promote the absorption of unconscious bodily memories into conscious self-narratives (van der Kolk and Fisler 1995). Expressing joins the hemispheres in building meaning and self-awareness.

CREATE: Adaptive Responses

Presenting personal difficulties through art-making is a novel, unexpected task for most people. Just as art-making in the presence of another invites expressivity and intimacy, it also invites stress. The art therapist and client have the joint opportunity to look at the individual's adaptation to the unexpected request.

Andrea Lewis, an art therapist, shared the following art therapy protocol in one of my classes: Chris, an artist, drew a series of four images about her diabetes, each of the drawings in a very different art style. First, she drew a realistic rendering of her insulin injections, followed by a naturalistic representation of her hand. She then presented an abstract image of her blood cells, culminating in a fragmented self-portrait. Jumping from one artistic style to another suggests that she is attempting to control her stress reaction.

Reflecting on Chris's anxiety, Andrea Lewis drew a Mandala of a blossomed flower within a circle. According to Jung, drawing within a circle is an effort to calm pain (Jung 1973). The dark, top petals of the flower are in red, whereas the underlying, triangular-shaped petals are in green. The symbolic meaning of red-stop and green-go colors is perhaps indicative of Andrea Lewis's attempts to balance her own excitatory sympathetic and rebalancing parasympathic responses (Figure 16.7).

Adaptive responses to new demands, such as drawing about health issues, require emotional flexibility as well as sympathetic and parasympathetic autonomic nervous system balance. Initially, there is a beneficial arousal of the sympathetic response that helps the client cope with the stressor, followed by protective dampening, mediated by the parasympathetic relaxation response (Sapolsky 1998). In the above art therapy protocol, Chris, the artist, was not able to calm herself and remained highly anxious. There are two main types of stress responses. The first, the short-term flight or fight stress response, activates adrenaline and the sympathetic nervous system readies the individual for action. Initially the flight-fight response increases immune function then diminishes it (Sapolsky 1998). The second, the long-term stress response, activates the hypothalamus-pituitary-adrenal axis (HPA), which results in an elevation of cortisol (Sapolsky 1998). A chronic stress response alters and diminishes long-term bodily projects, possibly damaging immune system function as it recruits all the individual's resources to adapt to the stressor (Sapolsky 1998; Figure 16.8).

Stress in art is frequently expressed as quick scribbles, spills and/or small, withdrawn representations. Structured art interventions can calm fear-based,

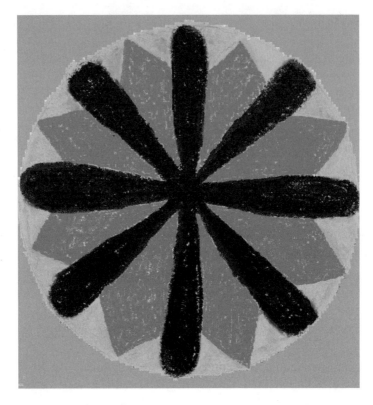

Figure 16.7 Two Mandala-like flowers. The dark is red and the light is green. By Andrea Lewis.

subcortical, right hemispheric, survival-based stress responses (Lusebrink 2004). The art therapist's invitation to use clear and simple forms, or structured media, can help mitigate the stress response. While the request to draw a problem can arouse stress and anxiety, it also affords the client antidotes, involving choices and a sense of control and dignity:

> Art-making as therapy can help people regain some measure of control in their lives by providing the freedom to choose materials, style and subject matter; to play freely with color, lines, forms, and textures; and to create what one wants to create. This element of choice can contribute to one's feelings of autonomy and dignity when other aspects of life seem out of control. (Malchiodi 1998, pp.174–175)

Prolonged cortisol release, associated with long-term stress response, can kill neurons in the hippocampus and affect memory function (Sapolsky 1998). When the HPA axis is enduringly active, the levels of cortisol are not regulated and the toll on the person's health can be significant. For example, a chronic stress response can amplify problems in insulin dependent-diabetes, such as Chris's, with hormones of the stress response causing more glucose and fatty acids to mobilize in the bloodstream, leading to elevated

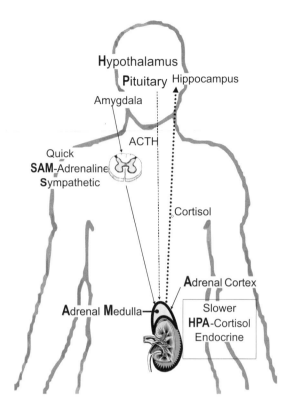

Figure 16.8 Stress response. *The adrenal cortex (the outer part) is activated by adrenocorticotrophic hormone (ACTH) sent out from the pituitary gland. The adrenal gland secretes two hormones collectively known as cortisol. The adrenal medulla (inner part) is an agent of the sympathetic nervous system and is activated by nerve impulses and adrenaline. Both parts of the adrenal gland's response help the body*

blood sugar levels and vascular damage. Cortisol can also suppress immune function and reduce the formation of new lymphocytes from thymic tissue (Sapolsky 1998). It would therefore be important to assist Chris in managing stress levels.

Art imagery can provide symbolic clues about immune system function (Ferencik, Novak, and Rovensky 1998; Ferencik and Stvrtinova 1997). These clues can assist in medical arts therapy practices (Achterberg *et al.* 1994; Brigham 1994; Hass-Cohen 2003; Kellogg 1992; Naparstek 1994). Clients may often compartmentalize their medical conditions and not bring them to therapy. Consequently, the art therapist is called upon to find creative ways to inform clients about the damage caused by stress. Stress and the inability to cope may also be associated with shame, which is important for both the art therapist and client to address since it adds to the effects of stress. Dissolving the boundaries between medical and mental health practices is part and parcel of the clinical-neuroscience-aware art therapist's repertoire of interventions (Galbraith, Subrin, and Ross 2008).

CREATE: Transformation and Empathy

Perhaps the loftiest goal of therapy is learning to trust and understand oneself and the other. Art visuals and narratives provide a window to the relational mind and the opportunity to understand one another through narratives, participation and art. There is an opportunity for knowing that another person means to connect through thinking, emoting and intuiting. Cortical and subcortical integration requires minds to read minds (Zimmer 2003). According to an analysis of 16 neuroimaging studies the superior temporal sulcus (STS), the anterior cingulate cortex (ACC), the parietal cortex and the prefrontal cortex are most likely involved (Brune and Brune-Cohrs 2006, review; Figure 16.5). Theory of mind (ToM) refers to the process of intuiting what others are thinking (Premack and Woodruff 1978), which is foundational to human social wiring and functioning (Frith 2007).

Developmental milestones set the stage for the neurobiological organization that allows most children by the age of four to mentalize and predict another person's behavior accurately (Frith and Frith 1999, review). ToM accounts for this phenomena. In psychology ToM is the cognitive capacity to assign mental states, beliefs, intents, desires, etc., to oneself and to others and to understand further that others may have quite different experiences, beliefs, desires and intentions (Frith and Frith 1999, review). Children's abilities to mind-read are easily observed by the art therapist. In my art therapy practice, I encourage children to layer their art pieces on the wall. This spatial, visual journal documents the therapy's journey and enhances the client's auto-biographical memory. The creation of the journal in the presence of another can put ToM into action. Evan, seven years old, asked to remove his *Playing in the Park* drawing from his wall journal, so we put it in his folder. The following week, his mother joined us for a session. Evan eagerly showed her the newly arranged wall journal. He was surprised and somewhat upset when she inquired about the whereabouts of the *Playing in the Park* drawing. Mindblindness, the inability to read another's mind (Baron-Cohen 1995), was demonstrated by his anticipation that his mother, without being there, would know that the drawing was put away.

Evan, who was diagnosed with an autistic spectrum disorder (ASD) acted upon what he deemed to be a correct belief. His failure to distinguish between his beliefs and that of others has been reported as typical of the ASD spectrum (Frith and Frith 1999, review). In response, I initiated verbal and non-verbal art therapy dual drawings between the two. Each took turns making a mark on the same page. Sometimes they discussed the topic before drawing; at other times, they were asked to draw without talking first. The task required both to focus on the other's intentions, which helped Evan practice, detect, and understand intentionality and cues involving mentalizing strategies. Mother and therapist also benefited from discussing some of the projective material that emerged (Gillespie 1994). The main advantage was that even though Evan and his mother were frequently mis-attuned to one another, they were able to participate in the art-making and relate to one another without their usual frustrations and anger. The dual work led them to ask questions about each other's art intentions and helped them practice understanding in a safe and contained environment. Shared attention and goal-directed activity utilized mentalizing abilities innate to dual-drawing experiences. Mother and child experienced their gazes locking and unlocking as they attended to an art-directed activity. In the art therapy room, this showed up as the ability to make dual drawing connections and links between ideas, feelings and events. Their increased ability to give form to feelings through symbolic representations allowed them to share interpersonally. Dual-drawings helped Evan's mother empathize with her child's ASD-related communication challenges. From a clinical neuroscience lens, dual drawings are a wonderful relational ToM activity.

Adult mind-reading skills are necessary for the appropriate understanding of socially constructed meaning. Therapy is essentially a reiterating narrative of mentalism: *he said, she said, they said* narratives. Mentalizing emerges from the desire to foresee, know, understand and move the other in relationship to the self. Figuring out what and how people think, intend and believe represent unique human abilities. Art therapy practices may enhance mentalizing when shared knowing of shapes and figurative marks emerge. Similar to comprehending conceptual art, the interpretation and understanding of art therapy expressions is socially constructed by therapists and clients who collaborate about relevant internal mental representations (Riley and Malchiodi 1994).

In 1918, the father of conceptual art, Kazimir, Severinovich Malevich, created "White on White," a white only painting. Malevich declared that behind the world of physical appearances exists a higher reality of artist-observer relationships. Malevich's white on white painting invites the observer to speculate and mind-read his intentions. Conceptual art focuses on how the final product can assist the observer in attuning to the artist's intentions and mental mind-set (Babcock 2003). Conceptual art and art therapy share a similar foundation, as art therapy expressions serve to transfer communication between minds. The sharing of symbolic meaning approximates real-life mind-reading of a metaphoric cultural language. Symbolic art metaphors require a second order level of reading others' mental states (Brune and Brune-Cohrs 2006). While artists' symbolisms are usually more associated with political and social meanings, clients' art will be more idiosyncratic to their culture and personal histories. Art therapy tasks require that the therapist and client assign meta-cognitions to the literal presentation of shapes, as well as pay attention to the corresponding action-oriented hand gestures. Art therapy offers the opportunity to activate neural integration and ultimately higher cortical functions that come from mentalizing personal idiosyncratic epistemologies (how we know who we are). On the page, as the client and therapist correspond about their mentalizing, new ways of knowing the self are co-constructed. Mindskills are associated with understanding false assumptions, motivating the other's mind and considering the other's expectations (Frith and Frith 1999, review). Non-verbal art actions and verbal interpretation synchronize to increase mind skills and shared mental representation.

Shared internal mental representations are not to be confused with empathic resonances. For example, most criminals have intact ToM abilities, but lack the emotional ability to put themselves in another's shoes (Dolan and Fullam 2004). Shared internal mental representations reflect shared social cognitions, whereas empathic representations evolve from experientially shared social resonances (Gallese 2006) that are crucial for therapeutic success. Observing actions, sensations, and emotions in others, as well as physically hearing their voices, activates the same brain areas that would be involved if the observer himself performed the actions, experienced the sensations and felt the emotions (Keysers and Gazzola 2006). Embodied empathic understanding of another's intentionality has been associated with mirror neuron system activations (Gallese 2006; Iacoboni and Dapretto 2006; review).

It is significant for art therapists to know that matching person to person experiences does not require verbalization (Gallese 2006; Milner and Goodale 1995). Furthermore, emotional experiences involving somatosensory touch, pain and attachment can all activate empathic resonances. Human neuroimaging shows that mirror systems activate during a wide variety of observed human body actions (Buccino *et al.* 2001; Gallese 2006; Watkins, Strafella, and Paus 2003). Here are several examples: (1) The neuroimaging of people who are observing the facial expressions of others experiencing disgust show activation in the same regions of the anterior insula as those who are actually experiencing the feeling (Wicker *et al.* 2003); (2) Watching a loved-one experiencing pain activates the same neural circuitry in the observer's brain as in the brain of the person in pain (Singer *et al.* 2004); (3) Distress at separation from loved ones activates parallel subcortical regions in both attached individuals (Watt 2005, review); and, finally, (4) Observing somebody being touched activates the same neural networks in one's own body as in the person being touched (Keysers *et al.* 2004).

Experiential simulation is a functional process that provides a window to the possible states of others. In my teaching practice, I role-play with students to show the difference between using art to trigger a conversation and to immerse oneself fully in the art therapy. I describe and demonstrate my heightened sensitivity to how hands pick up the media and to the specific sounds the first tentative scratches and the ensuing bold marks make on the paper. Body language alerts me to the person's emotional state. As the role-play imagery emerges, I am transported into the art and language. Direct observation gives a felt emotional sense that we are involved in the activities of those we observe (Gallese 2003). Observation of clients' art-making is an embodied simulation that contributes to the art therapist's fuller knowledge of the client's art processes.

The activation of parallel observer and observed neuron regions facilitates direct self-other experiences of actions, perceived communication, auditory sounds and intentionality. Perceived auditory and visual speech (Watkins *et al.* 2003) and a wide variety of other bodily actions such as communicative mouth movements (Buccino *et al.* 2001; Ferrari *et al.* 2003), activate mirror neurons in the "doer" and the observer.

For this reason, in my practice, I strive to attune to what tone of voice accompanies an art directive and how I ask for the title of the artwork. Whether I touch the client's art or not, my facial and my bodily expressions convey a sense of optimism that distress can be alleviated. "Empathy is more than an accurate perception of other's emotional state…[it] must involve some motivation for the relief of the other's distress" (Watt 2005, p.197). The felt sense of shared neural circuitry and the embodied understanding conveyed through the therapist's actions and implicit emotions transfer to the client. In short, art therapy practices provide concrete and plentiful opportunities to put empathy into action.

Summary

The six art therapy relational-neuroscience (ATR-N) principles of *CREATE* have emerged for the author as a helpful theoretical framework in the practice of successful art therapy. It is hoped that as theoretical constructs, they can function as holding markers for further art therapy dialogues, investigations and research.

CREATE (ATR-N) principles postulate that an integrated and attuned state of mind emerges during the novel sensory experience of making art in the therapist's presence. **C**reativity in action highlights how movement and action are art therapy therapeutic factors. The experience of actively matching inner states with corresponding visual expressions relieves stress. **C**reativity in action brings this concrete visual expression to the shared space of the art therapy table. The creative, action-oriented context uniquely shapes the therapist-client relational resonance. **R**elational studio art therapy experiences and concretized art-making call forth memories, emotions and cognitions, and have the potential to mend attachment ruptures. The inherent safety of the art-making context increases the capacity to tolerate emotional frustration and regulate ambiguity in one's art and life. **E**xpressive communication reflects on the duality of simultaneously expressing avoidant feelings such as fear while at the same time experiencing the positive affects of art-making. The experience of these two states helps therapists and clients contain the tangible art representation of their problems and let a new solution incubate through the art. **A**daptability is increased and the stress response reduced as expressive pleasure increases. **T**ransformations occur through interactive art therapy feedback loops that promote more flexible and stable responses. Art therapy experiences contribute to integrating both the mentalizing and empathic capacities necessary for the emergent relational self.

References

Achterberg, J., Dossy, L., Gordon, J. S., Hegedus, C., Herrmann, M. W., and Nelson, R. (1994). *Mind-Body Interventions:* Panel report to the National Institutes of Health on Alternative Medical Systems and practices in the United States. Washington, DC: U.S. Government Printing Office.

Ainsworth, M. D. S., Blehar, M. C., Waters, E., and Wall, S. (1978). *Patterns of Attachment: A Psychological Study of the Strange Situation.* Hillsdale, NJ: Lawrence Erlbaum Associates, Inc.

Alea, N. and Bluck, S. (2003). Why are you telling me that? A conceptual model of the social function of autobiographical memory. *Memory, 11*(2), 165–179.

Allen, G. and Courchesne, E. (2003). Differential effects of developmental cerebellar abnormality on cognitive and motor functions in the cerebellum: An fMRI study of autism. *American Journal of Psychiatry, 160*, 262–273.

Anderson, H. (1997). *Conversation, Language and Possibilities.* New York: Basic Books.

Babcock, C. (2003). Mentalism and mechanism: The twin modes of human cognition. In C. Crawford and C. Salmon (eds) *Human Nature and Social Values: Implications of Evolutionary Psychology for Public Policy.* London: Lawrence Erlbaum Associates.

Baron-Cohen, S. (1995). *Mindblindness: An Essay on Autism and Theory of Mind.* Cambridge, MA: MIT Press.

Beck, J. G., Palyo, S. A., Gudmundsdottir, B., Canna, M. A., and Blanchard, E. B. (2006). What factors are associated with the maintenance of PTSD after a motor vehicle accident? The role of sex differences in a help seeking population. *Journal of Behavior Therapy and Experimental Psychiatry, 37*(3), 256–266.

Beer, J. (2007). The importance of emotional-social cognition interactions for social functioning: Insights from orbitofrontal cortex. In E. Harmon-Jones and P. Winkielman (eds) *Social Neuroscience.* New York, London: Guilford Press.

Binkofski, F. and Buccino, G. (2004). Motor functions of the Broca's region. *Brain and Language, 89*, 362–369.

Birmes, P., Brunet, A., Carreras, D., Ducasse, J. L., Charlet, J. P., Lauque, D., *et al.* (2003). The predictive power of peritraumatic dissociation and acute stress symptoms for posttraumatic stress symptoms: A three-month prospective study. *American Journal of Psychiatry, 160*(7), 1337–1339.

Blair, H. T., Tinkelman, A., Moita, M. A., and LeDoux, J. E. (2003). Associative plasticity in neurons of the lateral amygdala during auditory fear conditioning. *Annals of the New York Academy of Sciences, 985*, 485–487.

Bluck, S. and Habermas, T. (2000). The life story schema. *Motivation and Emotion, 24*(2), 121–147.

Bowlby, J. (1988). *A Secure Base: Parent-Child Attachment and Healthy Human Development.* New York: Basic Books.

Brewin, C. R., Andrews, B., and Valentine, J. D. (2000). Meta-analysis of risk factors for posttraumatic stress disorder in trauma-exposed adults. *Journal of Consulting and Clinical Psychology, 68*, 748–766.

Bridges, M. R. (2006). Activating the corrective emotional experience. *Journal of Clinical Psychology, 62*(5), 651–668.

Briere, J. and Scott, C. (2006). *Principles of Trauma Therapy: A Guide to Symptoms, Evaluation and Treatment.* Thousand Oaks, CA: Sage Publications.

Briere, J., Scott, C., and Weathers, F. (2005). Peritraumatic and persistent dissociation in the presumed etiology of PTSD. *American Journal of Psychiatry, 162*(12), 2295–2301.

Brigham, D. D. (1994). *Imagery for Getting Well.* New York, London: W. W. Norton & Company.

Briggs, J. (2001). *Fractals: The Patterns of Chaos.* New York: Touchstone.

Brune, M. and Brune-Cohrs, U. (2006). Theory of mind-evolution, ontogeny, brain mechanisms and psychopathology. *Neuroscience Biobehavioral Review, 30*(4), 437–455.

Buccino, G., Binkofski, F., Fink, G. R., Fadiga, L., Fogassi, L., Gallese, V., *et al.* (2001). Action observation activates premotor and parietal areas in a somatotopic manner: An fMRI study. *European Journal of Neuroscience, 13*, 400–404.

Buccino, G., Binkofski, F., and Riggio, L. (2004). The mirror neuron system and action recognition. *Brain and Language, 89*, 370–376.

Camic, P. M. (1999). Chapter 2: Expanding treatment possibilities for chronic pain. through the expressive arts. In C. Malchiodi (ed.) *Medical Arts Therapy with Adults.* London and Philadelphia, PA: Jessica Kingsley Publishers.

Carr, R. (2007). Personal communication.

Carr, R. (2008). Sensory processes and responses. In N. Hass-Cohen and R. Carr (eds) *Art Therapy and Clinical Neuroscience.* London and Philadelphia, PA: Jessica Kingsley Publishers.

Carter, R. (1998). *Mapping the Mind.* Los Angeles, CA: University of California Press.

Damasio, A. R. (1994). *Descartes' Error: Emotion, Reason, and the Human Brain.* New York: Harper Perennial.

Demaree, H. A., Everhart, D. E., and Youngstrom, E. A. (2005). Brain lateralization of emotional processing: Historical roots and a future incorporating "dominance". *Behavioral and Cognitive Neuroscience Reviews, 4*(1), 3–20.

Dolan, M. and Fullam, R. (2004). Theory of mind and mentalizing ability in antisocial personality disorders with and without psychopathy. *Psychology Medicine, 34*(6), 1093–1102.

Eichenbaum, H. (2001). The long and winding road to memory consolidation. *Nature Neuroscience, 4,* 1057–1058.

Ferencik, M., Novak, M., and Rovensky, J. (1998). Relations and interactions between the immune and neuroendocrine systems. *Bratislavske Lekaraske Listy (Bratislava Medical Journal), 99*(8–9), 454–464.

Ferencik, M. and Stvrtinova, V. (1997). Is the immune system our sixth sense? Relation between the immune and neuroendocrine systems. *Bratislavske Lekarske Listy (Bratislava Medical Journal), 98*(4), 187.

Ferrari, P. F., Gallese, V., Rizzolatti, G., and Fogassi, L. (2003). Mirror neurons responding to the observation of ingestive and communicative mouth actions in the monkey ventral premotor cortex. *European Journal of Neuroscience, 17,* 1703–1714.

Fosha, D. (2005). Emotion, true self, true other, core state: Toward a clinical theory of affective change process. *Psychoanalytic Review, 92*(4), 513–551.

Fredrickson, B. L. (2001). The role of positive emotions in positive psychology: The broaden-and-build theory of positive emotions. *American Psychologist, 56,* 218–226.

Fredrickson, B. L. and Branigan, C. A. (2005). Positive emotions broaden the scope of attention and thought-action repertoires. *Cognition and Emotion, 19,* 313–332.

Fredrickson, B. L. and Levenson, R. W. (1998). Positive emotions speed recovery from the cardiovascular sequelae of negative emotions. *Cognition and Emotion, 12*(2), 191–220.

Frith, C. D. (2007). The social brain? *Philosophical Transactions of the Royal Society, 362,* 671–678.

Frith, C. D. and Frith, U. (1999). Interacting minds—a biological basis. *Science, 286*(5445), 1692–1696.

Gainotti, G. (2005). Emotions, unconscious processes, and the right hemisphere. *Neuro-Psychoanalysis, 7,* 71–81.

Galbraith, A., Subrin, R., and Ross, D. (2008). Alzheimer's disease: Creativity, art and the brain. In N. Hass-Cohen and R. Carr (eds), *Art Therapy and Neuroscience.* London and Philadelphia, PA: Jessica Kingsley Publishers.

Gallese, V. (2003). The roots of empathy: The shared manifold hypothesis and the neural basis of intersubjectivity. *Psychopathology, 36,* 171–180.

Gallese, V. (2006). Intentional attunement: A neurophysiological perspective on social cognition and its disruption in autism. *Brain Research. Cognitive Brain Research, 1079,* 15–24.

Gazzaniga, M. S. (2002). The split brain revisited. *Scientific American Special Edition, 12*(1), 27–31.

Gillespie, J. (1994). *The Projective Use of Mother-and-Child Drawings: A Manual for Clinicians.* New York: Brunner/Mazel Publishers.

Gonsalves, B. and Paller, K. A. (2000). Neural events that underlie remembering something that never happened. *Nature Neuroscience, 3,* 1316–1321.

Greenberg, L. S. and Pascual-Leone, A. (2006). Emotion in psychotherapy: a practice-friendly research review. *Journal of Clinical Psychology, 62*(5), 611–630. Review.

Harmon-Jones, E. (2007). Asymmetrical frontal cortical activity. In E. Harmon-Jones and P. Winkielman (eds) *Social Neuroscience, Integrating Biological and Psychological Explanations of Social Behavior.* New York, London: Guilford Press.

Hass-Cohen, N. (2003). Art therapy mind body approaches (2003). *Progress: Family Systems Research and Therapy, 12,* 24–38.

Hass-Cohen, N. (2006) Art therapy and clinical neuroscience in action. *GAINS Community Newsletter: Connections and Reflections, Premier Edition,* 10–12.

Hass-Cohen, N. (2007). Cultural arts in action: Musings on empathy. *GAINS Community Newsletter: Connections and Reflections, Summer 2007,* 41–48.

Hass-Cohen, N. (2008). Partnering of art therapy and clinical neuroscience. In N. Hass-Cohen and R. Carr (eds) *Art Therapy and Clinical Neuroscience.* London and Philadelphia, PA: Jessica Kingsley Publishers.

Henry, J. P. and Wang, S. (1999). Effects of early stress on adult affiliative behavior. *Psycho-neuroendocrinology, 23*(8), 863–875.

Hesse, E. (1999). The adult attachment interview: Historical and current perspectives. In J. Cassidy and P. R. Shaver (eds) *Handbook of Attachment: Theory, Research, and Clinical Applications* (pp.395–433). New York: Guilford Press.

Iacoboni, M. and Dapretto, M. (2006). The mirror neuron system and the consequences of its dysfunction. *Nature Reviews Neuroscience, 7*(12), 942–951.

Johnson, M. K. and Hirst, W. (1993). MEM: Memory subsystems as processes. In A. F. Collins, S. E. Gathercole, M. A. Conway, and P. E. Morris (eds) *Theories of Memory* (pp.241–286). East Sussex, England: Erlbaum.

Johnson, M. K., Raye, C. L., Mitchell, K. J., Greene, E. J., Cunningham, W. A., and Sanislow, C. A. (2005). Using fMRI to investigate a component process of reflection: Prefrontal correlates of *refreshing* a just-activated representation. *Cognitive, Affective, and Behavioral Neuroscience, 5,* 339–361.

Jung, C. G. (1973). *Mandala Symbolism.* Princeton, NJ: Princeton University Press.

Kalat, J. W. (2004). *Biological Psychology* (8th edition). Belmont, CA: Wadsworth/Thomson Learning.

Kandel, E. (1998). A new intellectual framework for psychiatry. *American Journal of Psychiatry, 155,* 457–469.

Kellogg, J. (1992). *Mandala: Path of Beauty.* Williamsburg, MA: Graphic Pub of Williamsburg.

Keysers, C. and Gazzola, V. (2006). Towards a unifying neural theory of social cognition. *Progress in Brain Research, 156,* 379–401.

Keysers, C., Wickers, B., Gazzola, V., Anton, J.-L., Fogassi, L., and Gallese, V. (2004). A touching sight: SII/PV activation during the observation and experience of touch. *Neuron, 42,* 1–20.

Konarski, J. Z., McIntyre, R. S., Grupp, L. A., and Kennedy, S. H. (2005). Is the cerebellum relevant in the circuitry of neuropsychiatric disorders? *Review of Psychiatric Neuroscience, 30*(3), 178–186.

Kourtzi, Z. and Kanwisher, N. (2000). Activation in human MT/MST by static images with implied motion. *Journal of Cognitive Neuroscience, 12*(1), 48–55.

Kramer, E. (1972). *Art as Therapy with Children.* New York: Schocken Books.

Lanius, R. A., Hopper, J. W., and Menon, R. S. (2003). Individual differences in a husband and wife who developed PTSD after a motor vehicle accident: A functional MRI case study (case conf). *American Journal of Psychiatry, 160,* 667–669.

Lezak, M. D., Howieson, D. B., and Loring, D. W. (2004). *Neuropsychological Assessment* (4th edition). New York: Oxford University Press.

LeDoux, J. (2002). *The Synaptic Self.* New York: Viking Penguin.

LeDoux, J. E. (2000). Emotion circuits in the brain. *Annual Reviews Neuroscience, 23,* 155–184.

Linehan, M. M. (1993a). *Cognitive-Behavioral Treatment of Borderline Personality Disorder.* New York: Guilford Press.

Linehan, M. M. (1993b). *Skills Training Manual for Treating Borderline Personality Disorder.* New York: Guilford Press.

Llinás, R. (2001). *I of the Vortex from Neurons to Self.* Cambridge, MA: MIT Press.

Lusebrink, V. B. (2004). Art therapy and the brain: An attempt to understand the underlying processes of art expression in therapy. *Art Therapy: Journal of the American Art Therapy Association, 21*(3), 125–135.

MacLeod, C. E., Zilles, K., Schleicher, A., Rilling, J. K., and Gibson, K. R. (2003). Expansion of the neocerebellum in Hominoidea. *Journal of Human Evolution, 44*(4), 401–429.

Macrae, C. N., Moran, J. M., Heatherton, T. F., Banfield, J. F., and Kelley, W. M. (2004). Medial prefrontal activity predicts memory for self. *Cerebral Cortex, 14*(6), 647–654.

Main, M. and Solomon, J. (1990). Procedures for identifying infants as disorganized/disoriented during the Ainsworth Strange Situation. In M. T. Greenberg, D. Cicchetti, and E. M. Cummings (eds) *Attachment in the Preschool Years: Theory, Research, and Intervention* (pp.121–160). Chicago, IL: University of Chicago Press.

Malchiodi, C. A. (1998). *The Art Therapy Sourcebook.* Los Angeles, CA: Lowell House.

Malchiodi, C. A. (ed.) (1999). *Medical Art Therapy with Adults.* London and Philadelphia, PA: Jessica Kingsley Publishers.

McNamee, C. M. (2003). Bilateral art: Facilitating systemic integration and balance. *The Arts in Psychotherapy, 30,* 283–292.

Mead, M. (2001). *Growing Up in New Guinea: A Comparative Study of Primitive Education* (1st Perennial Classics edition). New York: Harper Perennial.

Miller, M. M. and McEwen, B. S. (2006). Establishing an agenda for translational research on PTSD. *Annals of New York Academy of Sciences, 1071,* 294–312.

Milner, A. D. and Goodale, M. A. (1995). *The Visual Brain in Action.* New York: Oxford University Press.

Naparstek, B. (1994). *Staying Well with Guided Imagery.* Boston, MA: Warner Books.

Neborsky, R. J. (2006). Brain, mind, and dyadic change processes. *Journal of Clinical Psychology, 62*(5), 523–538.

Ogden, P. and Minton, K. (2000). Sensorimotor psychotherapy: One method for processing traumatic memory. *Traumatology, VI*(3), article 3.

Ogden, P., Minton K., and Pain, C. (2006). *Trauma and the Body: A Sensorimotor Approach to Psychotherapy.* New York: W. W. Norton.

Parkin, A. J. (1996). *Explorations in Cognitive Neuropsychology.* Malden, MA: Blackwell Publishing.

Pennebaker, J. W. (1997). *Opening Up: The Healing Power of Expressing Emotions.* New York: Guilford Press.

Petrides, M., Alivisatos, B., and Frey, S. (2002). Differential activation of the human orbital, midventrolateral, and mid-dorsolateral prefrontal cortex during the processing of visual stimuli. *Proceedings of the National Academies of Science, 99*(8), 5649–5654.

Phelps, E. A., Delgado, M. R., Nearing, K. I., and LeDoux, J. E. (2004). Extinction learning in humans: Role of the amygdale and vmPFC. *Neuron, 43*, 897–905.

Premack, D. and Woodruff, G. (1978). Does the chimpanzee have a theory of mind? *Behavioral and Brain Sciences, 1*(4), 515–526.

Riley, S. (2004). The creative mind. *Art Therapy Journal of the American Art Therapy Association, 21*(4), 184–190.

Riley, S. and Malchiodi, C. A. (1994). *Integrative Approaches to Family Art Therapy.* Chicago, IL: Magnolia Street Publishers.

Rimé, B., Finkenauer, C., Luminet, O., Zech, E., and Philippot, P. (1998). Social sharing of emotion: New evidence and new questions. *European Review of Social Psychology, 9*, 145–189.

Rizzolatti, G., Fadiga, L., Gallese, V., and Fogassi, L. (1996). Premotor cortex and the recognition of motor actions. *Cognitive Brain Research, 3*, 131–141.

Robbins, A. (1999). *Between Therapists: The Processing of Transference/Countertransference Material* (2nd edition). London: Jessica Kingsley Publishers.

Rueda, M. R., Posner, M. I., and Rothbart, M. K. (2004). Attentional control and self-regulation. In R. F. Baumerister and K. D. Vohs (eds) *Handbook of Self-regulation: Research, Theory, and Applications* (pp.283–300). New York: Guilford Press.

Sapolsky, R. (1998). *Why Zebras Don't Get Ulcers.* New York: W. H. Freeman & Company.

Sapolsky, R. (2003) Taming stress. *Scientific American, 289*(3), 86–95.

Schmahmann, J. D. (1996). From movement to thought: Anatomic substrates of the cerebellar contribution to cognitive processing. *Human Brain Mapping, 4*, 174–198.

Schmahmann, J. D. and Sherman, J. C. (1998). The cerebellar cognitive affective syndrome. *Brain, 121*, 561–579.

Schore, A. (1999). *Affect Regulation and the Origin of the Self.* London: Lawrence Erlbaum Associates.

Schore, A. (2007) The Science of the Art of Psychotherapy [Conference]: Skirball Cultural Center, Los Angeles, CA, February.

Singer, T., Seymour, B., O'Doherty, J., Kaube, H., Dolan, R. J., and Frith, C. F. (2004). Empathy for pain involves the affective but not the sensory components of pain. *Science, 303*, 1157–1162.

Tamietto, M., Adenzato, M., Geminiani, G., and de Gelder, B. (2007). Fast recognition of social emotions takes the whole brain: Interhemispheric cooperation in the absence of cerebral asymmetry. *Neuropsychologia, 45*, 836–843.

Tronick, E. (2007). *The Neurobiology and Social-Emotional Development of Infants and Children.* New York: Norton & Company.

Tugade, M. M., Frederickson, B. L., and Barrett, L. F. (2004). Psychological resilience and positive emotional granularity: Examining the benefits of positive emotions on coping and health. *Journal of Personality, 72*(6), 1161–1190. Review.

Turken, A. U. and Swick, D. (1999). Response selection in the human anterior cingulate cortex. *Nature Neuroscience, 2*(10), 920–924.

Vance, R. and Wahlin, K. (2008). Memory and art. In N. Hass-Cohen and R. Carr (eds) *Art Therapy and Clinical Neuroscience.* London and Philadelphia, PA: Jessica Kingsley Publishers.

van der Kolk, B. A. and Fisler, R. (1995). Dissociation and the fragmentary nature of traumatic memories: Overview and exploratory study. *Journal of Traumatic Stress, 8*(4), 505–525.

Vasterling, J. J. and Brewin, C. R. (2005). *Neuropsychology of PTSD: Biological, Cognitive, and Clinical Perspectives.* New York: Guilford Press.

Voges, M. A. and Romney, D. M. (2003). Risk and resiliency factors in posttraumatic stress disorder. *Annals of General Hospital Psychiatry, 2*(1), 4.

Wager, T. D, Phan, K. L., Liberzon, I., and Taylor, S. F. (2003). Valence, gender, and lateralization of functional brain anatomy in emotion: A meta-analysis of findings from neuroimaging. *Neuroimage, 19*(3), 513–531.

Watkins, K. E., Strafella, A. P., and Paus, T. (2003). Seeing and hearing speech excites the motor system involved in speech production. *Neuropsychologia, 41*(8), 989–994.

Watt, D. F. (2005). Social bonds and the nature of empathy. *Journal of Consciousness Studies, 12*(8–10), 185–209.

Weiner, I. B. (2003). *Principles of Rorschach interpretation* (2nd edition). Mahway, NJ: Erlbaum.

Wicker, B., Keysers, C., Plailly, J., Royet, J.-P., Gallese, V., and Rizzolatti, G. (2003). Both of us disgusted in my insula: The common neural basis of seeing and feeling disgust. *Neuron, 40*, 655–664.

Winnicott, D. W. (1971). *Playing and Reality.* London: Routledge.

Wright, T. M., Pelphrey, K. A., Allison, T., McKeown, M. J., and McCarthy G. (2003). Polysensory interactions along lateral temporal regions evoked by audiovisual speech. *Cerebral Cortex, 13*(10), 1034–1043.

Zimmer, C. (2003). How the mind reads other minds. *Science, 300*, 1079–1080.

Glossary

Acetylcholine (ACh). ACh is an excitatory neurotransmitter that supports learning and memory functions. It stimulates arousal and attention circuits in the central nervous system and motor circuits in the peripheral nervous system.

Action Potential. An electrical impulse generated only when a neuron's cell body is sufficiently stimulated by presynaptic neurons. The "on" or "off" aspect of the action potential allows the neuron's signaling to be easily read by another neuron.

Adrenocorticotropic Hormone (ACTH). The pituitary gland secretes ACTH as part of the endocrine system's stress response. ACTH subsequently stimulates the adrenal glands above the kidneys to secrete cortisol into the bloodstream.

Affect. Emotion and/or subjectively experienced feeling.

Afferent. An afferent nerve conveys sensory information from a sensory source towards a processing center in the central nervous system. Afferent refers to the direction of movement.

Allostasis. Body processes that counteract the influence of internal or environmental challenges or stressors. These bodily changes restore normal functioning, stability and viability to the organism.

Allostatic Balance. A state or pattern of balance achieved through allostasis that is retained in memory. This memory allows quicker generic responses in the future when similar homeostatic challenges or stressors are encountered.

Allostatic Load. Allostatic load is a burden borne by the body. The burden results when incomplete transitions back to normal functioning occur during allostasis.

Allostatic Overload. Allostatic overload is the accumulated effects of allostatic load over time. It leads the body towards a condition of chronic stress and promotes disease.

Amygdala. Two almond-shaped, limbic system structures that initiate the sympathetic nervous system's stress response. Amygdala reactions shape implicit processing of emotion (especially fear) and memory. Amygdale refers to one of the amygdala pair.

Anterior. In the direction of the nose or the front of a designated biological structure.

Anterior Cingulate Cortex (ACC). A structure in the cerebral cortex that mediates affect and mind-body conflicts like anxiety. The ACC helps detect cognitive and emotional processing errors and facilitates visuospatial and memory processing, reward-based learning and social awareness. It connects the limbic brain with cortical regulation. (See Cingulate Cortex.)

Arousal. The excitation and energizing of neural networks or structures and consequently their respective functions.

Association Areas and/or Pathways. Cortical areas in the occipital, parietal, temporal and frontal regions whose circuitry carries multimodal sensory or motor information to other cortical areas in order to facilitate complex integration functions.

Attachment. The propensity of infant mammals and humans to seek their mothers in establishing a safe, secure base of exploration. Patterns of attachment formed establish a template for intimate relationships throughout life.

Attunement. A developmental or attachment theory term. It indicates a person's emotional capacity to identify with another's state of being. Attunement happens before having actually interacted with the other person as well as during any subsequent interactions.

Auditory Cortex. Temporal lobe areas that process auditory information from the hearing organs.

Autobiographical Memory. Episodic memory that connects a sense of one's self to his or her past, present and future.

Autonoetic Memory. Memories triggered by self-awareness or self-perception of sensory information and episodic events. (See Implicit/Non-Declarative Memory.)

Axon. Neuron fiber that conducts the action potential or nerve impulse from the neuron's cell body to the axon terminal.

Axon Terminal. The end of the axon containing neurotransmitter vesicles where the action potential or nerve impulse causes neurotransmitter release into the synapse.

Basal Ganglia. Subcortical structures in the central brain region that provide feedback to the cortex and modulate voluntary motor movements. Interface with emotional-motor areas supports flexible emotional function.

Blood Brain Barrier. A semi-permeable membrane facilitating the free flow of blood to the brain while protecting it from damaging or toxic blood-borne substances.

Bottom-Up Processing. Experiential learning that uses awareness of low order sensory or emotional features to progress, step by step, to higher-order perceptions. (See Top-Down Processing.)

Brainstem. The brainstem governs basic involuntary body functions like heart and breathing functions. It connects the spinal cord with subcortical brain regions. The brainstem and thalamus co-regulate sensory information moving upward from the body as well as motor information moving downward towards the body.

Broca's Area. An area of the left frontal lobe associated with language processing as well as speech production and comprehension.

Catecholamines. A neurotransmitter category that includes dopamine, norepinephrine (noradrenaline) and epinephrine (adrenaline).

Caudate. A basal ganglia structure in the limbic system associated with multimodal information processing and inhibition.

Central Nervous System (CNS). Consists of the brain and spinal cord.

Cerebellum. A brain lobe that helps control complex motor movements and procedural learning and analyzes visuospatial signals corresponding to self and/or others' movements. It is located at the back of the brain beneath the visual cortex adjacent and behind the brainstem.

Cingulate Cortex. A neocortical structure located above the corpus callosum that divides into anterior (front) and posterior (back) sections. Its functions integrate a multitude of sensory, memory and executive functions. (See Anterior Cingulate Cortex.)

Circuitry. Neural pathways that connect and facilitate communication between various structures or regions in the brain and/or the body.

Consolidation. The process of stabilizing internalized representations and short-term memories with pre-existing long-term memories.

Corpus Callosum (CC). A wide band of nerves connecting and facilitating communication between the right and left hemispheres.

Cortex. Outer layer of any organ or structure. In the brain, it often refers to the cerebral or neocortex ("new" cortex), which is the most recently evolved and most human brain structure.

Corticotropin-Releasing Hormone (CRH). A hormone released by the hypothalamus. CRH initiates the endocrine system's HPA stress response. It stimulates the pituitary to release adrenocorticotropin (ACTH) into the bloodstream. (See Andreocorticotropic Hormone; Stress Response.)

Cortisol. An endocrine stress hormone released from the adrenal gland that helps stop the HPA stress response. It travels through the vascular system to the pituitary and hypothalamus, where it stimulates reduced ACTH and CRH secretions. Cortisol increases glucose metabolism producing additional energy and shifts in immune responses. (See Adrenocorticotropic Hormone; Stress Response.)

Critical (Sensitive) Periods. Vulnerable developmental stages when biological structures and functions are sensitive to experiential and environmental influences that permanently define and change their structure and functioning. (See Experience-Dependent Maturation.)

Cytokines. Proteins that mediate immune and inflammatory reactions. Cytokines are produced by macrophages and T cells during innate and adaptive immune responses.

Decay Theory. The idea that forgetting results from passive degeneration or deterioration of memory traces. Forgetting happens over time when information is not rehearsed or practiced.

Dendrites. Branches extending from the neuron cell body. Provided with sufficient stimulation from presynaptic neurons, dendrites convey excitation to the neuron's cell body.

Dentate Gyrus. A small crescent-shaped part of the hippocampus associated with neurogenesis, new memories and regulating happiness.

Dopamine (DA). DA, a central nervous system neurotransmitter/neuromodulator, is associated with feelings of reward, pleasure and salience. DA is critical to motor functions, motivation, learning and memory.

Dorsal. A direction indicating the upper or top region of a referenced biological structure.

Dorsal Stream (*Where-How* or Parietal Stream). Parietal circuitry that quickly integrates vision with action. It is sensitive to motion and implied motion and facilitates rapid reactions to the environment.

Dorsolateral Prefrontal Cortex (DLPC). A portion of the frontal lobe that organizes working and contextual memory, focuses attentional processes, manages spatial information, and guides and inhibits behavior based upon left hemisphere reasoning. It also manages cognitive conflicts, sets goals, makes plans, perseveres, monitors and self-regulates.

Dysregulation. The disorganizing or interruption of necessary functions. Dysregulation results in diminished ability to maintain or re-establish homeostatic functioning.

EEG N170 Response. A typical electroencephalogram response activated during the viewing of low spatial frequency or low and high spatial frequency facial images.

EMDR. Eye movement desensitization and reprocessing is a psychotherapeutic technique used in treating people suffering from trauma and distressing event impacts.

Encoding. Putting information in a new or suitable form for memory storage and retrieval, especially sensory information.

Endogenous Opiates/Opioids. The body's natural produced painkillers.

Entorhinal Cortex. Input from the entorhinal cortex to the hippocampus contributes to learning and long-term memory. The entorhinal cortex is a central brain structure separating the cortex and the hippocampus.

Entrainment. Bringing into synchrony various functions and the structures that regulate them.

Epinephrine/Adrenaline (E). A neurotransmitter released by sympathetic nerves and the adrenal gland's medulla. E mobilizes flight or fight responses by accelerating body responses that facilitate emergency functioning while decelerating non-emergency functions. (See Short-Term Stress Response.)

Episodic Memory. Long-term mental maps of personally experienced past events that contain specific time and context: what, when, how and where. Episodic memories can be explicit/conscious or implicit/unconscious. (See Implicit and Explicit Memory.)

Experience-Dependent Maturation. Genetic/environmental influences impact exceptionally vulnerable developing areas of brain growth during critical periods. Morphology, volume, density and function are easily enhanced or diminished by environmental impacts only during these times. (See Critical Periods.)

Explicit/Declarative Memory. Conscious, intentional recall of previously learned information from past experiences and/or facts for conscious exposition and task performance.

Fear Response. An amygdala-based reaction to an unconsciously or consciously perceived threat that initiates a fight, flight, or freeze response.

Flashbulb Memory. Long-lasting, unusually vivid, detailed memory for circumstances related to an emotionally intense event or trauma.

Feedback. A system response regulated or modified by additional input once the system's response has begun (learning or allostatic responses). For example, moving the hand proceeds from a general movement to a finer movement based upon feedback during the process.

Feed-forward. A learned, preset nervous system response to a stimulus that ensures the sequence of actions that follows. Learned or homeostasis responses are examples. (See Feedback.)

Flight or Fight Response. Fast sympathetic nervous system reaction to potential threats or stressors. Norepinephrine and epinephrine are released which ready the body for fleeing or fighting.

Fractals. Similar patterns in progressively smaller parts, which echo or reproduce the characteristics of the whole.

Frontal Lobe. The brain's primary executive area responsible for assimilating and integrating perceptual, volitional, cognitive, motor and emotional processes. It helps plan, coordinate, control, and execute behavior.

Fusiform Face Area (FFA). A color, word, number, and especially sensitive face processing area (fusiform gyrus) in the temporal cortex near the occipital lobe. The FFA perceives face configurations and similarities. There is a processing bias for familiarity in its ventral portion.

Gamma-Amino Butyric Acid (GABA). The brain's major inhibitory neurotransmitter. Released into a synapse, GABA prevents the postsynaptic neuron from activation.

Glucocorticoids. Corticosteroids secreted by the adrenal gland's cortex in response to serious injury or stressors. They shift fat metabolism, regulate blood pressure and have inflammatory effects. (See Cortisol.)

Glutamate (Glu). The main excitatory neurotransmitter in the brain and sensory portion of the peripheral nervous system. While easily made and essential to long-term potentiation, prolonged neuron exposure to Glu is toxic.

Gray Matter. Gray unmyelinated tissue in neuron cell bodies, axons and dendrites in the brain and spinal cord. (See Myelination.)

Habituation. Decreased responsiveness to or increased tolerance of a stimulus through repeated exposure.

High Road Response (Indirect Path). Sensed, potentially threatening stimuli are sent through the thalamus to cortical areas that facilitate slower, detailed processing and that moderate more immediate low road responses. (See Low Road Response.)

High Spatial Frequency. Visual objects with sharp or crisp edges or contours.

Hippocampus. A stress-sensitive, seahorse-shaped, limbic structure in the central brain region. It is responsible for spatial navigation, learning, and initiating and consolidating explicit memory processes.

Hormones. Chemicals produced by endocrine glands and used by the endocrine system to transmit messages through fluid-based systems in the body.

Hypothalamus-Pituitary-Adrenal (HPA) Axis. Endocrine glands that release stress hormones. The HPA axis regulates the nervous, immune and endocrine management of bodily needs during prolonged or recurrent stressors. (See Hypothalamus; Pituitary Glands; Corticotropin-Releasing Hormone, Adrenocorticotropic Hormone and Cortisol.)

Hypothalamus (HY). A lower brain endocrine structure that bridges nervous system and endocrine functioning, especially autonomic functions. It strongly influences body functioning during developmental and stress states.

Immune System. A defensive bodily system that differentiates organism cells from foreign cells and debris. Innate immune responses provide general protection from invaders. Adaptive immune responses, which develop later, involve specific immune responses to invaders.

Implicit/Non-Declarative Memory. Memory used during tasks not requiring conscious recall, like walking or talking. Sometimes referred to as automatic, non-declarative or procedural memory, implicit memories are free of time or place of origin references.

Inferior Parietal Lobes. Lower regions of the parietal lobes.

Inhibit. In neurons or brain structures, inhibit means to stop or block activation or functioning.

Insula or Insular Cortex. Processes interoceptive stimuli and tracks self and others' ongoing body conditions. It helps mediate extreme emotions, awareness, and expressions of bodily states like pain. Insula function contributes to theory of mind and empathic functioning.

Interleukin I-2. Immune messenger, a type of cytokine.

Intrusion. Insertion of new information that interferes with new learning, and conflicts with, or alters older information. For example, saying a list of words interferes with depositing a new word into memory. Traumatic memories can intrude on current experiences.

Isomorphism. Shared form or function resemblance. An assumed correspondence between mental events and their underlying neural events.

Kindling. A progressively increasing neuronal response to a stimulus that affects memory and is associated with trauma. Traumatic kindling may reflect amygdala and hippocampal conditioning that results in flashbacks.

Lateral Geniculate Nuclei (LGN). Bilateral lobes in the thalamus that receive input from the opposite half of each eye's visual field. The LGN sends and receives visual information to and from the primary visual cortex.

Lateralization. Refers to the localization of a function within a brain hemisphere or brain structure. For example, most language functions are lateralized to the left hemisphere.

Left Hemisphere. The brain hemisphere associated with cognitive and language functions, sequential processing, explicit awareness, and conscious functions.

Limbic System. A conceptual, rather than anatomical, designation used to group central brain structures that regulate, evaluate and integrate emotion into motivational states, survival responses and memories.

Locus Coeruleus (LC). A brainstem structure implicated in anxiety and fear reactions that secretes norepinephrine (NE) and serotonin (5-HT). It is also part of the brain's reward circuitry.

Longitudinal Fissure. A crevice anatomically separating the right cerebral hemisphere from the left. It defines the boundary between the right and left hemisphere.

Long-Term (Chronic) Stress Response. A slow, more sustainable endocrine response to threats and stressors. It modifies body functioning so that prolonged stress or survival challenges are manageable. (See Hypothalamus-Pituitary-Adrenal Axis.)

Long-Term Depression (LTD). Long-lasting weakening of a synaptic response to specific stimuli between two neurons that causes "forgetting" at a synaptic level. (See Decay Theory.)

Long-term Memory. A type of memory that holds needed information from 30 seconds to decades. By comparison, *short-term memory* holds limited information from 20 to 30 seconds, unless the information is kept longer by being mentally rehearsed.

Long-Term Potentiation (LTP). Long-lasting enhancement of neuronal communication about specific stimuli. LTP is created through repeated activation of synaptic connections that strengthen and speed reactivity. It forms the basis for long-term learning and memory, especially in hippocampal neurons.

Low Road Response (Direct Path). Sensed, potentially threatening stimuli are sent through the thalamus directly to the amygdala that activate the sympathetic nervous system's flight or fight reaction. (See High Road Response.)

Low Spatial Frequency (Low Frequency Visual Perceptions). Visual objects whose edges or contours are not sharp or crisp.

Lymphocytes. Cells in the adaptive immune system that combat invaders. Lymphocytes are the only immune system cells with receptors that can distinguish between foreign substances delineating different invading microbes. T-lymphocytes function within infected cells, whereas B-lymphocytes travel in the blood and lymph systems.

Magnocellular (M) Cells. Large, fast-acting neurons that receive retinal perceptions of motion, depth, and coarse outlines, which are analyzed and interpreted before being sent to the primary visual cortex. They are found throughout the visual system.

Medial Frontal Lobes. Anterior sections of the frontal lobes closest to the midline that separates the hemispheres.

Medial Temporal Lobe. The inner surface of each temporal lobe, which includes the hippocampal area, entorhinal cortex and amygdala. These carry on multi-functional processing and serve memory functions.

Medulla. A structure's internal portion, like the adrenal medulla of the adrenal cortex, or the medulla (oblongata) in the brainstem. The medulla is involved in autonomic life functions (breathing and blood pressure) and facilitates sensory and motor signals to and from higher brain centers. The adrenal medulla cortex is involved in the short-term stress response.

Mirror Neurons. Activated when a purposeful task is performed, observed being performed, or viewed as the intent in a person. Non-purposeful actions don't stimulate them.

Mirror Neuron Systems. Located in the parietal cortex, frontal premotor cortex, and the superior temporal sulcus (STS), they contribute to mimicry, imitation, simulation, and perhaps empathy. The specific region activated depends on what is being observed.

Motivation. The force felt within a person that initiates and energizes the pursuit, direction, persistence and vigor of goal-directed behavior.

Motor Strip (Primary Motor Cortex). Anterior to the central sulcus in the frontal lobe, the motor strip contains distinct areas for most body parts. Cortical neurons connect from those areas to specific body parts, like a hand.

Myelination. A white sheath that develops over neuronal axons as they mature. Myelin enables faster, more efficient communication and delineates white matter from gray matter (unmyelinated neurons).

Natural Killer (NK) Cells. Cells in the innate immune system that kill microbe-infested cells and activate other immune cells called phagocytes to remove cellular debris.

Negative Feedback. Negative feedback tends to cause a decrease in the behavior or the process of which it is a part. A reaction to or an effect of an activity that attenuates or inhibits an activity.

Neocortex. This uppermost brain is the newest to evolve. It enables complex stimulus analysis, precise motor control, enhanced learning and memory and abstract and rational thought.

Neurogenesis. The formation of new neurons, either during prenatal development or later in the hippocampus, a brain structure highly involved in learning as well as explicit and spatial memory.

Neuromodulators. Chemicals released by a neuron that enhance or dampen neurotransmitter effects over a region of neurons. Neuromodulators do not perform neurotransmitter functions themselves.

Neuron. The basic functional unit in the nervous system. It receives information through specialized receptor sites and conveys information to other neurons and cells using electrical impulses and chemical messengers. (See Axon and Dendrites.)

Neuropeptides. Neuropeptides function as either neurotransmitters or hormones. Many cross the blood brain barrier linking brain activities to bodily functions.

Neuroplasticity or Plasticity. A neuron's ability to increase, decrease or shift synaptic connections can strengthen, renew and to a certain degree rewire neural networks. Neuroplasticity can ease or complicate neural network functioning.

Neurotransmitters. Messenger chemicals that transfer information across a synapse allowing synaptically connected neurons to communicate.

Nodes of Ranvier. Short, unmyelinated gaps that occur at regular intervals between myelinated sections on a neuron's axon.

Norepinephrine/Noradrenaline (NE). Crucial to maintenance of alertness, drive and motivation states. NE is released from the adrenal medulla during the SAM axis stress response and from the brainstem's locus coeruleus. (See Locus Coeruleus.)

Nucleus. The center core of a structure that determines the cell or structure's behavior. In cells and neurons, it contains most of the genetic material.

Occipital Face Association Area (OFA). A visually face-sensitive processing area in the visual cortex. The OFA responds to isolated, inverted, or upright facial parts in images.

Occipital Lobe. Where visual stimulation from the retina is processed into what we see and forwarded to other cortical structures for further integration. Also called the visual cortex.

Olfactory Lobes. The forebrain's olfactory bulb, tract and cortex. They create the sense of smell. Utilizing this quick route to the brain, smell stimuli bypass the thalamus, and connect directly to the amygdala, thereby influencing emotional processing.

Ontogeny. The developmental sequence an individual organism follows from conception to death. By comparison, phylogeny is about the course of a species development over evolutionary time. (See Polyvagal Theory.)

Orbital Frontal Cortex (OFC). A ventral prefrontal area associated with integrating and regulating emotional processes, along with holding and processing of autobiographical memory. The right OFC helps regulate affective decision-making.

Oxytocin (OXY). A peptide hormone active in breastfeeding, sex, bonding, affiliative responses, stress reduction, and neural development. OXY is produced in the hypothalamus and released into circulation by the pituitary.

Parietal Lobes or Cortex. The parietal lobes facilitate cohesive and multi-level awareness of one's body-self within the environment. Located in the posterior cerebral cortex, they process multi-modal sensory inputs from somesthetic, kinesthetic, and proprioceptive senses as well as motivationally significant visual stimuli.

Parvocellular (P) Cells. Small, slow acting neurons that receive perceptions of color, shades of gray, low contrast and fine detail. Found throughout the visual system, they engage in meaning-making before activating the primary visual cortex.

Peripheral Nervous System. Consists of the autonomic and somatic nervous systems and facilitates mind/body functions through connections with the central nervous system.

Pituitary Gland. The body's master endocrine gland is connected to the hypothalamus. Hypothalamic releasing factors stimulate pituitary hormones to circulate and alter the body's glandular functioning. (See Adrenocorticotropic Hormone, Oxytocin, Hypothalamus-Pituitary-Adrenal Axis).

Plaques. Circular sticky structures outside of the neuron associated with the progression of Alzheimer's disease.

Polyvagal Theory. A social engagement theory that correlates body immobilization, motivation and social communication. The vagus nerve enables self-soothing, calming, and sympathetic adrenal inhibition. The theory proposes a biological basis for social behavior based upon phylogenic stage-based activation of the vagus nerve. (See Ontogeny.)

Positive Feedback. Positive feedback tends to cause an increase in the behavior or process of which it is a part. Positive feedback is a reaction to or effect of an activity, which amplifies that activity.

Posterior. A direction indicating a region toward the back or rear of a designated biological structure.

Posterior Cingulate Cortex. The rear cingulate cortex area. It activates during emotion and memory retrieval functions, especially during autobiographical memory retrieval. (See Cingulate Cortex.)

Postsynaptic Neuron. The receiving neuron. Its dendrites transfer information from the presynaptic neuron.

Prefrontal Cortex (PFC). Located in the frontal lobe behind the forehead. The PFC significantly directs executive functions, problem-solving and anticipating impactful events. It helps configure and reconfigure perceptions; maintain attention; and coordinate and control affect and behavior.

Presynaptic Neurons. The neuron that releases neurotransmitters into the synapse, i.e. sends its message to the postsynaptic neuron, muscle or gland.

Priming. Using contextual cues to facilitate or inhibit recall of another response.

Projection Pathways. Neuronal fibers that connect cortical and subcortical structures to form top-down and bottom-up axes of communication.

Psychoneuroimmunology (PNI). Interdisciplinary study of the interactions between psychological processes and the nervous, immune and endocrine systems of the body.

Pulvinar Nucleus. A thalamic region that receives auditory, somatosensory, visual and superior colliculus inputs. It influences visual attention, especially suppressing attention to irrelevant stimuli.

Raphe Nucleus. A source of serotonin in the brainstem, the raphe nucleus is associated with motivation, affect processing and slow wave sleep.

Recall. Spontaneous retrieval of information from memory with or without cues.

Recognition. When retrieved memory information matches external experiences or other internal representations.

Reconsolidation. The updating of specific long-term memories with current information. Perceptions in the present may combine with these internal representations from the past.

Regulation. The ability to inhibit or control processes that would otherwise disorganize or derail well-being and healthy functioning.

Rehearsal. Visual, phonological, and emotional repetition of events and internal representations in order to refresh, maintain or elaborate upon memory or understanding.

Reticular Activating System (RAS). A brainstem area regulating basic life functions like breathing, heartbeat, and blood pressure. The RAS is considered the center of arousal and motivation.

Right Hemisphere (RH). The brain hemisphere associated with global, non-verbal and affective processing; preconscious and visual spatial awareness; feelings and intuitions; and how more immediate stress and emotions impact bodily change.

Salience. The state or quality of a stimulus' prominence or conspicuousness relative to nearby stimuli. Saliency guides attention and learning.

Self-Similarity. Similar forms of self or relationships on smaller or larger scales.

Semantic Memory. Long-term memory of facts not related to specific episodic events and/or to autobiographical memories.

Sensory System. Neurons, called afferent neurons, and central nervous system structures like the thalamus or parietal area that convey and/or process sensory information. (See Afferent Neurons.)

Septal Nuclei or Septum Pellucidum. One of the limbic system pleasure centers that when stimulated creates sensations of well-being. It extends down from the corpus callosum.

Serotonin (5-HT). A neurotransmitter that generally has a calming effect and produces a sense of well-being. Underactivation is associated with depressive and OCD disorders.

Sex Hormones. Gonad (ovaries or testes) produced hormones that control development of primary or secondary sexual characteristics: estrogens, progestagens, and androgens.

Short-Term (Acute) Stress Response. Quick flight, fight or freeze reactions to threats and/or stressors that energize the body for immediate action. It contextually halts unnecessary bodily functions. (See Sympathetic Adrenal Medulla Axis.)

Somatosensory Cortex or Area (Somatosensory Strip; SSA). Posterior to the central sulcus in the parietal lobe, the SSA maps sensory input from the whole body onto sections representing those body areas before sending its input for further processing.

Spinal Cord. Part of the central nervous system within the backbone, or vertebral column. It connects the central nervous system to the peripheral nervous system.

Stress Response. Mind-body arousal that ensures survival and/or manages stressors, so that homeostasis or normal functioning can be re-established. (See Hypothalamus-Pituitary-Adrenal Axis, Sympathetic Adrenal Medulla Axis and Amygdala.)

Striatum. A forebrain region near the thalamus involved mainly in movement planning and control. It reacts to salient, reward and adverse stimuli in order to facilitate cognitive executive functions.

Subcortical. Areas of the brain below the cerebral cortex that regulate and create involuntary and/or automatic functions less accessible to conscious awareness. Their functions reflect adaptations from earlier periods of evolutionary development.

Superior Colliculus (SC). A subcortical, visual system structure that helps localize attention to quick, peripheral movements, and aspects of the spatial environment. It receives visual stimuli independently of the thalamus.

Superior Frontal Gyrus. A gyrus or raised fold in the cerebral cortex running along the upper frontal lobe activated along with other areas during self-face processing.

Superior Temporal Sulcus (STS). Temporal lobe juncture where visual, somatosensory and auditory inputs converge. The STS delineates salient stimuli and facilitates reading facial emotions, emotional learning; and knowing another person, all of which are theory of mind functions. The right STS area detects motion.

Sympathetic Adrenal Medulla (SAM) Axis. The acute stress response axis. The sympathetic nervous system stimulates the medulla of the adrenal glands to release adrenaline and noradrenaline. The SAM response rapidly mobilizes the body to manage survival threats or stressors.

Synapse. A junction or gap between neurons or a neuron and a muscle or a gland. Neurotransmitters cross synapses in order to transfer information and facilitate continued activation of postsynaptic neurons.

Tangles/Neurofibrillary (NFTs). The outcome of proteins breaking within neurons. Tangles/NFTs are associated with the progression of Alzheimer's disease.

Temporal Lobes. Located in the cerebral cortex, they process inputs leading to memory and complex visual, auditory, linguistic, emotional, and motivational functions. These contribute to forming language, evaluating, interpersonal interaction, and non-verbal response-oriented activities. The right temporal lobe is associated with non-verbal response-oriented activities.

Temporoparietal Junction (TPJ). A boundary area between the temporal and parietal lobes that facilitates processing of self and multi-sensory body-related information. TPJ helps build representations of one's body in space along with specifically facilitating reasoning about the contents of another person's mind (Theory of Mind).

Thalamus. A pair of egg-shaped structures in the central brain area. It functions as a sensory gateway and relays nearly all sensory and motor information between the body/brainstem and cortical/subcortical areas.

Thymus. Tree-shaped, lymphoid organ where immune system T cells are produced. The thymus is located just below the thyroid gland at the base of the neck.

Top-Down Processing. Information processing utilizing complex cortical, often cognitive, functions. These cortical functions enlist and regulate subcortical sensory or affect-based, limbic processes. (See Bottom-Up Processing.)

Vagus Nerve. The most important nerve in the parasympathetic nervous system. It connects body organs with the brainstem. Excessive vagal activation during emotional stress causes it to compensate for overly strong sympathetic nervous system reactions by slowing heart rate and creating a freeze response or faint.

Vasopressin. A hypothalamic peptide hormone released by the pituitary gland that helps regulate water retention and blood pressure. In the brain, it may improve attention, concentration and memory as well as promote aggression and relationships in male rats and humans.

Ventral. A direction indicating the underneath region of a biologically designated structure.

Ventral Stream (*What* or Temporal Stream). A pathway carrying visual information from the visual cortex to the temporal lobe that integrates shape, color and significance with object recognition and meaning. Connections between the temporal lobe and the limbic system allow emotion, recognition and memory to influence the meaning ascribed to visual attributes.

Ventral Tegmental Area (VTA). A midbrain structure in the brainstem that releases dopamine into the limbic and prefrontal circuits. VTA activation releases dopamine, which helps facilitate motivation and emotional responsiveness.

Visual Cortex. Area in the occipital lobe responsible for decoding, encoding and distribution of visual stimuli. (See Occipital Lobe.)

Visual System. Nervous system structures involved in processing vision. Included are two pathways that aid integration of visual information in the temporal and frontal lobes. (See Ventral and Dorsal Stream.)

Von Economo Neurons (Spindle Cells, VEN). Cingulate neurons that coordinate input from diverse brain regions. VEN cells facilitate solving intricate problems with fast intuitive assessments of complex situations, especially psychosocial situations. (See Cingulate Cortex.)

Wernicke's Area. An area in the left temporal lobe area associated with understanding language and syntax.

White Blood Cells/Lymphocytes. Immune cells that form into B cells, T cells and natural killer cells.

White Brain Matter. White tissue seen in the brain and spinal cord. It looks white due to the myelin coating on the neuron's axon. (See Myelination.)

Working Memory. Temporary memory storage of information that supports the performance of current tasks only.

Notes on Contributors

Noah Hass-Cohen, PsyD, MA, ATR-BC, LMFT, is the founder and Chair of the Art Therapy/MFT Department at Phillips Graduate Institute (PGI) Encino, California, USA. Originally from Israel, Noah became fascinated in describing art therapy in action when she was exposed to systems theory and neurobiology in the United States. The mother of three grown children, she is vested in understanding the diversity of child art expressions. Noah publishes on art therapy clinical neuroscience approaches and has presented locally, nationally and internationally on the topic. She likes to work in pastels and her clinical interests include neuropsychological and psychodiagnostic testing (noah@pgi.edu).

Richard Carr, PsyD, MA, faculty in the Art Therapy/MFT Department, Phillips Graduate Institute, and Assistant Professor at Cleveland Chiropractic College, Los Angeles, USA, has provided over 30 years of counseling to parents, individuals, and couples. College interests in marine biology, anthropology, and child development ultimately led him to neuroscience and attachment theory. A ten-year member in Dr. Allan Schore's Developmental, Affective Neuroscience and Clinical Practice Group, Richard has published and presented statewide and nationally about neuroscience and its clinical applications, human development, and relationships. Richard, an outdoor enthusiast who loves skiing, sailing, kayaking, snorkeling, and hiking, is married with two grown children (plusmed@aol.com).

Terre Bridgham, MA, IMFT, artist and art therapist, practices at Family Service Agency of Burbank, California, USA. She provides individual and group art therapy at the agency and in schools. Terre is also associated with Wonderland Center, Los Angeles, an addictions treatment facility where she specializes in substance abuse. A PGI graduate, she is interested in neurobiology, attachment, and mindfulness practices.

Darryl B. Christian, MA, ATR-BC, LMFT, specializes in working with adolescents. Previously core faculty in the Art Therapy/MFT Department, Phillips Graduate Institute, Encino, California, USA and Clinical Director at North Hills Prep School, a special education school, Darryl provides clinical supervision at PGI California Family Counseling Center. Darryl enjoys drawing, painting, and ceramics, as well as playing the piano and oboe.

Joanna Clyde Findlay, MA, ATR-BC, LMFT, artist and certified MARI® Mandala trainer, was former faculty at the Art Therapy Department, Phillips Graduate Institute, Encino, California, USA. English by birth, Joanna now lives in France and is the Director of the Centre de Psychothérapie et Art Thérapie de Provence. The mother of two school-age children, Joanna integrates family therapy, art therapy and mindfulness practices; working with physical health challenges, childbirth and parenting. She conducts trainings in the Jungian based MARI® Mandala assessment tool and her clinical interests include the neurobiology of imagery for healing (www.cpatp.com).

Anne Galbraith, MA, ATR, LMFT, is an artist and art therapist. Faculty in the Art Therapy/MFT Department at Phillips Graduate Institute, Encino, California, USA, she is assistant director at OPICA Adult Day Service/Counseling Center in West Los Angeles. Anne is also associated with the MS Achievement Center at UCLA. Anne is interested in understanding how creative self-expression can enhance a sense of well-being for people living with chronic and terminal illness. She continues to study and integrate the latest research in neurobiology, and mindful awareness into her clinical practice (anne@opica.org).

Erin King-West, MA, ATR-BC, LMFT, is an artist and art therapist. She is core faculty in the Art Therapy/MFT Department, Phillips Graduate Institute, Encino, California, USA. She most enjoys the intimate teaching environment involved in academic and clinical art therapy supervision and consultation. Erin is in private practice in Burbank, specializing in working with women with anxiety disorders, post-traumatic stress disorder and dissociative identity disorders. Erin's creative endeavors include photography and photo collage, quilting, ice skating and gardening (Ekingwest@pgi.edu).

Kathy Kravits, RN, MA, has had a 30-year career in health care with experience in critical care, emergency, surgical and oncology nursing practice. She is Director of Clinical Supportive Care and Spiritual Care Services at City of Hope National Medical Center, Duarte, California, USA and faculty in the Phillips Graduate Institute Art Therapy/MFT Department. Ms. Kravits is the Primary Investigator on a research project funded by the Unihealth Foundation, Inc., Self-Care Strategies for Health Care Professionals, an interventional study of health promotion behaviors and stress management techniques incorporating art therapy (kkravits@coh.org).

Margarette Erasme Lathan, MA, LMFT, practices at the Los Angeles Child Guidance Clinic, USA, specializing in the Zero to Five Population. Previously involved with the Early Childhood/Parenting Centers at Cedars Sinai Medical Center in Los Angeles, she conducts school-based, art therapy and grief support groups for Our House, Los Angeles. A Phillips Graduate Institute board member and licensed Marriage and Family therapist, she is a strong advocate of art therapy as a professional discipline. A strong believer in the value of family, Margarette nurtures a blended family of five. The oldest is 35, the youngest ten and the newest member a one-year-old grandchild. Margarette enjoys photography, kite running, swimming, hiking and singing (maggylathan@yahoo.com).

Nicole Loya, MA, PLMHP, is an artist and art therapist who practices at the Child Saving Institute in Omaha, Nebraska, USA. She works as an early childhood mental health consultant serving Omaha community childcare, providing therapy for young parents and expecting young parents. Nicole has also worked with elementary schools in the Los Angeles Unified School District as well as with older adults afflicted with Alzheimer's disease. A PGI graduate, Nicole has developed an interest in neuropsychology, infant mental health, and therapeutic photography (nloya@childsaving.org).

Drew Ross, MA, LMFT, draws on his background as a professional musician to blend relational therapies with creative arts therapy. A graduate of PGI, he trained at OPICA, Adult Day Service. He also provides consulting for elder care providers and is the former chairman of the Sonoma County Alzheimer's Task Force. Currently he is director of *Creative Counseling for Elders and Families*, offering psychotherapeutic services, case management and assessment.

Ruth Subrin, MA, LMFT, artist, and art therapist is associated with the Psychological Trauma Center/Cedars Sinai Hospital where she works with traumatized children from South LA elementary schools. A PGI graduate, she was previously at OPICA Adult Day Service, West Los Angeles and The

Center for Healthy Aging in Santa Monica and now also works at the UCLA MS Achievement Center. Ruth enjoys working with baby boomer women helping them to recognize the joy and wisdom of aging. Ruth has been an active yoga practitioner and mediator for over 25 years, and applies those practices to her clinical practice (subrinart@msn.com).

Jessica Tress Masterson, MEd, artist and photographer, is completing her master's degree in psychology/art therapy at Phillips Graduate Institute, Encino, Californina, USA. Adding to her expertise in art history and art education, her current research focuses on understanding the creative process from a neuroscientific point of view, specifically related to gender differences and their implications for couples art therapy. She has previously worked with Psychotherapy Perspectives, Sojourn Services for Battered Women, the Los Angeles County Museum of Art, the Los Angeles Unified School District and the International School of Lusaka in Zambia, Africa (jessica.masterson@hotmail.com).

Robin Vance, MA, ATR-BC, LMFT is an exhibiting fine artist and art therapist. She is a faculty member of the Art Therapy/MFT Department at Phillips Graduate Institute, Encino, California, USA. Robin maintains a private practice where she uses a body/mind approach to work with health, anziety and women's issues. Robin's artwork is a narrative exploration of the real and the imagined, via the female figure and landscape. Her artwork may be viewed at robinbvance.com.

Kara Wahlin, MA, IMFT, is an artist and art therapist who infuses her art therapy practice with postmodern collaborative therapies. Kara is the program coordinator of Daybreak, a transitional living program for adolescents, for Youth and Family Enrichment Services of San Mateo County. A graduate of PGI, she is interested in culturally under-represented topics such as women's reproductive issues, the prison system, resistance movements, language and race. Kara works with multiple medias to create imagery that elicits a sense of both nostalgia and the abject in the viewer. (k.wahlin@hotmail.com).

Subject Index

ACC *see* anterior cingulate cortex
acetylcholine (ACh) 81–2, 311
acquired immune deficiency syndrome
    (AIDS) 270–81
    development of secondary medical
        problems 272
    protocols for therapeutic intervention
        272–5
    therapeutic directions 275–81
acrylic paint media 38
ACTH *see* adrenocorticotropic hormone
    (ACTH)
action potential 77, 311
adaptive responses 299–301
ADD *see* attention-deficit disorder (ADD)
adolescents
    attachment styles 140, 142
    attention and executive performance 29,
        152–3
adrenal cortex 78
    stress responses 118–19, 208, 301
adrenal medulla 84–5, 166, 318, 319
    stress responses 116–21, 208, 229, 276,
        301
adrenaline 84–5, 314
adrenocorticotropic hormone (ACTH) 78,
    88, 118–19, 208, 301, 311, 313
    placental response 132
affect, defined 311
affect dysregulation 227–31, 293–9
    neurobiology 230
affect expression 31–3, 274
    role of amygdala 51–6
affect regulation 30–1, 33–6, 56, 67, 74,
    295, 311
    and hemisphere functions 35, 293–5
    mediation through relationships 36–9
    neural pathway hypothesis 72
    role of amygdala 51–6
    role of prefrontal cortex 70–2
    role of temporal lobes 67
afferent neurones 22–4, 64, 311
AIDS (acquired immune deficiency
    syndrome) 270–81
    development of secondary medical
        problems 272
    protocols for therapeutic intervention
        272–5
    therapeutic directions 275–81
alerting systems 150
alertness problems 154
allostasis 111–12, 311
allostatic balance 111–12, 311
allostatic load 111–12, 311
allostatic overload 111–12, 311
Alzheimer's disease 254–67
    language problems 260
    memory and attention deficits 257–9
    mild cognitive impairment (MCI) 255–7
    mood changes 260–2
    neuropathology 266–7
    protective factors 30
        brain reserve capacity (BRC) 262–4
        cognitive reserve (CR) 262–4
        and neurogenicity 254
    therapeutic interventions 254, 256–64
    visuospatial deficits 259
amygdala 25–6, 31–3, 51–6, 311

basic emotional responses 33, 51–4
    gender biases 55, 175–6, 177
    and memory 52–3, 160–2, 166,
        169–70
    right and left responses 53, 55
    stress responses 113–15, 229–30,
        296–7
    visual ventral stream functions 98–9
anger responses 32–3, 228–9
anterior, defined 311
anterior cingulate cortex (ACC) 32, 34–5,
    56–8, 71, 230–1, 295–9, 311
    gender biases 175
anterior executive system 151
anxiety responses 30–2, 35, 112
    direct and indirect response pathways
        113–15
    role of amygdala 54–6
    role of anterior cingulate cortex 56–8
    role of serotonin 86–7
    see also complex post-traumatic-stress
        disorder (C-PTSD); fear responses
apathy, therapeutic interventions 260–2
arousal 296–7, 311
    problems 154
art appreciation, neurobiological responses
    33–4
art media, choice considerations 37–8
art therapy
    definitions 21
    principles of imagery 214–15
        case study 215–20
            re-imprinting the cerebral cortex
                274–5
    through affect regulation 33–6
    through mediation of stress responses 26
    through memory and learning reward
        processes 82–3
    through relational empathy 36–8
    use of CREATE principles 283–305
Art Therapy Relational Neuroscience
    (ATR-N) principles 283–305
association cortex 64–6, 66–7, 68, 312
    visual pathways 95
attachment 131–44, 191–3, 236, 312
    developmental events 132–9
        conception to birth 134, 132–3
        birth to two months 133–6
        two to seven months 135, 136–7
        seven to 36 months 137–8
        36 months/bilateral communication
            139
        adult responses 140–3, 193
    emotional resonance 131
    neurocorrelate correspondences 274
    over the lifespan 140–3
    and relational empathy principles
        289–91
    and the stress response 122–5
    styles and categories 140–1, 192–3
    theory 192–3
    therapy interventions 193–205
attention 124–5
    anatomical structures 149
    bottom-up and top-down regulatory
        systems 148–54
    deficit problems 147–8, 154–6
    development and maturation 152–4

attention-deficit disorder (ADD) 154–6
attunement 71–2, 106, 132–3, 135, 139,
    312
    problems 132–3, 137, 141
auditory cortex 65, 67, 149, 261, 312
auditory processing 67
authorship 35
autistic spectrum disorder (ASD) 28, 302–3
autobiographical consciousness 71
autobiographical memory 165–8, 290–3,
    312
autogenic training 214
autonoetic memory 165–6, 312
autonomic nervous system (ANS), described
    22–3
axon 26–7, 63, 77, 152, 312
axon terminal 26–7, 77, 312

babies, art-making activities 29
basal ganglia 31–2, 149, 287, 312
beliefs, and memory 167
bipolar disorder 72
blindsight 45
blood brain barrier 78, 312
body language 304
bottom-up processing 31–2, 50, 63, 74,
    99, 147–8, 151, 153
    defined 312
brain
    anatomical structures (overview)
        central and limbic system 25–6,
            31–3, 317
            cortex and brain stem 25–6, 47
            lateralization of structures 51
    development 26–9
    evolutionary development 45–7
    functional map areas 34
        hemispheres 35–6
    maturation and growth 28–9
    neurophysiology 25–38
        chemical messenger systems 76–89
        neural pathways and connections
            26–7, 63–6, 76–7, 79
    plasticity 30–1, 264
    weight 30
brain lateralization 35, 46–7, 65–6, 317
    bi-lateral integration 32, 34–5, 65,
        293–5
    fetal development 132–3
        gender biases 174–5, 176–7
        infant development 139
    of emotional processing 293–4
        dominance theory 293–4
    of memory functions 160
    split-brain surgery studies 295–6
    therapeutic interventions, facial
        recognition work 103–5
brain reserve capacity (BRC) 262–4
brainstem 34, 312
Broca's area 34, 36, 37, 67, 312

C-PTSD *see* complex post-traumatic-stress
    disorder (C-PTSD)
cancer
    and chemotherapy responses 112, 115
    psychoneuroimmunology 209–10
        case study 215–20

Cannon, Walter 24
Capgras's syndrome 98
catecholamines 80, 116–17, 132–3, 274, 312
caudate 63–4, 83, 312
cave paintings 44–5
central nervous system 23, 119, 313
cerebellum 25, 284, 286–8, 313
cerebral cortex, anatomical structures 25–633–5, 43–4, 62–4, 70, 284
chemotherapy, conditioned stress responses 112, 115
child development
   attachment 131–44
      event timeframes 132–9
      ruptures and repairs 139
      and the stress response 122–5
      vulnerability factors 139
   attachment styles 140–1
   impact of trauma and abuse 241
   mind—body connectivity 26–9
   and mind-reading 302–3
   visual systems 99
childhood experiences
   abuse survival 223–49
   impact on brain development 28–9, 50, 241
choice-making, neurobiology 34, 37–8, 57
chronic stress responses 55, 126, 176, 183, 207–8, 229, 264, 272, 279–80, 299–300
   neurobiology 24–6, 30, 31, 116–19
cingulate cortex 32, 34–5, 56–8, 153, 295, 313
circle drawings, and attachment states 191–202
circuitry, defined 313
clinical neuroscience, definitions 21
cloth albums 195–203
cognitive behavioural therapies, and brain plasticity 30
cognitive reserve (CR) 262–4
collages 28, 92, 97
   landscape (without movement) 97
   and portraits 105–6
color symbolism 228
complex post-traumatic-stress disorder (C-PTSD) 16–17, 225–36, 241, 246
   affect dysregulation expressions 227–31
   attention and consciousness alterations 232–3
      and primary dissociation 233–6
      and secondary dissociation 236–7
      and tertiary dissociation 237–8
   neurobiology 230
   working with the parts 238–45
      developing intimacy and trust 240–5
      maintaining empathy 246–8
      treatment opportunities 240
consolidation, of memories 52–3, 58 313
corpus callosum 32, 34–5, 64–5, 313
   fetal development 132–3
   gender biases 174–5, 176
cortex, definitions 313
cortical dampening reactions 32
corticotrophin-releasing hormone (CRH) 117–19, 208, 313
cortisol 78, 118–19, 207–9, 226–7, 229–31, 313
   maternal 132–3
   and trauma memories 234
countertransference 248
couples art therapy 16, 174–87
   neurobiological biases
      females 174–6
      males 176–7
   study directives 177–83
      Abstract of the Marital Relationship Drawing 179–81

Non-Verbal Joint Drawing 178–9
Two-Dimensional Bridge Drawing 181–3
   seating arrangements 184–5
   therapeutic inquiry 185–6
   relational stages 186–7
CREATE principles 283–305
   Creativity in Action 285–9
   Relational Resonance 289–93
   Expressive Communication 293–9
   Adaptive Reponses 299–301
   Transformation and Empathy 302–5
crisis events, neurobiological responses 31
critical periods 29, 152, 313
culture, and fear responses 54–5
cytokines 119, 207, 211, 313

dance movements, and memory 159–61
decay theory 160, 313
decision-making
   gender biases 177
   neurobiology 34, 37–8, 57
   role of chemical messengers 85–6
   role of prefrontal cortex 68–72
declarative memory 53, 314
dendrites 27, 30, 76–7, 79, 133, 313
dentate gyrus 264, 313
depression
   neurochemical responses 81, 86–7
   therapeutic interventions 260–2
dis-integration (attention deficits) 154–6
   treatment considerations 155–6
Disorders of Extreme Distress (DES) 225
dissociation reactions 231–8
   primary 233–6
   secondary 236–7
   tertiary 237–8
   working with the parts 238–40
Dissociative Identity Disorder 237–8
dominance theory (brain lateralization) 293–4
dopamine (DA) 82–4, 97, 314
   and attachment responses 122, 124
   dysfunctions 84, 154
dorsal, defined 314
dorsal stream 314
dorsal vagal complex (DVC) 120–1
dorsal "where—how" stream 95–7
   purposes 96
dorsolateral prefrontal cortex (DLPFC) 71–2, 314
drama work 261
drawing characteristics, analysis 273
dreams, trauma responses 232–8
Dual Representation Theory (DRT) 233–5
DVC see dorsal vagal complex (VVC)
dysregulation 314

earned attachment 193–4
EEG N170 response 314
efferent nerves 23–4
EMDR (eye movement desensitization and reprocessing) 26, 314
emotion regulation 30–1, 33–6, 57, 295, 297
   and hemisphere functions 35, 293–5
   mediation through relationships 36–9
   neural pathway hypothesis 72
   role of amygdala 51–6
   role of prefrontal cortex 70–2
   role of temporal lobes 67
emotional arousal 296, 296–7
emotional awareness 72, 298
emotional learning 67
emotional memory 176
emotional processing 293–9
   key mechanisms 293
   see also affect expression

emotional stress
   gender biases 176–7
   see also stress responses
emotions see affect expression
empathy 302–5
   neurobiological basis 36–8, 73–4
   role of insula cortex 68
   in the therapeutic relationship 246–8, 302–5
encoding 52, 81, 160, 163, 167, 213, 314
endocrine responses 31–2
endogenous opiates 116, 314
endorphins 116–17
entorhinal cortex (EC) 32, 168, 284, 291, 314
entrainment 283–4, 314
epinephrine (E) 84–5, 116–17, 314
episodic memory 165, 258, 314
evolution see human evolution
excitatory glutamate (Glu) 79–81
excitotoxicity 80–1
executive attention 151
executive function 256
experience-dependent maturation 28, 94, 133, 161, 314
experiential simulation 394–5
explicit memory 164–8, 314
exposure techniques 240
expressive communication 293–9
eye contact 99

facial recognition 68, 99–106
   and portraits 101–2
   therapeutic considerations 103–6
family support 261–2
fear responses 31, 33, 229–30, 296–7, 315
   role of amygdala 51–6, 229–30
feed-forward linkages 79, 81–3, 315
feedback loops 47–8, 50, 54, 78, 226–7, 283–4, 287, 305, 315
feedback learning 79, 82–3
female brains 55, 133, 174–6, 178–80, 182–3
FFA see fusiform face area (FFA)
"fight or flight" response 23, 31, 51–6, 84–5, 299, 315
finger tapping 240
flahbulb memory 166, 315
flashbacks, trauma responses 232–8
forgetting 81, 161
fractals 285, 315
frameworks ATR-N (art therapy relational neurobiology principles) 21
frontal lobes 25–6, 29, 34, 315
fusiform face area (FFA) 96, 99–105, 315

GABA see gamma-amino butyric acid (GABA)
gamma-amino butyric acid (GABA) 81, 87–8, 315
gender
   and amygdala functioning 55
   neurobiological biases
      females 55, 133, 174–6, 178–80, 182–3
      males 133, 142, 174, 176–7
gestures 288–9
Glu see excitatory glutamate (Glu)
glucocorticoids 118–19, 207–9, 315
glutamate 80, 162, 315
gray matter 62–3, 152, 315
"Greebles" studies 102–3
Grice's Maxims 203–4
group art therapy 264
group discussions 259
guided imagery 115
"gut feelings" see intuitive feelings

habituation 54, 58, 97, 235, 315
hand gestures 68
    evolutionary development 44
Harm Avoidance 86
hemispheric differences *see* brain
    lateralization
high road response (indirect path) 52–3, 54,
    315
high spatial frequency 314, 315
hippocampus 25, 30, 32, 72, 213, 227,
    235, 258, 264, 267, 274–6, 316
    gender biases 176–7
    and imagery 213
    and memory 161–2, 166, 283–4, 291,
        300–1
    neurogenesis 30
hormones 77–8, 316
HPA response *see*
    hypothalamus—pituitary—adrenal
    (HPA) response
human evolution
    brain development 45–7, 57
    role of neocortex 43–5
hypothalamus 31–2, 47, 52, 78, 117–8,
    123–4, 316
    attentional systems 149
    gender biases 176
    stress responses 113–18, 123–4, 132,
        207–9, 210
hypothalamus—pituitary—adrenal (HPA)
    response 83, 116–19, 121–2, 207–9,
    210, 226–7, 229–31, 299–301, 316
    and imagery 213

imagery research 212–14
    see also visual imagery
imitation 288–9
    neurobiology 36–7, 288
immune function
    background overview 211
    and AIDS 270–281
    and cancer 209–10
        case study 215–20
    definitions 316
    enhancing immune function 210–20,
        283–4
        background and rationale 210–12
        use of imagery 212–15, 215–20
    and stress 119, 207–10
implicit meanings 97
implicit memory 162–3, 259, 316
infant development *see* child development
infant experiences, impact on brain
    development 28–9
information processing pathways 62–6
inhibit, defined 316
insular cortex 34–5, 51, 62, 68, 316
    gender biases 175, 316
interleukin-2 209, 316
internal imagery 212–14
interpersonal relationships *see* couples art
    therapy; interpersonal social
    functioning; relationships
interpersonal social functioning
    role of prefrontal cortex 68–72
    stress responses 179–83
    see also attachment; couples art therapy
intimacy 290
intrusion 160–1, 240, 316
intuitive feelings 46, 175
isomorphism 316

kindling 240, 316

language
    deficits 260
    neurobiology 34, 36, 67

see also non-verbal communication
lateral geniculate nucleus (LGN) 49, 93,
    94–5, 316
lateralization, defined 317
lateralization of the cortex *see* brain
    lateralization
learning
    and attention 153–4
    gender biases 176–7
        under stress 178–9
    neurobiology 27–9, 35, 55–6
        chemical messenger systems 79–81,
            81–8
        empathic imitation and observation
            36–9
left-brain hemisphere 35, 51–4, 65–6, 317
    see also brain lateralization
left-brain lesions 92
    see also brain lateralization
LGN *see* lateral geniculate nucleus (LGN)
limbic system 25–6, 30–1, 32, 63, 317
    deficit problems 148
    regulatory mechanisms 35–6
    and attention 149
    and stress responses 113–15
locus coeruleus (LC) 149, 317
long-term depression (LTD) 81, 227–9,
    231, 317
long-term memory 30, 169–72, 257–9,
    317
long-term potentiation (LTP) 79–81,
    161–2, 317
    mechanisms 162, 229–30
long-term stress responses 55, 126, 176,
    183, 207–8, 229, 264, 272, 279–80,
    299–300
    neurobiology 24–6, 30, 31, 116–19
longitudinal fissure 62, 317
low road response (direct path) 52–3, 54,
    56, 317
low spatial frequency 99, 317
lymphocytes 118–19, 207, 211, 301, 317,
    323

Macaque monkey research 36–7, 288
magnocellular (M) cells 94, 96, 317
male brains 55, 133, 174, 176–8, 182
Mandala drawings 155, 191, 196–203,
    299
marital relationships
    stages of development 186–7
    see also couples art therapy
mastery
    and dorsal stream reactivity 97
    imagery 214–15, 217, 220, 225,
        274–5, 286, 298
meaning-making 125, 138, 298–9
meaningful memory 290–1
media in art therapy
    choice consideration 37–8, 100
        safety—mastery continuum 100
        ventral stream studies 98–9
medial frontal lobes 101, 153, 317
medial temporal lobes 67, 96, 105–6, 160,
    164, 170, 265, 318
meditation techniques *see* visual imagery
medulla 318
    see also adrenal medulla; sympathetic
        adrenal medulla (SAM) response
memory 16–17, 25–6, 27, 159–72
    background and overview 159–61
    consolidation mechanisms 291
    deficits 256–9
    formation processes 30, 161–2, 258
        neurochemical pathways 79–88
        role of amygdala 52–3, 160–2, 166,
            169–70
    role of anterior cingulate cortex 57

role of hippocampus 30, 160–2, 164,
    166, 168–70
role of prefrontal cortex 68–72
role of temporal lobes 67
    fragmentation 232–3
    and dissociation 233–8
    gender biases 175–7
    hemispheric lateralization 46, 160
    and learning 81–3
    and movement 159–61
    neurocorrelate correspondences 274
    and sensory processing 152
    and stress 119
    types
        autobiographical 68–72, 165–8,
            290–3
        declarative memory 53
        emotional 176
        episodic 165
        explicit 164–8
        implicit 162–3
        long-term 30, 169–72, 291
        semantic 164–5
        short-term 30–2, 168–9
        working 70–2, 168–9
mentalizing 303–4
metaphors and symbolism 270–2, 301
mimicry 288–9
mind—body connectivity 13–14, 15, 21–6
    anatomical and physiological structures
        21–6
    development and learning 26–9
    therapeutic intervention principles 21–6,
        38–9, 283–305
mind-reading 301–2
mindblindness 302
mindfulness, neurobiological basis 36–8
mirror gestures 288–9
mirror neurones 288–9, 318
mood disorders, neurobiology 30–1
mother—infant interactions 28–9, 55
    attachment 192–3
        conception to birth 132–3, 134
        birth to 2 months 133–6
        2 to 7 months 135, 136–7
        7 to 36 months 135, 137–8
    key features 139
        and the stress response 122–5
    therapeutic interventions 193–205
        relational resonance principles 289
    visual systems 99
    vulnerability factors 139
motivation 84–6, 122, 123–4, 152, 154,
    293–4, 318
    and reward systems 82–3, 288, 298
    and targeted visualizations 214
motor cortex 34, 68, 286–8, 318
movements 284, 285–9
    and memory 159–61
    repetitive activities 240
music 254, 261
myelin sheath 27
myelination 28, 67, 318

narratives 303–4
National Research Council of Medicine 29
natural killer (NK) cells 209–10, 318
negative emotional responses, effects of
    talking 36
negative feedback loops 114, 117–18, 284,
    318
neglect (childhood) 29, 50, 133
    thalamus feedback loops 50
neocerebellum 287–9
neocortex 25, 318
    anatomical structures 25
neural connections 26–7, 76–7, 79
neural pathways 63–6

neurofibrillary tangles (NFTs) 265–7, 322
neurogenesis 30–1, 133, 241, 264, 318
    inhibition 133, 241, 264
neuroimaging studies, definitions 21
neuromodulators, described 76–8, 318
neurons, anatomical structure 26–7, 76–7,
    318
neuropeptides 123, 132, 318
neurotransmitters 27, 76–89
    described 76, 319
    and forgetting (LTD) 81
    and learning (LTP) 79–81
    acetylcholine (ACh) 81–2
    dopamine (DA) 82–4
    epinephrine/adrenaline (E) 84–5
    excitatory glutamate (Glu) 79–81
    gamma-amino butyric acid (GABA) 87–8
    norepinephrine/noradrenaline (NE)
        85–6
    serotonin (5-HT) 86–7
NMDA receptors 79–80, 162
Nodes of Ranvier 27, 319
non-declarative memory 162–3, 259, 316
non-verbal communication 99, 133, 155,
    175, 262, 302–5
    neurobiology 33, 35, 133, 185
    relationship therapy exercises 177,
        178–9
noradrenaline 85–6, 116–17, 319
norepinephrine (NE) 85–6, 116–17, 319
nucleus 319

obsession 125
obsessive compulsive disorders,
        neurochemical imbalances 87
occipital face association area (OFA) 96, 99,
    319
occipital lobes 25, 34, 66–7, 93–7, 319
OFA see occipital face association area (OFA)
OFC see orbital frontal cortex
ontogeny 47, 319
opiates 116
orbital frontal cortex (OFC) 33–5, 54, 56,
    58, 71–2, 293–9, 319
orienting systems 150
oxytocin 78, 122–3, 186, 217, 319
    and gender 176, 181

pain responses 48, 57, 248
    affective responses 248
    control 212
    distraction 160–1
panic disorder 87
parasympathetic nervous system (PNS)
        described 22–3
    and stress responses 116–19
parietal lobes 25, 50, 316, 319
    visual spatial processing 67–8
parvocellular (P) cells 94, 319
peripheral nervous system 319
        described 22–3
personality, role of prefrontal cortex 70–2
personality disorders, neurochemical
        imbalances 87
photographs 92
    of faces 105
pituitary gland 31–2, 320
    stress responses 117–19
pituitary neurohormones 78
plaques 265–7, 320
plasticity 30–1, 264, 319
play 139, 289
    and art therapy 300, 302
pleasure, neurobiology 31, 82–4, 298
Polyvagal Theory 120–1, 229–30, 320
portraits 101–3
positive feedback loops 136, 284, 320

post-traumatic stress disorder (PTSD)
        responses 50, 112
    see also complex post-traumatic-stress
        disorder (C-PTSD)
posterior cingulate cortex 32, 34–5, 56–8,
    153, 295, 313, 320
posterior orienting systems 150
postsynaptic neurones 76–7, 79, 320
preconscious processes see unconscious
        processes
prefrontal cortex (PFC) 34–6, 37–8, 62,
    68–72
    anatomical structures 33–5, 43–4, 63
    sensory processes and responses 43–58
primary visual cortex (V1–V3) 95–7
priming 168–9, 320
procedural memory 162–3, 259
    and fear responses 55
projection pathways 64–6, 320
psychoneuroimmunology (PNI) 21–2, 320
    and cancer 209–10
psychosocial stress responses see stress
        responses
pulvinar nucleus 93–4, 320

Raphe nucleus 113, 123, 288, 320
RAS see reticular activating system (RAS)
recall (memory) 229–30, 320
recognition 26, 52, 56, 73, 81, 95–6, 98,
    320
    faces and expressions 99–106
recollection processes 168
reconsolidation 58, 296, 321
redundancy mechanisms 66
reflex actions 45–7
regulation, defined 321
rehearsal 166, 168–9, 170, 321
relational resonance (CREATE principles)
    17, 283, 289–91, 305
relationships
    couples
        stages of development 186–7
        stress responses 178–81
    neurobiological impact 36–9
    see also attachment; couples art therapy
relaxation therapies 115, 217
repetitive art activities 240, 254
    and rituals 259
resilience 132, 134, 139, 140, 142, 286
reticular activating system (RAS) 124–5,
    149, 321
reward systems 82–3, 288, 298
    role of dopamine 82–4, 97
right hemispheres (RH) 35, 51–4, 65–6,
    159, 181, 295, 321
    see also brain lateralization
right-brain lesions 92, 104
risk tolerance 176–7
rituals 259
rock art 44–5
Romanian child care 131–2, 144

salience, defined 321
SAM response see sympathetic adrenal
        medulla (SAM) response
SAM-DRT see situational accessible memory
        system (SAM-DRT)
SC see superior colliculus (SC)
scaffolding techniques 155–6
schizophrenia 72
seating positions 184–5
self see sense of self
self-control 68
self-portraits 101
self-regulation 73–4, 150
self-similar fractals 285
self-similarity 285, 321
semantic memory 164, 258, 321

sense of self 71–2, 98, 125, 290–3
    and autobiographical memory 165–8,
        290–3
sensory processes and responses 24, 35–6,
    45–8, 45–58
    development and maturation 133–4
    evolutionary perspectives 45–7
    and meaning 125
    and memory 147–8
    neural pathways 63–6, 147–9
    role of amygdala 51–6
    role of anterior cingulate cortex 56–8
    role of thalamus 48–50, 113–15
    stress responses 113–15
    top-down processing 151–2
sensory system, defined 321
septal nuclei 124, 321
sequencing, and memory 166
sequencing (therapeutic) interventions 156
serotonin (5-HT) 86–7, 122, 124, 321
sex drive 177
sex hormones 186, 321
sexual abuse 224, 226, 229, 232, 241
    see also complex post-traumatic-stress
        disorder (C-PTSD)
sexual atraction 187
short-term stress response 208, 321
situational accessible memory system
    (SAM-DRT) 233–5, 239–40
social affects 32
social interactions see interpersonal social
        functioning
somatic nervous system, described 22–3
somatosensory cortex (SSA) 34–5, 47, 50,
    68, 321
sound processing 67
spatial awareness 177
speech production 36
spinal cord 321
spindle cells see Von Economo neurons
    (VENs)
split brain experiments 65–6
startle reflexes 46–7, 53
stress responses 23–6, 31–3, 52–6,
    111–26, 301, 322
    adaptive responses 299–301
    brief overview 111–12, 208
    gender biases 178–81
    impact on immune function 207–9
    neurocorrelate correspondences 274
    protective factors 210
        role of creative actions 285–9
    regulation mechanisms 78, 83–4,
        210–12
        allostatic balance 111–12
        direct and indirect pathways 113–16
    Polyvagal Theory 120–1
        short- and long-term control 116–19
    role of attachment theory 122–5
    see also anxiety responses; complex
        post-traumatic-stress disorder
        (C-PTSD)
striatum 160, 322
STS see superior temporal sulcus (STS)
subconscious see unconscious processes
subcortical, defined 322
superior colliculus (SC) 45–6, 49, 93–5,
    322
superior frontal gyrus 101, 322
superior temporal gyrus 34–5
superior temporal sulcus (STS) 67, 99–101,
    293–5, 322
survival reactions 26
symbolism and metaphors 270–2, 301
sympathetic adrenal medulla (SAM)
    response 116–21, 122–3, 208, 274,
    276, 301, 322
sympathetic nervous system (SNS)
        described 22–3, 51–6

and stress responses 116–19
    Polyvagal Theory 120–1
synapse 77, 322
synaptic plasticity 79, 81
synaptic pruning 28

talking about art *see* verbalization effects
tangles 265–7, 322
Tau proteins 265
tempera paints 38
Temporal Binding Theory 233
temporal lobes 25–6, 34, 36, 67, 322
    emotional regulation 67
    gender biases 175, 177
    language function 67
    and ventral stream 98–9
temporoparietal junction (TPJ) 67, 322
testosterone 176–7
thalamus 31–2, 48–50, 93–5, 287, 322
    cortical feedback 48–50
    response to trauma 50
    role in visual processing 93–5
theory of mind 73–4, 302
therapeutic relationship 26–7, 123, 193,
    285, 289, 297
    and countertransference 248
    empathy 246–8
    qualities 142
    trust development 240–5
    see also empathy
thymus 118–19, 207, 210–11, 322
tool use, motor responses and mimicry
    36–7, 288–9
top-down processing 31–2, 50, 63, 74,
    147–8, 151–3, 156, 323
Tourette's syndrome 84
trauma responses 50, 227–31
    trauma-based clusters 227
trust development 240–5

unconscious processes
    evolutionary advantages 45–8
    memory processes 162–3
    trauma reactions, dreams and flashbacks
        232–8

vagus function 24, 120–1
vagus nerve 120–1, 323
VAM-DRT *see* verbally accessible memory
    system (VAM-DRT)
vasopressin 123, 323
ventral stream 98–9, 323
purposes 96
ventral tegmental area (VTA) 83, 113, 288,
    323
ventral vagal complex (VVC) 120–1
verbalization effects 36, 181, 185–6, 235,
    298–9
    gender biases 176–7
    group discussions 259
verbally accessible memory system
    (VAM-DRT) 233–5, 239–40
violence, childhood experiences 241
visual association pathways 96
visual cortex 65, 66, 323
    see also visual systems
visual imagery 212–14
    and art therapy 214–15
    case study 215–20
    key principles 215
visual information processing *see* visual
    systems
visual spatial processing 67–8
    deficits 259
visual systems 33–4, 64–7, 92–107, 255,
    317, 319, 322, 323
    background and overview 92–5

and attachment 274
and facial recognition 96, 99–106
role of association cortex 66–7
role of dorsal "where—how" system
    95–7
role of occipital lobes 66–7
role of ventral stream 98–9
see also attention
visualization training 213–14
    see also visual imagery
Von Economo neurons (VENs) 57, 323
vulnerability, and insecure attachments 139
VVC *see* ventral vagal complex (VVC)

Wernicke's area 34, 36, 67, 323
white blood cells 207, 211, 323
white matter 63–4, 152, 323
"White on White" painting (Kazimir) 303
women, neurobiological biases 174–6
working memory 168–9, 256–7, 323

Author Index

Abitz, M. 28
Achterberg, J. 21, 26, 210, 214, 216, 219, 270, 272–3, 301
Adcock, R.A. 82
Adelman, G. 78
Adolphs, R. 52–3, 98, 103, 104–5
Ahlander, N.R. 29
Ainsworth, M.D.S. 192, 196, 289
Albert, M.S. 254
Aldridge, D. 261
Alea, N. 290–1
Aleman, A. 105
Alivisatos, B. 290
Allen, G. 287
Allen, I.G. 240
Allen, J.P. 140, 142
Allen, J.S. 30
Allison, T. 105
Allman, J.M. 56–7, 71, 274
Alloway, T.P. 168–9
Altmann, E.M. 160
Alvisatos, B. 33–4
Amassian, V.E. 210
Amitai, Y. 81
Andersen, S.L. 227
Anderson, H. 290
Andrade, J. 240
Andrews, B. 230, 286
Angelucci, A. 94
Appleton, J.P. 185
Arbib, M.A. 73
Aron, A. 82, 84, 97, 186
Atkinson, A.P. 52
Atri, A. 81
Avrahami, D. 115, 225, 233
Awh, E. 57
Azad, I. 241

Baars, B.J. 150
Baas, D. 105
Babcock, C. 303
Bach, S. 212, 275, 278
Backman, L. 254
Baddeley, A. 159, 240
Banfield, J. 37, 68, 70, 72
Barkley, R.A. 148
Barlow, B. 25
Bar, M. 105
Baron-Cohen, S. 175–7, 182, 302
Barrett, L.F. 31, 32–3, 298
Bartels, A. 187
Basso, M.A. 95
Bateson, G. 278
Battino, R. 214
Batty, M. 99
Baumeister, R.F. 31
Bear, M.F. 28–9, 95, 174
Bechara, A. 56
Beck, J.G. 286
Beck, J.S. 212, 270
Becker, J.T. 254, 256
Beeman, M.J. 67
Beer, J. 297
Bellinger, D.C. 131
Bell, S. 267
Bentin, S. 104
Berninger, V.W. 62–7, 72

Berns, G.S. 57
Berntson, G.G. 85
Besson, C. 102
Biedeman, J. 154
Biederman, I. 159
Binkofski, F. 36–7, 288
Birmes, P. 286
Bishop, C.M. 27
Bjartmar, L. 94
Blair, H.T. 296
Blakemore, S.J. 73
Bluck, S. 290–2
Blum, D. 174
Boesiger, P. 99
Bond, A.J. 86
Bookheimer, S.Y. 235, 274
Booth, J.R. 153
Bowlby, J. 192, 289
Bradshaw, J.L. 44
Brake, W. 86
Branigan, C.A. 298
Braun, B. 240
Braver, T.S. 82
Bremner, J.D. 26, 30, 85, 226, 229–31, 240
Brewin, C.R. 224, 226–7, 230, 233, 235, 239–40, 286, 296
Bridges, M.R. 293, 298
Briere, J. 224–5, 227, 231–2, 241, 247–8, 286, 295–6
Briggs, J. 285
Brigham, D.D. 301
Brittain, W.L. 104
Brizendine, L. 175–6, 181–3
Brown, J.W. 82
Brown, T.E. 148
Brune, M. 302–3
Brune-Cohrs, U. 302–3
Bruno, J.P. 150
Bruss, J. 30
Buccino, G. 36–7, 288, 304–5
Buitelaar, J.K. 86
Bullier, J. 98
Buonocore, M.H. 57
Burbridge, J.A. 232
Buron, V. 94
Burrow, G.N. 132
Bushman-Wiggs, A. 95–8
Byrnes, J.P. 160–1, 172

Cahill, L. 55, 174–8
Calcagnotto, M.E. 47–50
Camic, P.M. 21, 285
Cannon, W.B. 24, 121
Carli, G. 98
Carlson, N.R. 22, 24, 159, 162
Carr, R. 286, 295
Carter, C.S. 132
Carter, R. 35, 67, 71, 159, 294
Casagrande, V.A. 95
Casey, B.J. 152–3
Caspers, K.M. 140, 142
Caspi, A. 183
Castellanos, F.X. 154
Castro, A.J. 76
Castro-Alamancos, M.A. 47–50
Cauli, O. 80

Chambers, R.A. 124
Changeux, J.P. 83
Chapman, L. 33, 225, 234, 240–1
Chavanon, M.L. 83
Cheng, P. 147
Chiarello, C. 67
Chiu, S. 152
Christopher, M. 111, 125–6
Chun, M.M. 99
Church, R.P. 155
Cicchetti, D. 139
Cinotta, C.M. 82
Clark, D.M. 232
Cleveland, A. 99
Clyde Findlay, J. 273
Coe, C.L. 133
Cohen, J.A. 97
Cohen, J.D. 85
Cohen, S. 212
Cohn, J. 99, 137
Colcombe, S.J. 30
Collette, F. 256
Collie, A. 254
Collie, K. 33
Collins, M.P. 213
Colonius, H. 95
Cone-Wesson, B. 184
Conklin, C.A. 213
Connors, B. 29, 81, 95, 174
Conway, M.A. 213
Corbetta, M. 148, 150
Cordova, M. 212
Courchesne, E. 28, 287
Cousins, N. 21
Cox, R. 147
Cozolino, L. 29, 50, 62, 68, 72, 163, 166, 184, 186, 257–8, 264, 279
Craighero, L. 73
Crandell, L.E. 99
Critchley, H.D. 57
Crommelinck, M. 102
Cromwell, H.C. 95–8
Cummings, J.L. 255, 260

Dalgleish, T. 226
Damasio, A. 22, 35, 56, 283, 298
Damasio, H. 30, 56
Daniels, M. 210
Dapretto, M. 37, 246, 304
Darlington, R.B. 43
Daruna, J. 78, 207, 210, 270
Davis, E.P. 133
Dawkins, R. 43
Day, J. 152
De Bellis, M. 85–6
De Gasperi, R. 30
De Graaf Peters, V.B. 133
de Kloet, C.S. 226
De Leon, M.J. 265
De Wolff, M.S. 132, 141, 143
Dean, L. 272
Decety, J. 73–4, 246, 248
Dehaene, S. 83
deJong, J.T. 240–1
Demaree, H.A. 294
Denburg, N. 52
Derbyshire, S.W.G. 57

Dermietzel, R. 78, 82, 84
DEsposito, M. 168
Destexhe, A. 50
Detillion, C.E. 62
Devan, B.D. 168
DeVries, A.C. 62
Diamond, A. 152, 154
Diamond, M. 26
Diedrich, A. 95
Diego, M. 86
Dietrich, A.M. 233
DiGirolamo, G.J. 150
Dolan, M. 304
Dolan, R.J. 57
Donaldson, V.W. 213–14
Dossey, B. 210, 270, 272–3
Downing, P.E. 97
Drachman, D.A. 254
Draganski, B. 30
Dufresne, M.M. 83
DuHamel, K.N. 115
Dunn, L.F. 213
Durkin, D.G. 210

Eagly, A.H. 174
Edelman, G.M. 47
Edwards, B. 103
Egeland, B. 193
Ehlers, A. 232
Eichenbaum, H. 170, 291
Eisenberger, N.I. 57
Ekman, P. 104–5
Elder, G.A. 30
Eldridge, L.L. 277
Eliot, L. 28–9
Elliott, R. 57
Elzinga, B.M. 169
Emmerling, M. 263, 265–7
Eriksson, P.S. 30
Esch, T. 122–3
Esiri, M.M. 265–7
Everhart, D.E. 294

Fan, J. 148, 150, 152
Farone, S.V. 154
Faw, B. 37, 97
Feldman, R. 86
Ferencik, M. 301
Fernandez-Duque, D. 150
Ferrari, P.F. 305
Field, T. 86
Figueiredo, H. 87
Fink, G.R. 276
Finley, B.L. 43
Fisher, B.C. 147–8, 150, 152–4
Fisher, D.A. 132
Fisher, H.E. 177, 186–7
Fisler, R. 232, 299
Fogassi, L. 68
Folkman, S. 125–6
Fonagy, P. 195
Ford, J.D. 225, 227
Forhead, A.J. 133
Forssberg, H. 151
Fosha, D. 298
Fowden, A.L. 133
Fraley, R.C. 192
Fredrickson, B.L. 298
Frewen, P.A. 229, 234
Frey, J. 33–4
Frey, S. 290
Frith, C. 57, 67, 73, 302–4
Frith, U. 67, 73, 302–4
Fullam, 304

Gabrieli, J.D. 275
Gage, F.H. 264

Gainotti, G. 293
Galbraith, A. 301
Gallese, V. 36, 68, 73, 288, 304
Galvin, J.E. 254
Gama Sosa, M.A. 30
Ganis, G. 92–3, 98, 212–13
Gardner, H.E. 104
Garrett, A.S. 57
Gaser, C. 30
Gathercole, S.E. 168–9
Gauthier, I. 99, 102–4
Gazzaniga, M.S. 97, 185, 294
Gazzola, V. 246, 288, 304
Gegelashvili, G. 80
Gehring, W.J. 57
Geiger, J.F. 176
George, C. 192, 195, 197
Ghosh, A. 79
Giedd, J.N. 29
Giese-Davis, J. 212
Gil, Z. 81, 87
Gill, K.M. 78
Gillespie, J. 29, 302
Givens, B. 150
Gladding, S.T. 177, 181
Glascher, J. 53, 105
Glaser, R. 207–10, 212, 239
Glover, N.S. 133
Gloviczki, P.J. 131
Goffaux, V. 104
Gogtay, N. 152
Gold, P.E. 81
Goldberg, E. 254–6, 262, 264
Goldstein, S. 148
Goldwyn, R. 193, 280
Gonsalves, B. 291
Goodale, M.A. 304
Gordon, N.S. 139
Gore, J.B. 168
Gould, E. 132, 256, 264
Goulven, J. 35
Gracon, S.I. 263, 265–7
Grafman, J. 71–2, 74
Gratton, A. 86
Gray, W.D. 160
Greenberg, D.L. 168
Greenberg, L.S. 293, 297
Greenspan, S.I. 62
Greer, S. 125
Gregg, M. 214
Grice, H.P. 193–4, 203–5, 272
Grossberg, S. 147
Gunstad, J. 261
Guntrip, H.J.S. 238
Gurian, M. 174, 175–6, 177, 182–3, 185

Habermas, T. 292
Hadar, U. 55
Hadders-Algra, M. 133
Haines, M.E. 260
Haist, F. 168, 170
Halgren, E. 99
Hall, C. 214
Hall, G.B. 176–7
Haman, S.B. 52
Hammer, E.F. 104, 280
Hannan, A.J. 39
Hannesdottir, K. 255, 260–1
Hariri, A.R. 235, 274
Harmon-Jones, E. 35, 294
Harrington, C.R. 256
Hartzell, M. 192, 195
Hass-Cohen, N. 21, 24, 26, 37, 39, 97,
    191, 204–5, 212, 214, 219, 246–7,
    270, 273, 285, 289–92, 301
Haxby, J.V. 95, 99
Hellawell, S.J. 233, 240

Hendler, T. 55
Hendren, R.L. 152
Henley, D. 155
Hennessy, R.G. 235
Henry, J.P. 26, 117–18, 270, 298
Herek, G. 272
Herlitz, A. 254
Herman, J.L. 225, 227
Herman, J.P. 88
Hernandez-Reif, M. 86
Hesse, E. 140, 142, 193, 201, 203, 289,
    291
Hirst, W. 290
Hobson, R.P. 99
Hodges, D.A. 261
Holmes, E.A. 213, 224, 235–6, 240
Hong, N.S. 168
Hopper, J.W. 230, 234–5, 286
Hopson, J. 26
Horner, P.J. 264
Horng, S.H. 94
Horowitz, H.A. 142
Howard, P.J. 76
Howieson, D.B. 92
Huizink, A.C. 86
Hull, A. 33

Iacoboni, M. 37, 68, 246, 304
Iidaka, T. 105
Irwin, M. 210
Ishai, A. 99
Itier, R.J. 99
Izquierdo, A. 52

Jackson, P.L. 73, 246
Jacobsen, E. 214
Jacobvitz, D. 201
Janov, A. 176
Jansari, A. 103–4
Jensen, E. 39, 155
Jessel, D. 176
Jia, H. 272
Johnson, M. 152, 167, 290
Joseph, S. 226
Jung, C. 299

Kaas, J.H. 94
Kabat-Zinn, J. 214
Kahn, R.S. 105
Kalat, J.W. 36, 93, 97–8, 162, 164, 286
Kalocsai, P. 159
Kandel, E. 30, 166, 283
Kandler, K. 87–8
Kane, J. 272–3
Kanwisher, N. 73, 97, 99, 101–3, 105, 288
Kaplan, F. 15
Kaplan, H.H. 26
Kaplan, H.I. 78
Kaplan, N. 192, 195, 197
Kapoor, A. 133
Karus, D. 272
Kastner, S. 94
Kaufman, J. 226, 231
Kavanagh, D. 240
Kazui, H. 259
Kellogg, J. 191, 195–6, 198–200, 202,
    293, 301
Kemeny, M.E. 218
Kerzberg, M. 83
Keysers, C. 36, 246, 288, 304
Kiecolt-Glaser, J.K. 207–10, 212, 239
Kim, M.J. 81
Kimura, D. 175–7, 182
Kitayama, N. 230
Klingberg, T. 151
Klorer, G.P. 227
Klorer, P.G. 33

Knickmeyer, R.C. 176
Knox, D. 85
Kobiella, A. 99
Kolkmeier, L. 210, 270, 272–3
Konarski, J.Z. 288
Kosinski, R.J. 51
Kosslyn, S.M. 92, 92–3, 95, 98, 105,
    212–13
Kourtzi, Z. 97, 288
Koyama, T. 48
Kozorovitskiy, Y. 256, 264
Kramer, E. 286
Kravits, K. 24
Kwiatkowska, H.Y. 174

Lakatos, K. 142
Lamm, C. 74, 248
Landes, A.M. 260–1
Landgarten, H.B. 174, 177, 181, 270
Lanius, R.A. 50, 229–31, 233–4, 286
Lark, C. 38
Larsen, P.R. 132
Lasley, E.N. 30
Lathan, M. 191
Lathrope, J. 202
Lazar, S.W. 30
LeDoux, J.E. 31, 33, 113–15, 163, 166,
    168–9, 178, 185, 229, 256, 258,
    296–7
Lekander, M. 207–8
Lemche, E. 55
Lennart, N. 209
Leserman, J. 272, 281
Letinic, K. 80, 87
LeVay, S. 174, 176
Levenson, R.W. 298
Levitin, D.J. 261
Levy, J.A. 81
Lewis, A. 299
Lezak, M.D. 92, 295
Liang, K.C. 85
Lichtenberg, P.A. 261
Lieberman, M. 36, 57
Lipton, S.A. 80
Litvan, I. 71, 74
Litwiller, R.M. 176
Li, X. 95
Llinas, R. 47–50, 285
Lopez, O.I. 267
Loring, D.W. 92
Louilot, A. 102
Lowenfeld, V. 104
Loya, N. 101
Lulbach, G.R. 133
Luna, B. 152
Lusebrink, V.B. 21, 26
Lutchmaya, S. 176
Lydiard, R.B. 229
Lyons, C.A. 124
Lyons-Ruth, K. 201

McCarthy, G. 103, 105
McDermott, J. 99
McDermott, K.B. 87
McDonagh, A. 241
McDonald, R.J. 168
McEwen, B. 30, 112, 296
McFarlane, A.C. 225, 227
McGeown, K. 131, 144
McIntyre, C.K. 81
McKenzie, C.D. 226
McKinney, M. 43
MacLean, K. 144
MacLeod, C.E. 283, 287
McNamee, C.M. 35–6, 295
MacNeill, S.E. 260
Macrae, C.N. 291
Maddock, R.J. 57

Main, M. 140, 142, 192–3, 195, 201, 203,
    280, 289
Malberg, J.E. 30
Malchiodi, C.A. 21, 33, 38, 98, 155, 212,
    214, 225, 254, 286, 289, 297, 300,
    303
Mao, H. 168
Markowitsch, H.J. 52–3
Marmar, C.R. 233, 236
Marriott, L.K. 81
Maruff, P. 254
Mast, B.T. 261
Mateer, C.A. 151, 156
Mather, M. 167
Mather, N. 148
Matthews, A.M. 213
Matthews, S.C. 57
May, A. 30
Mazziotta, J.C. 235, 274
Meador, K.J. 274
Meaney, M.J. 86
Mechelli, A. 30
Meldrum, B.S. 80–1
Meltzoff, A.N. 73
Menon, R.S. 230, 286
Michael, G.A. 94
Miller, L.J. 35
Miller, M.M. 296
Milner, A.D. 304
Minton, K. 225, 285–6
Mirescu, C. 132
Mishkin, M. 185
Mizumori, S.J.Y. 78
Moffit, T.E. 183
Moir, A. 176
Montogomery, G.H. 115
Morelli, M. 80
Morris, J.C. 254
Morris, R.G. 254, 261, 265–7
Moshel, Y.A. 210
Moskowitz, J.T. 125
Mueller, N.K. 87
Mulder, E.J.H. 86
Muller, J. 113–15
Munakata, Y. 152
Murray, E.A. 52, 112, 115

Nainis, N. 212
Nakayama, K. 103
Naparstek, B. 21, 212, 214, 285, 290, 301
Neal, C. 133
Neborsky, R.J. 290
Nemeroff, C.B. 85–7
Newport, D.J. 227
Nicastro, N. 43
Nickerson, C. 131–2, 144
Nieuwenhuis, S. Aston-Jones, G. 85
Nigg, J.T. 148, 150, 154
Nijenhuis, E.R. 225–6, 233, 238
Nithianantharajah, J. 39
Nomura, M. 99
Norris, M.P. 260
Northoff, G. 87
Novak, M. 301

Oatley, K. 163
OConnor, D.H. 94
OConnor, T.G. 132–3
ODoherty, J. 71
Ogawa, J.R. 140
Ogden, P. 225, 285–6
Overman, A.A. 256

Pain, C. 225, 285–6
Paller, K.A. 291
Panksepp, J. 31, 33, 46, 76, 78, 81, 85–6
Paradiso, M. 29, 95, 174

Parkin, A.J. 294
Pascual-Leone, A. 39, 293, 297
Patrick, M.P. 99
Paulus, M.P. 58
Paus, T. 304
Pennebaker, J.W. 217, 239, 298
Perry, B.D. 26, 29, 132–3, 241
Pert, C.B. 207
Peters, J.D. 132
Petersen, R.C. 254, 265
Petersen, S.E. 150
Petrides, M. 33–4, 290, 297
Peuskens, H. 97
Phelps, E.A. 33–4, 185, 296
Phillips, D.P. 55, 72
Phillips, M.L. 152
Pillemer, D.B. 166, 212–13
Pinsk, M.A. 94
Pitman, R.K. 227
Platek, S.M. 99, 101
Porges, S. 24, 114–15, 120–1, 123, 229
Posner, M.L. 148, 150–3, 295
Postle, B.R. 168
Potenza, M.N. 124
Potts, R.B. 44–5
Pourtois, G. 99
Premack, D. 302
Proverbio, A.M. 177, 185
Putnam, F. 226, 238

Quinn, S. 230

Rakic, P. 80
Ramachandran, V.S. 45, 98
Rauch, S.L. 227, 229
Raz, A. 56, 81, 82, 84–5
Raz, N. 256
Redd, W.H. 115
Repa, J.C. 51
Resnick, H.S. 226
Ressler, K.J. 85–7
Ribary, U. 50
Richards, T.L. 62–7, 72
Richmond, B.J. 112, 115
Riggio, L. 36, 288
Riksen-Walraven, J.M. 122, 125
Riley, S. 27, 92, 98, 174, 248, 254–6, 261,
    285, 289
Rime, B. 298
Rivas-Vasquez, R.A. 254–5
Rizzolatti, G. 36, 68, 73, 288
Robbins, A. 289
Robertson, E.M. 72
Robin, R.W. 183
Rodrigues, S.M. 229
Roelofs, K. 169
Rogosch, F.A. 139
Roisman, G.I. 193
Romney, D.M. 286
Roseann, C. 35
Rosenberg, P.A. 80
Rosenkranz, M.A. 125
Rosenstein, D.S. 142
Ross, C. 226, 238
Ross, D. 254, 261, 301
Rossion, B. 102, 104–5
Rossman, M. 212
Rothbart, M.K. 148, 150, 153, 295
Rothstein, P. 55
Rovensky, J. 301
Royal, D.W. 95
Rubin, D.C. 168
Rueda, M.R. 148, 150, 153, 295
Ryff, C.D. 208

Sabbagh, L. 152–3
Sadock, B.J. 78

Safran, D.S. 148, 155
Sagiv, N. 104
Salm, A.K. 55, 133
Sandman, C.A. 133
Sapolsky, R. 24, 26, 43–4, 52, 86, 91, 111,
    125, 161, 168–9, 207, 210, 213,
    227, 285, 296, 299–301
Sarter, M. 85, 150
Sary, G. 95
Satz, P. 30, 255, 262
Saunders, J. 224, 240
Saxe, R. 73
Scaer, R.C. 227
Scarmeas, N. 255, 262, 264
Schaaf, R.C. 35
Schafe, G.E. 229
Schechter, L.E. 30
Schelling, G. 226, 234
Schiltz, C. 102
Schmahmann, J.D. 287–8
Schmidt, C.F. 99
Schneider, M.L. 133
Schoenemann, P.T. 43
Schore, A.N. 26, 29, 33, 43, 46, 50, 52,
    55, 58, 67, 71, 99, 131–4, 136–9,
    183, 185, 192, 236, 241, 273, 290,
    297–8
Schousboe, A. 80, 87
Schrauf, R.W. 168
Schupp, H.T. 55–6
Schweizer, K. 147
Scott, C. 224–5, 227, 231–2, 247–8, 286,
    295–6
Seger, C.A. 82
Serences, J.T. 148, 151
Shafir, E. 167
Sharma, J. 94
Shatz, C.J. 94
Shaw, P. 98
Shaw, W.A. 214
Shea, A. 227
Shea, E. 137
Sheng, M. 81
Shepherd, D. 98
Sherman, J.C. 287
Shima, K. 57
Shin, L.M. 227, 229–31, 248
Shipp, S. 150
Shi, S.-H. 79
Shors, T.J. 176, 178, 181
Shulman, G.L. 148, 150
Siegel, D.J. 21, 36, 65, 71–3, 139–44, 147,
    153, 155, 163, 166, 168–70, 192–3,
    195, 197–8, 200, 213, 226, 240,
    246, 258, 261, 272, 275
Singer, B.S. 208
Singer, T. 248, 304
Sininger, Y.S. 184
Slotnick, S.D. 98
Small, B.J. 254, 256
Smith, B.H. 78
Smitheman-Brown, V. 155
Smyke, A.T. 131–2, 144
Snowdon, D. 255, 262, 264
Sohlberg, M.M. 151, 156
Solomon, J. 192, 289
Southwick, S.M. 275
Spangler, G. 133, 139–41, 143
Sperry, S.D. 260–1
Spiegel, B.S. 210, 212
Spitznagel, M.B. 261
Sprengelmeyer, R. 105
Spring, D. 227
Sroufe, L.A. 192–3, 280
Staff, R.T. 262–3
Steele, K. 225–6, 233, 238
Stefano, G.B. 122–3
Stein, M. 30
Stern, Y. 255, 262–4

Stevens, K. 175, 177, 185
Strafella, A.P. 304
Strauss, M.E. 260–1
Striano, T. 99
Stvrtinova, V. 301
Subrin, R. 301
Sugiura, M. 99, 101
Sullivan, R.M. 83
Sur, M. 94
Suslow, T. 52
Suzuki, J. 232
Swanson, R.A. 81
Sweeney, J.A. 152
Swick, D. 71, 295
Szpunar, K.K. 87

Talge, N.M. 133
Tamietto, M. 31, 293
Tamminga, C.A. 56
Tanji, J. 57
Tannock, R. 154
Tarr, M. 102
Taylor, J.R. 124
Taylor, M.J. 99
Taylor, S.E. 182
Teicher, M.H. 227, 241
Theuring, F. 256
Thompson, W.L. 92–3, 98, 212–13
Tiffany, S.T. 213
Tomita, H. 277
Tomoda, A. 227
Tong, F. 103
Tononi, G. 47
Tranel, D. 52, 103–4, 178
Tremont, G. 261
Trevarthen, C. 138
Tronick, E. 29, 99, 137, 289
Tugade, M.M. 298
Tulving, E. 167, 178
Tuohy, V.K. 210
Turken, A.U. 71, 295
Tyzio, R. 87
Tzourio-Mazoyer, N. 35

Ullman, S.E. 226
Underwood, M.K. 174
Ungerleider, L.G. 95, 99
Urgesi, C. 97
Uvnas Moberg, K. 78

Valentine, J.D. 230, 286
Van Bakel, H.J.A. 122, 125
Van der Hart, O. 225–6, 233, 238
Van der Kolk, B. 166, 225, 227, 232–5,
    239–41, 299
Van der Linden, M. 256
Van Essen, D.C. 95
Van Ijzendoorn, M.H. 131–2, 141, 143
Vance, R. 27, 159, 161, 164–5, 167,
    170–1, 288
Vasterling, J.J. 296
Vermetten, E. 85, 226, 229, 231
Virshup, E. 98
Voges, M.A. 286
Vohs, K.D. 31
von Bohlen and Halbach, O. 78, 82, 84
Vuilleumier, P. 99

Waagepetersen, H.S. 87
Wadeson, H. 174, 177–9
Wager, T.D. 293
Wahlin, K. 27, 288
Waldinger, R.J. 140
Wald, J. 92
Walrond-Skinner, S. 246
Walter, H. 159
Wang, S. 26, 117–18, 270, 298

Wang, X. 84
Watkins, K.E. 304
Watson, J.M. 87
Watt, D. 74, 246, 304–5
Weathers, F. 286
Weiner, H. 210
Weiner, I.B. 285
Weinfield, N.S. 193
Weisaeth, L. 225, 227
Weiss, B. 131
Weisz, C. 152
Weller, A. 86
Westerberg, H. 151
Whalen, P.J. 99, 104–5
Wicker, B. 68, 246, 304
Williams, K.D. 57
Windhorst, C. 167
Wingfield, J.C. 112
Winnicott, D.W. 293
Wischik, C.M. 256
Wolf, H. 255
Wood, G.E. 176, 178, 181
Wood, S. 147
Wood, W. 174
Woodruff, G. 302
Wright, J.C. 174
Wright, L.S. 226
Wright, T.M. 293

Yaha, H. 209
Yamada, H. 136
Yan, S.D. 265
Yantis, S. 148, 151
Yehuda, R. 227
Youngstrom, E.A. 294
Yovel, G. 99, 100, 101, 103, 105
Yucel, M. 230

Zaidel, D.W. 92, 97
Zakriski, A.L. 174
Zald, D.H. 52
Zeanah, C.H. 36
Zeki, S. 187
Zimmermann, P. 133, 139–41, 143
Zoncu, R. 80